IF YOU ARE LIVING WITH DIABETES, YOU ARE NOT ALONE.

In the United States, over 27 million people—9% of the population—have diabetes, and 1.5 million people are diagnosed every year.

IF YOU ARE LIVING WITH DIABETES, WHAT YOU EAT IS THE KEY TO GOOD HEALTH.

Here is the one-stop guide for managing diabetes and reducing complications.

THE DIABETES CARBOHYDRATE AND CALORIE COUNTER

is a one-of-a-kind book that lists thousands of brand name, take-out, and restaurant foods, providing counts for carbohydrates, calories, sugar, and fat—all the information you need to set up a healthy eating plan. Use this reliable meal-planning guide to customize your diet to fit your food likes and dislikes, your culture, and your life's demands.

Managing diabetes has never been easier!
It's up to you.

Books by Annette B. Natow and Jo-Ann Heslin

The Calorie Counter (*Fourth Edition*)

The Cholesterol Counter (*Sixth Edition*)

The Complete Food Counter (*Second Edition*)

The Diabetes Carbohydrate and Calorie Counter
(*Third Edition*)

Eating Out Food Counter

The Fat Counter (*Sixth Edition*)

The Healthy Heart Food Counter

The Most Complete Food Counter (*Second Edition*)

The Protein Counter (*Second Edition*)

The Ultimate Carbohydrate Counter

The Vitamin and Mineral Food Counter

Available from POCKET BOOKS

THE
DIABETES CARBOHYDRATE AND CALORIE COUNTER

Third Edition

Annette B. Natow, Ph.D., R.D.

Jo-Ann Heslin, M.A., R.D.

With the assistance of Karen J. Nolan, Ph.D.

POCKET BOOKS
New York   London   Toronto   Sydney

The authors and publisher of this book are not physicians and are not licensed to give medical advice. The information in this book has been collected for the convenience of the reader. The nutrient values for prepared foods are subject to change and may now differ from listings herein, which are based on research conducted prior to spring 2006. Such information does not constitute a recommendation or endorsement of any individual, institution, or product, nor is it intended as a substitute for personalized consultation with your physician. The authors and publisher disclaim any liability arising directly or indirectly from the use of this book.

An *Original* Publication of POCKET BOOKS

 POCKET BOOKS, a division of Simon & Schuster, Inc.
1230 Avenue of the Americas, New York, NY 10020

Copyright © 1991, 2003, 2007 by Annette Natow and Jo-Ann Heslin

All rights reserved, including the right to reproduce this book or portions thereof in any form whatsoever. For information address Pocket Books, 1230 Avenue of the Americas, New York, NY 10020

ISBN-13: 978-1-4165-0983-7
ISBN-10:   1-4165-0983-6

This Pocket Books paperback edition January 2007

10   9   8   7

POCKET and colophon are registered trademarks of Simon & Schuster, Inc.

Cover design by Heather Kern, photo by Dennis Gottlieb/Jupiter Images

Manufactured in the United States of America

For information regarding special discounts for bulk purchases, please contact Simon & Schuster Special Sales at 1-800-456-6798 or business@simonandschuster.com.

To our families, who support us through every project: Harry, Allen, Irene, Sarah, Meryl, Laura, Marty, George, Emily, Steven, Rebecca, Joseph, Kristen, Brian, Karen, and John.

ACKNOWLEDGMENTS

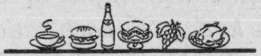

For graciously sharing her knowledge, Karen J. Nolan, Ph.D.

For all her continuous support and help, our agent, Nancy Trichter.

For her suggestions and editing skills, Sara Clemence.

Without the tireless cooperation of Stephen Llano and the production department at Pocket Books, *The Diabetes Carbohydrate and Calorie Counter*, Third Edition, would never have been completed.

A special thank you to our editor, Micki Nuding.

And, we'd like to thank all our readers for their suggestions and questions. Your input helps us to provide you with the most useful information.

"The regulation of the diet is the most important consideration in the treatment of diabetes mellitus."

"While certain general principles in regard to diet for diabetes can be laid down, each patient presents an individual problem. . . ."

Mary Swartz Rose, Ph.D.
Feeding the Family
The Macmillan Company, 1919

CONTENTS

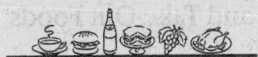

PART ONE
Brand Name, Nonbranded (Generic),
and Take-Out Foods

67

PART TWO
Restaurant Chains

399

INTRODUCTION

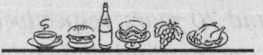

You've just been told by your doctor
that you have diabetes.

OR

Someone in your family or someone
close to you has diabetes.

OR

Your doctor said you have a cluster of risk factors
that signals a higher chance of getting diabetes
in the near future.

Every 24 hours, 4,100 new cases of diabetes are diagnosed in the U.S. At first, most people feel devastated—being told to change the way they eat, lose weight, exercise, and take medication is overwhelming. But there is good news. Diabetes is a condition over which you, as an individual, have a great deal of control. And the more control you exercise, the healthier and more complication-free your life will be. Most important, you can look forward to a very long life.

YOU SHOULD KNOW

Exercise, diet, and compliance pay off
Gerald and Robert, brothers who have had diabetes for 85 and 70 years, respectively, credit their long lives to conscientious daily attention to their condition. Diabetes experts say these brothers—and others like them—are living proof that careful control can ensure long, healthy, and productive lives for people with diabetes.

There is no question that being diagnosed with diabetes is a jolt—emotionally, physically, and even socially. It is a condition that requires constant attention and modifications to how you lead your life. It isn't unusual to feel down. If you do, talk with your doctor about how you are feeling. Depression can be caused by feeling that you can no longer control your body and your life. But you can.

With some adjustments, life will be normal again, and sooner than you think. Initially it is going to take work on your part, a commitment to follow your doctor's orders. But the commitment will pay off. Your body will respond to your new diet, exercise, and medication plan in ways that may amaze you.

UNDERSTANDING DIABETES

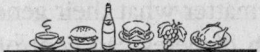

What Is Diabetes?

When you have diabetes, there is too much sugar in your blood. After you eat, your food is broken down into a sugar called *glucose*, which is carried by your blood to cells throughout your body. *Insulin*, a hormone, helps the glucose move from the bloodstream into cells, where it is burned as energy to keep your body functioning. People with diabetes either don't make enough insulin or their cells don't recognize insulin. The result in both cases is that glucose in the bloodstream can't get into cells to be used for energy, and too much glucose builds up in the blood.

What Causes Diabetes?

In most cases, it's your genes. Nine percent of the U.S. population (over 27 million people) have diabetes. It's estimated that a person born in 2000 has a 1 in 3 chance of developing diabetes in his or her lifetime. But the good news—are you getting the picture, that there is always good news?—is that lifestyle choices can alter the action of your genes. Just because you carry the *risk* for diabetes doesn't mean you will *get* diabetes. People who stay slim, exercise regularly, don't smoke, and eat generally healthy diets decrease their odds of developing diabetes, no matter what their genetic profiles say. And people with diabetes can control the condition, and in some cases even reverse it, with lifestyle changes.

What Puts a Person at Risk for Diabetes?

The risk of developing diabetes increases with each of the following:

- Being 45 or older
- Being overweight
- Having a parent or close relative with diabetes
- Being African American, American Indian, Asian American, Pacific Islander, or Hispanic/Latin American
- Having diabetes during pregnancy
- Giving birth to a baby weighing more than 9 pounds
- Having high blood pressure
- Having high cholesterol
- Exercising very little or not at all

YOU SHOULD KNOW

Knowledge is power

The more you know about diabetes, the better you can take care of yourself and the healthier you will be.

What Are the Symptoms of Diabetes?

Diabetes often goes undetected for a long time, because many people have no symptoms, or they ignore symptoms because they seem harmless. See your doctor if you experience any of the following problems:

- Being very thirsty
- Needing to urinate frequently
- Being very hungry
- Weight loss without any effort
- Feeling tired and weak
- Blurry vision
- Cuts and bruises that heal very slowly, or do not heal at all
- Tingling or numbness in your hands or feet
- Recurring or hard-to-heal infections
- Annoying itching

How Is Diabetes Diagnosed?

Your doctor screens for diabetes and other health issues when you have blood tests. Everyone over the age of 45 should be screened. If everything is normal, screenings should be repeated every 3 years. Younger individuals need to be tested earlier if they have a number of the risk factors noted above. Children who are overweight should be tested periodically, too.

YOU SHOULD KNOW

About screening tests for diabetes

Random Blood Glucose—*Your doctor checks your blood glucose without regard to when you last ate. A normal result is less than 200.*

Fasting Blood Glucose—*Your doctor tests your blood after you have not eaten for at least 8 hours. Results below 100 are normal. Between 100 and 125 you have a condition known as prediabetes, which signals your risk of developing diabetes in the future. If the results are 126 or higher, the test is usually repeated on another day. If the numbers stay high, this confirms a diagnosis of diabetes.*

Oral Glucose Tolerance Test—*Your blood is tested in the morning after you have not eaten for at least 10 hours; then it is tested a second time, 2 hours after you drink a sweetened beverage. Results of 139 or below are normal. Between 140 and 199, you have prediabetes. Results over 200 indicate diabetes. Some doctors repeat the results on another day to confirm the diagnosis.*

How Do I Manage My Diabetes?

Diet, exercise, and medication all play roles in managing diabetes. Once you've been diagnosed, your primary care doctor will help you organize your health care team—a group of health professionals who help manage all aspects of your condition. The most important member of the team is YOU. Only you know how you feel. You will be the first to notice any problems. And you will set the pace for what you are willing and able to do. The rest of the team depends on you to be honest and to thoroughly report on your home care.

YOUR HEALTH CARE TEAM

Health Professional	Seen How Often	To Help You With
Primary care doctor	Every 3 months	To provide general care
		To monitor blood sugar
		To refer you to other specialists
Certified Diabetes Educator (CDE); may be a nurse with special training in diabetes management	As needed	To help put your drug, diet, exercise, and daily care plan in place
		To help you manage problems such as sick days
		To answer all questions about your self-care routine

(continued)

Health Professional	Seen How Often	To Help You With
Registered Dietitian (RD); may also be a CDE	As needed	To help you set up a meal plan tailored to your treatment goals and personal choices
Eye doctor	Yearly	To monitor the health of your eyes To prevent and treat complications from diabetes
Podiatrist	As needed	To care for your feet and lower legs To treat corns, calluses, and sores
Dentist	Twice yearly	To monitor the health of your mouth To prevent or treat gum disease and infections

TYPES OF DIABETES

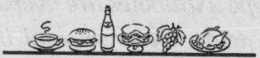

Diabetes or, more correctly, *diabetes mellitus* is a group of similar conditions all resulting in the same outcome—too much sugar in the blood. Why one person develops diabetes and another does not has to do with complicated interaction between genes and environment.

Researchers classify diabetes into 4 main groups—type 1, type 2, pregnancy diabetes, and from other causes. This last group accounts for a very small percentage of cases and the development of diabetes is usually secondary to another condition, such as Down's syndrome.

Type 2

This is the most common form: 90% to 95% of people with diabetes have type 2 and the number of people with this condition is increasing daily. Experts believe that as time goes on, more and more people—even children—will develop type 2 diabetes because so many people are overweight and inactive. Couple this with the fact that our population is aging (type 2 is most common in those over 30) and the number of new cases is overwhelming. The total number of people with diabetes is estimated to reach over 77 million in the next 10 years.

YOU SHOULD KNOW

Approximately 50% of men and 70% of women who develop type 2 diabetes are overweight. Weighing less could delay the onset and in some cases prevent the condition entirely.

Type 2 diabetes begins when your body is unable to use the insulin it produces. The cells don't recognize insulin, so it isn't allowed to enter cells to deliver glucose, needed for energy. To solve this problem, the pancreas—which makes insulin—produces more. At first this works, but after a while the pancreas gets exhausted from all the extra work, and it loses its ability to make enough insulin.

Type 2 is managed by lifestyle changes, diet, losing weight, and, when needed, medication and possibly insulin. In some cases the disease can even be reversed with conscientious attention to diet, exercise, and weight control.

Type 1

In the past this form of diabetes was called *juvenile diabetes* because most people developed it in childhood or early adulthood, but it can occur at any age. Only 5% to 10% of people with diabetes have type 1. It develops when something happens to destroy the cells in the pancreas that produce insulin. A person with type 1 cannot make any insulin, and must supply it daily by injection, through an insulin pump, or by a newly approved inhaled form. The amount of insulin taken daily must be balanced with diet and exercise. There is no known way to prevent type 1 and it cannot be reversed.

Pregnancy Diabetes

Gestational diabetes mellitus occurs only during pregnancy and usually disappears after the baby is born. Being overweight or having a family history of diabetes can increase a woman's risk. To prevent problems, all pregnant women are tested for pregnancy diabetes. If their blood sugar levels are too high, they are taught to adjust their food intake and they may be given insulin until their baby is delivered. Having pregnancy diabetes increases a woman's risk of developing type 2 diabetes in the next 5 to 10 years.

YOU SHOULD KNOW

Diabetes is a serious condition
Terms such as "a touch of diabetes," "mild diabetes," or "my sugar is a little high" shouldn't be used, because they minimize a serious health problem.

Complications

The key to being healthy and avoiding complications from diabetes is working with your health team to keep your blood sugar down, your blood pressure down, and your blood fats low, and taking your medication or insulin as prescribed.

Regardless of the type, when diabetes is not well controlled you are at risk for complications—heart disease, stroke, eye disease, kidney disease, nerve damage, gum disease, tooth loss, and even amputations. It's a pretty scary list. But, as we said before, with the bad news comes some really good news: *Serious complications are not inevitable.*

- Keeping blood sugar levels within the normal range can reduce eye, kidney, and nerve problems by as much as 40%.

- Reducing your systolic blood pressure (the top number) by 10 reduces the risk for all complications by 12%.

- Lowering blood fats (triglycerides and cholesterol) can reduce the risk of heart disease and stroke by 20% to 50%.

- Visiting your eye doctor regularly can reduce the risk of vision problems by 50% to 60%.

- Visiting your podiatrist regularly can reduce amputation rate by 45% to 85%

The most important thing you need to know about diabetes is that *you* are in control. By keeping your condition under control, *you* control your risk for complications and serious health problems.

A Word About Prediabetes

Prediabetes, also known as metabolic syndrome, is not a disease but a cluster of symptoms that doubles your risk for heart disease and quadruples your risk for diabetes.

It is estimated that 41 million people, including 2 million children, have prediabetes. Of those over age 60, 50% have prediabetes. The guidelines for this condition were set by experts to cast a wide net, to catch and treat as many people as possible to prevent more serious problems like heart attack, stroke, and type 2 diabetes.

Having 3 of the following risk factors classifies you as someone with prediabetes:

- Being 30 or more pounds overweight (men with waists larger than 42 inches and women with waists greater than 35 inches)

- Having HDL cholesterol of less than 40 for men and less than 50 for women

- Having triglycerides of 150 or higher after fasting, or 400 or higher without fasting

- Having a blood pressure of 130/85 or higher or taking high blood pressure medication

- Having a blood sugar level of 100 or higher after fasting, or 140 or higher 2 hours after eating (these values are higher than normal, but not high enough for a diagnosis of diabetes)

If untreated, people classified with prediabetes are likely to develop diabetes within 10 years. But the good news is that this is not inevitable. With treatment, prediabetes can be reversed and may never develop into diabetes.

YOU SHOULD KNOW

If you have prediabetes, losing 5% to 7% of your current weight and walking 2.5 hours a week can reduce your risk of developing diabetes by 58%. For people over age 60, the risk goes down over 70%.

SETTING YOUR WEIGHT LOSS GOALS

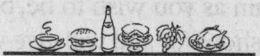

How Much Weight Do I Have to Lose to Control My Diabetes?

Your health care team will help you set your specific weight loss goals, but any weight loss is beneficial—even just a few pounds can be significant. A loss of between 10 and 20 pounds, which can be accomplished in 3 to 4 months, will improve type 2 diabetes remarkably. Your blood sugar will drop, your cholesterol and triglycerides will go down, you'll have more energy, and you'll look and feel better. You may even find you're able to reduce or possibly eliminate medication.

How Much Should I Weigh?

There are many ways to determine your best weight or target weight—weight charts, equations, even guesstimates. Your doctor, diabetes educator, or dietitian may help you with this step. But a very easy way to "guess" at a good target weight is:

Multiply your weight at age 20 × 1.2 = Target Weight
For example, if you weighed 135 pounds in your early 20s
$$135 \times 1.2 = 162 \text{ pounds}$$

Your target weight should be 162 pounds or less. This may not be as thin as you wish to be, but it is a reasonable estimate to shoot for and will give you health benefits.

YOU SHOULD KNOW

10% IS GREAT!
Losing 10% of your body weight—15 pounds for someone who weighs 150 pounds, 20 pounds for a person weighing 200 pounds, or 30 pounds if the scale tips in at 300 pounds—is all that is needed to significantly improve your health. Lose 10% of your current body weight and you'll have:
Lower blood sugar
Lower blood pressure
Improved cholesterol levels
Better sex

How Many Calories Should I Eat Every Day?

As with target weight, your doctor may give you a daily calorie intake to aim for. But here's a way to determine how many calories to eat each day. First, you need to know your target weight, which you get by using the equation above. Second, select an activity factor that fits your current activity level.

1. Your target weight is: _____

2. Your activity factor is: _____
    20 = Very active men
    15 = Moderately active men or very active women
    13 = Inactive men, moderately active women, and
       people over 55
    10 = Inactive women, repeat dieters, seriously
       overweight people
3. Target Weight × Activity Factor = Calories needed
    each day

For example, if your target weight is 162 and you are an inactive woman (factor 10), you need about 1600 calories a day.

$$162 \text{ pounds} \times 10 = 1620 \text{ calories}$$

Eating approximately 1600 calories each day will guarantee weight loss because you are getting only enough calories to support your target weight, not your current heavier weight. Add some exercise and the weight will come off even faster.

YOU SHOULD KNOW

Your weight loss goals
   Your target weight is: _____
   Your daily calorie intake is: _____

Why Is Exercise So Important?

Daily exercise helps to control your blood sugar and maintain your target weight. Everything counts—window shopping, gardening, housework, bowling.

- Try to be active every day
- Aim for 30 minutes of activity each day; you can accumulate this by doing short periods of activity (10 minutes or less) throughout the day
- Start walking—even short walks, like from the edge of the parking lot or up and down the aisles of the supermarket

LET'S TALK ABOUT FOOD

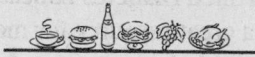

We know that when you are first diagnosed, it's over-whelming. There are so many things to manage—your weight, your blood sugar, your food, your medication, how much you exercise. So, when it comes to food, let's take it slowly. We'll go step by step, and before you know it you'll be a pro at planning meals and choosing the right foods.

The first question everyone asks is, "What can I eat, now that I have diabetes?" The simple answer is "every-thing." No foods are off-limits. It's when you eat and the amount you eat that needs to be watched.

Meal Planning

At first, the idea of planning all of your meals and snacks can be stressful. But relax, it really isn't that hard. Start slowly. First, become accustomed to regular serving sizes, which are probably smaller than what you now eat. Stick with the smaller, regular sizes as often as you can. Next, work on spacing out meals and snacks throughout the day, and try to keep to this schedule daily. Now, work on making the best selections each time you eat. You may need to count calories and carbohydrates. In the beginning, counting carbs is smart because it will help you learn a great deal about the foods you eat, and you'll become very skilled at making choices. Your Certified Diabetes Educator or Registered Dietitian will be a great resource for meal planning and carb counting. We'll help get you started with both, as well.

Meal Planning Hints

Do: Eat regular meals: aim for the same amount of food at about the same time each day

Choose regular serving sizes

Eat moderately sized meals

Choose foods with carbohydrate and fiber at each meal and each snack

Choose foods low in fat

Bring food with you so that you don't miss a meal or snack

Go easy: On foods containing sugar

On foods containing saturated fat

On alcohol

Don't: Skip meals or snacks

Overeat

YOU SHOULD KNOW

When researchers compared people who ate on an irregular schedule to those who ate meals at regular times each day, they found that those with the regular meal pattern had lower blood sugar, lower cholesterol, and lower LDL (bad) cholesterol.

The American Diabetes Association (ADA) recommends the following approach to managing diabetes:

Lose weight, if needed
Be active daily
Eat a healthy diet

The ADA further recommends that lifestyle changes be individualized for each person. To do that, you need to consider:

Your life's circumstances
Your culture
Your heritage
Your food likes and dislikes
Your willingness to make changes

As we said earlier, *you* are the most important part of your health care team. Only you can decide what you can and will do to manage your diabetes.

Let's look at some good advice for healthy living. Most of this applies to everyone, whether they have diabetes or not. If you haven't paid too much attention to what you ate or how much you exercised in the past, these general guidelines will help you begin to make better choices.

Carbohydrates

- Include whole grain breads and cereals, fruits, vegetables, and lowfat milk in your meals and snacks

- Keep track of the amount of carbohydrates you eat each day; include carbs at every meal and snack

- It's OK to use low calorie and no calorie sweeteners

- It's OK to eat sugar and foods containing sugar, but eat small amounts and count sugar as part of your day's total carbohydrate amount

- Eat sugar and sugary foods with meals or snacks, not alone

Fat

- Eating less fat will help you lose weight and reduce your cholesterol

- Eat more of the foods that contain good (monounsaturated) fats—olive oil, canola oil, seeds, nuts

- Eat moderate amounts of the foods that contain polyunsaturated fat—margarine, corn oil, vegetable oil, salad dressing

- Eat less of the foods that contain saturated fat—meat, whole milk, butter, cheese

Regular Serving Sizes

Often the portions of food you make at home or that are served in restaurants are much too large. At first, use measuring cups, measuring spoons, or a kitchen scale to get used to the size of a regular portion. The following information will get you started.

What Is a Serving?

Food	Serving Size

Breads, cereals, high-carb foods

Food	Serving Size
bread	1 slice
roll, bun, or pita pocket	½
crackers	4 to 6
tortilla	1 (6 inches)
cereal, cooked	½ cup
cereal, ready-to-eat	¾ cup
rice, cooked	⅓ cup
pasta, cooked	½ cup
popcorn	3 cups

Vegetables and fruits

Food	Serving Size
raw or cooked vegetables	½ cup
raw or cooked leafy greens	1 cup
green peas	½ cup
beans	¼ cup
potato	1 small
mashed potatoes	½ cup
french fries	10 pieces
fresh fruit	1 small
banana	½ regular or 1 very small
dried fruit	2 tablespoons
canned fruit	½ cup
juice	½ cup

Milk, yogurt, cheese

Food	Serving Size
nonfat or lowfat milk	1 cup
nonfat or lowfat yogurt	1 cup
cheese	1 ounce or 1 slice
cottage cheese	½ cup

(continued)

Meat, poultry, fish

cooked	3 to 4 ounces
egg, cooked	1

Fats

butter or margarine	1 teaspoon
cream cheese	2 tablespoons
salad dressing	2 tablespoons
oil	1 tablespoon

Sugar

sugar	1 teaspoon
honey	1 teaspoon
syrup	2 tablespoons

YOU SHOULD KNOW

Seeing is believing

These visual cues will help you keep portion sizes reasonable.

computer mouse = 4-ounce portion of meat, chicken, seafood

        or

        1 medium baked potato

yo-yo = a mini bagel or 100 calories. How many yo-yos fit into your bagel, muffin, or pastry?

tennis ball = medium piece of fresh fruit

ping-pong ball = 2 ounces cheese

        or

        2 tablespoons salad dressing, gravy, sour cream

thumbnail = 1 pat butter

LET'S TALK ABOUT COUNTING CARBS

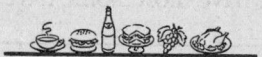

Everyone who has diabetes should know how to count carbs. Some people do it every day, some do it a few days a week to check on how they are doing, and others do it occasionally. Your Certified Diabetes Educator or Registered Dietitian will be your resource for which system is best for you. When you are first diagnosed, counting carbs is an excellent way to become more familiar with how to manage your condition.

You've got a great resource right in front of you. *The Diabetes Carbohydrate and Calorie Counter* has the carb counts for over 11,000 foods. You can look up any food you eat and know exactly how many carbs are in a serving.

The goals of carbohydrate counting are to:

- Learn which foods have carbs
- Know how much carb is in each food
- Count up the carbs in each meal
- Count up the carbs in each snack
- Aim to eat the same amount of carbs each day

Finding Carbohydrate Foods

You know that bread, pasta, cereal, and potatoes have carbs. But are you aware that fruits, vegetables, cakes, ice cream, candy, jelly, cookies, sugar, milk, and beans have carbs, too? Some have more, some have less.

YOU SHOULD KNOW

Which has more carbs?
Whole milk or skim milk?
White bread or whole wheat bread?
White sugar or brown sugar?
The carb count in each pair is the same. The color of a food or the amount of fat it has does not change the amount of carbs.

Most people eat about 35 foods regularly. We are all creatures of habit and we tend to pick the same foods over and over again. A simple way to get familiar with the carb counts in the foods you usually eat is to list your favorites on the following chart, and then look up how much carb is in each food. You may find the amount you usually eat is more than you should. Go back to pages 23-24 to find out what a normal portion size is and adjust your list.

This might seem time-consuming at first, but it is a truly valuable exercise. This sheet will serve as a quick reference when you are planning meals and snacks. You may eventually make a number of these sheets, one for each group of foods you eat. We've also had people tell us they make a list of possible choices before they go out to eat, so they can make the best choices from a restaurant menu. There are many uses for a tool like this. You'll probably come up with your own inventive ways of using it.

CARBS IN MY FAVORITE FOODS			
Food I Often Eat	My Typical Serving Size	Normal Serving Size	Grams of Carbohydrate

Your Daily Carb Budget

Thinking about the amount of carb you can eat each day as if it's a budget is an easy way to help you divide up carbs into meals and snacks. If you had $30 a day and were told to buy 3 meals and 2 snacks, you would budget your money to cover all your food. It's the same idea with carbs. Your Certified Diabetes Educator or Registered Dietitian will help you set up your carb budget.

We recommend that 45% to 60% of your daily calories come from carbs. But people don't think in terms of percentages. You want to know what foods you can eat, and when. First we have to determine how many carbs you can eat each day, based on the amount of calories you are eating daily. On page 17 you figured out how many calories you needed each day. Find that number on the following chart, "My Daily Calories and Carbs," and you'll find a target amount of carbs to eat. This number may vary slightly if you have already set up a carb budget with a diabetes educator, but the concept will remain the same.

YOU SHOULD KNOW
Your Daily Carb Budget
Each day I can eat:
Calories _____
Carbs _____

MY DAILY CALORIES AND CARBS

Calories Each Day	Grams of Carbs Each Day
1200	150
1300	160
1400	175
1500	190
1600	200
1700	215
1800	225
1900	240
2000	250
2100	265
2200	275
2300	290
2400	300
2500	315
2600	325
2700	340

* Carb recommendations are based on 50% of daily calories as carbohydrates.

Carbohydrate-containing foods have the greatest impact on your blood sugar. Eat too many carbs and your blood sugar goes up; eat too few and your blood sugar may drop too low; eat the right amount, and your diabetes will be well controlled.

YOU SHOULD KNOW

Counting carbs counts toward managing your diabetes and keeping you healthy.

LET'S EAT—
PUTTING IT ALL TOGETHER

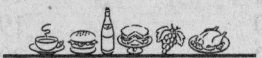

You should try to eat your meals and snacks at the same times each day. This timing helps your body use the carbs you eat and keeps your blood sugar normal. If there is a long time between meals, your blood sugar could drop very low. If you eat fewer, large meals, your blood sugar may go up too high.

Carb Choices

> 1 carb choice = 15 grams of carbohydrate
> 1 slice of bread = 15 grams of carbohydrate

The easiest way to understand carb choices is to relate everything to a slice of bread, which is 15 grams of carb or 1 carb choice. If you look up a food, such as a slice of apple pie, and you see that it has 45 grams of carb, that equals 3 slices of bread or 3 carb choices. You can make this choice work if you eat half a slice of pie, or pick something similar like a baked apple, which is lower in carb. Some typical carb choices, all of which have 15 grams of carb, are on the following chart, "Carb Choices."

CARB CHOICES

1 CARB CHOICE = 15 GRAMS OF CARBOHYDRATE

Breads & Cereals	Fruits	Vegetables
⅓ cup cooked rice	½ banana	⅓ cup beans
½ roll	1 small apple, orange, peach	½ cup green peas
1 (4-inch) pancake		½ cup corn
½ cup cooked cereal	4 fresh apricots	½ cup plantain
¾ cup ready-to-eat cereal (unsweetened)	1 cup cut-up melon	½ cup boiled or mashed potato
	12 cherries	1 cup winter squash
	18 grapes	
½ cup ready-to-eat cereal (sweetened)	½ papaya	
	½ cup unsweetened canned fruit	
8 animal crackers	¾ cup fresh berries	
6 saltines	1 cup fresh strawberries	
3 cups popcorn		
½ cup pasta	1¼ cup cubed watermelon	
	½ cup fruit juice	
	⅓ cup prune juice	

Planning Your Day

At this point, you know a lot! You know how many calories to eat each day. You know how many grams of carb to eat each day. You know which foods contain carb. And you know what a carb choice equals and you have some typical examples to use. So, let's plan a sample day.

Let's assume you can eat 1800 calories a day. A person eating 1800 calories a day can eat 225 grams of carb each day. (See chart on page 29, "My Daily Calories and Carbs.") If you divide 225 by 15, you will find out how many carb choices you can eat.

$$225 \div 15 = 15$$

Daily Carbs ÷ 1 Carb Choice = Number of Carb
Choices allowed daily

The rest is simple. Here are some basic meal-planning tips to help you get started.

- Divide your carb budget for the day between your meals and snacks

- Eat some carb at every meal
  Women: at least 2 to 3 carb choices at each meal
  Men: at least 3 to 4 carb choices at each meal

- Eat at least 1 carb at every snack; eat at least 2 snacks a day

- Include a protein choice or a fat choice at each meal or snack

- Do not eat carb alone because this causes blood sugar to rise too high

- Don't skip meals

The following sample day uses the example we started above for a person eating 1800 calories a day, including 15 carb choices.

SAMPLE DAY

Dividing Your Daily Carb Budget Between Meals and Snacks

For a woman:

Daily Carb Budget: 15 Carb Choices or 225 grams Carb

Breakfast	_3_	*Carb choices*	=	_45_ grams Carb
AM Snack	_1_	*Carb choices*	=	_15_ grams Carb
Lunch	_4_	*Carb choices*	=	_60_ grams Carb
PM Snack	_1_	*Carb choices*	=	_15_ grams Carb
Dinner	_4_	*Carb choices*	=	_60_ grams Carb
Night Snack	_2_	*Carb choices*	=	_30_ grams Carb
Total	_15_	**Carb choices**	=	_225_ total grams Carb

For a man:

Daily Carb Budget: 15 Carb Choices or 225 grams Carb

Breakfast	_4_	*Carb choices*	=	_60_ grams Carb
AM Snack	_1_	*Carb choices*	=	_15_ grams Carb
Lunch	_4_	*Carb choices*	=	_60_ grams Carb
PM Snack	_1_	*Carb choices*	=	_15_ grams Carb
Dinner	_4_	*Carb choices*	=	_60_ grams Carb
Night Snack	_1_	*Carb choices*	=	_15_ grams Carb
Total	_15_	**Carb choices**	=	_225_ total grams Carb

Use the following box to divide your daily carb budget into a pattern you can follow for meals and snacks. Your diabetes educator may have you change this pattern depending on your medication and your blood sugar values. Or you may adjust the pattern if you know you will be eating out or if your activity schedule changes. The goal is to evenly divide the carbs you eat throughout the day and never go without food for long periods.

Dividing Your Daily Carb Budget Between Meals and Snacks			
Daily Carb Budget: ____ Carb Choices or ____ grams Carb			
Breakfast	_____	*Carb choices* =	_____ *grams Carb*
AM Snack	_____	*Carb choices* =	_____ *grams Carb*
Lunch	_____	*Carb choices* =	_____ *grams Carb*
PM Snack	_____	*Carb choices* =	_____ *grams Carb*
Dinner	_____	*Carb choices* =	_____ *grams Carb*
Night Snack	_____	*Carb choices* =	_____ *grams Carb*
Total	_____	**Carb choices** =	_____ total grams Carb

To take this planning one step further, here is an example of the possible foods choices for 1800 calories and a carb budget of 225 grams.

SAMPLE MENU FOR A WOMAN

1800 Calories
Carb Budget: 225 grams or 15 Carb Choices

Food	Portion	Calories	Carbs
Breakfast Goals			**45**
Pink grapefruit sections	½ cup	37	9
Cottage cheese, 1% fat	½ cup	82	3
Cornflakes	¾ cup	100	24
Nonfat milk	1 cup	86	12
Coffee + sugar substitute	as desired	0	0
Breakfast Subtotals		**305**	**48**
Morning Snack Goals			**15**
Apple	1 small	63	16
Morning Snack Subtotals		**63**	**16**
Lunch Goals			**60**
Tuna salad	½ cup	192	10
Rye bread	2 slices	130	24
Swiss cheese	1 oz	107	1
Tossed salad	1½ cups	32	7
Low cal Italian dressing	2 tbsp	32	2
Diet cola	1 can	0	0
Light flavored yogurt	1 pkg	100	16
Lunch Subtotals		**593**	**60**
Afternoon Snack Goals			**15**
Graham crackers	2 squares	60	10
Lowfat cream cheese	1 tbsp	60	2
Tea + sugar substitute	as desired	0	0
Afternoon Snack Subtotals		**120**	**12**
Dinner Goals			**60**
Roast chicken w/skin	½ breast	142	0
Rice	⅔ cup	137	30
Cracked pepper	sprinkle	0	0
Butter	1 tablespoon	108	tr
Broccoli, cooked	1 cup	46	8

(continued)

Vanilla ice cream (no sugar added)	¾ cup	165	21
Sparkling water	as desired	0	0
Dinner Subtotals		**598**	**59**
Evening Snack Goals			30
Popcorn	2 cups	62	12
Nonfat milk	1 cup	86	12
Sugar free chocolate syrup	2 tbsp	15	5
Evening Snack Subtotals		**163**	**29**
Day's Totals		**1842**	**224**

If the sample day above was being planned for a man, the food choices would be very similar. Simply adjust the carb choices to reflect the way your individual carb budget is set up for the day. When you are first getting used to carb counting and learning to manage your condition, it is helpful to keep daily food records. Your diabetes educator may have already suggested this. It's also smart to check yourself regularly, to see if you are eating the calories and carbs that meet your treatment goals. The following sample menu planning sheet will be a useful tool. Share the days you record with your diabetes educator to get feedback and fine tune the management of your condition.

SAMPLE MENU

Date _____

_____ **Calories Per Day**

Daily Carb Budget: _____ grams or _____ Carb Choices

Food	Portion	Calories	Carbs
Breakfast Goals			_____
Breakfast Subtotals		_____	_____
Morning Snack Goals			_____
Morning Snack Subtotals		_____	_____
Lunch Goals			_____
Lunch Subtotals		_____	_____
Afternoon Snack Goals			_____
Afternoon Snack Subtotals		_____	_____
Dinner Goals			_____
Dinner Subtotals		_____	_____
Evening Snack Goals			_____
Evening Snack Subtotals		_____	_____
Day's Totals		_____	_____

LET'S TALK ABOUT EATING OUT

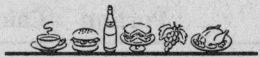

Whether it's a business lunch with clients, take-out on the way home from work, or a quick burger with your kids, eating out is part of the way we live. It's easy, quick, and fun, and it can even be healthy. Eating out, even regularly, can definitely fit into your diabetic meal plan.

You walk into a restaurant, you're shown to a table and handed a menu. Believe it or not, your key to a successful evening of eating out is right there in your hands. Read the menu carefully. Don't be afraid to ask for special options or substitutions. Many restaurants cater to diners' health needs. Some even offer "healthy" choices regularly.

Menu selections that tend to have fewer calories and fat are:

au jus (in its own juice)	cooked with lemon juice
baked	cooked with wine
boiled	deviled
broiled	fresh

garden fresh	poached
grilled	roasted
julienne	steamed
lean	stir fry
marinara	without skin

Menu choices that are more calorie dense are:

au gratin	gravy
battered	hollandaise
buttered	kiev
breaded	parmesan
casserole	parmigiana
cheese sauce (morney)	pastry
cream sauce (à la king)	pot pie
creamy (béchamel)	prime
creamed	remoulade
crispy	rich
deep fried	scalloped
escalloped	thermidor
fried	

Simply apply the meal-planning skills and carb-counting strategies you use every day to eat at home. All restaurants have low calorie and no calorie sweeteners. Most carry sugar free syrups and jelly, lowfat or nonfat salad dressings, nonfat milk, and diet drinks. Menu choices such as salads, fish, broiled lean meats, vegetables, fresh fruit, and whole grain breads are readily available. Do not be afraid to take control: ask questions, suggest substitutions, and be creative in putting together a meal you'll enjoy that fits into your daily carb and calorie budget.

YOU SHOULD KNOW

Before you order a predinner drink

Alcohol has no nutrients but it does have calories, and beer, wine, and mixed drinks contain carbs. Always drink alcohol with food because drinking on an empty stomach can make your blood sugar drop too low.

- *Good News: Light to moderate use of alcohol lowers the risk for diabetes.*
- *Bad News: Heavy drinking increases the risk for prediabetes and diabetes.*

Let's Order

- *Don't be afraid to ask*

  Can you split a dinner between two?

  Can your choice be broiled instead of fried?

  Can you skip the potato and order double vegetables?

  Can you swap French fries for sliced tomato?

  Can the chef leave off the salt?

- *Avoid temptation*

  Stay away from all-you-can-eat buffets; it's too tempting to overeat

  Don't supersize your choice; large portions mean more carbs and calories

  Take a roll and then ask that the bread basket be removed from the table

  Request no butter for the bread

Keep the vegetable tray and give back the chips and dip

- *"Something to drink?" "Water, thank you."*
  Choose calorie-free drinks—water, mineral water, club soda, unsweetened iced tea
  Choose lower calorie drinks—wine, wine spritzers, fruit juice with club soda, diet soda
  Limit alcohol; many drinks are packed with calories and carbs

- *Make an "appetizer" a meal*
  Order an appetizer portion as an entrée
  Ask if a luncheon portion can be ordered at dinner
  Share a main dish and order extra vegetables

- *Play with your food*
  Trim away excess fat
  Remove skin from poultry

- *On the side*
  Butter, gravy, salad dressing, sauce, sour cream, syrup, guacamole, grated cheese
  Use very small portions to enhance flavor and avoid piling on calories
  Try dipping your fork into the "extra" and then spear a piece of food, rather than dunking each bite

- *Eat slowly*
  Enjoy the company—talk more, eat less
  Enjoy the ambiance of the restaurant

- *Eat till you feel fine, not full*
  You don't have to clean your plate
  Ask for a "doggie bag" to take home

- *Split dessert*
  Share with another person, or better yet with the
     whole table
  Order fresh fruit
  End the meal with a richly flavored coffee or inter-
     esting tea instead of dessert

YOU SHOULD KNOW

The Diabetes Carbohydrate and Calorie Counter *is a
great eating out resource. In addition to the 89
restaurant chains listed in Part Two, there are over
600 take-out choices listed.*

LET'S TALK ABOUT SUGAR

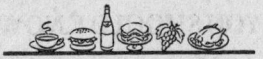

You are probably wondering why we haven't talked much about sugar up to now. In the past, people with diabetes were told they could not eat sugar because it would make their blood sugar go up too high. In fact, there is a long-standing myth that eating too much sugar causes diabetes. It's not true.

Research has shown that sugar has the same effect on blood sugar as *any* other carbs you eat. Calorie for calorie, sugar raises blood sugar about the same amount as bread, pasta, or potatoes. You can eat sugar and foods with sugar, as long as you count them in your total carb budget for the day.

Counting Sweets

As you choose different sweets, you need to know how each affects your carb budget for the day.

Let's start with the simplest sugars and sweeteners.

Sugars include table sugar, honey, brown sugar, molasses, fructose, corn syrup, raw sugar, and powdered sugar. Each contains carb, which needs to be counted as part of your daily carb budget.

YOU SHOULD KNOW
Sugar counts
1 teaspoon sugar = 4 grams carb

Reduced calorie sweeteners are often found in low calorie and low sugar foods like chewing gum, candy, cookies, and desserts. They appear on labels as *Sorbitol, Mannitol, Xylitol, Isomalt, Lactitol, Maltitol,* and *Trehalose.* These sugar substitutes, called *sugar alcohols,* are absorbed slowly by the body, so they have less impact on blood sugar levels. But they still contain carbs and calories, about half the calories of sugar. If you regularly eat foods with sugar alcohols, you need to count them in your carb budget for the day.

YOU SHOULD KNOW
How to carb count sugar alcohol
Sugar alcohol is listed on the nutrition label. Subtract half the sugar alcohol from the total carbohydrate. Count the answer in your carb budget for the day.

For example:
1 energy bar = 15 grams of carb and
6 grams of sugar alcohol
Half the sugar alcohol = 3 grams
15 – 3 = 12

Count 12 grams of carb in your daily carb budget when you eat this energy bar for a snack.

No calorie sweeteners or artificial sweeteners don't contain calories or carbs, and they don't affect your blood sugar. They are often referred to as "free foods" and you can use them as often as you wish. Brand names you may be familiar with are *Sweet'N Low, Sweet Twin, Equal, Sugar Twin, Sunette, Sweet One,* and *Splenda.*

YOU SHOULD KNOW

Color Counts
Tabletop sweetener comes in different-colored packages.
> *No calorie sweeteners: pink, blue, or yellow*
> *Sugar: white*
> *Raw sugar: tan*

Everyone loves desserts. Just because you have diabetes does not mean you have to give up desserts. Instead of "give it up," think "downsize and negotiate." Eat a smaller portion, or trade dessert for a meal carb. Many desserts, like custard, rice pudding, or fruit-based sweets, are good for you, and can be part of a healthy meal. Purely indulgent choices are not off-limits either; in those cases just think small. Instead of a large candy bar, have a snack size. Try mini-cupcakes. With a little creative planning, there is a way to fit in your favorites.

- Small amounts of dried fruit can satisfy a sweet tooth
- Eat smaller amounts of your favorites—a ½ cup of ice cream instead of a soup bowl-full

- When you eat out, split dessert with someone, or better yet, share with the whole table
- Try lower calorie, lower sugar recipes
- Buy lower sugar versions of favorites, but remember that low sugar doesn't always equal low calorie
- Use diet soda, sugar free drinks, and no calorie sweeteners in coffee and tea

---

Instead of Apple Pie, Try:

In a microwave safe serving dish, place
1 small apple, peeled and sliced
1 tablespoon raisins
1 teaspoon chopped walnuts
Pinch of cinnamon
1 pkg artificial sweetener*

Cover with plastic wrap or wax paper and microwave on high for 1 minute 45 seconds.

Calories: 106   Carb: 23

A la mode with ¼ cup light vanilla ice cream and the total is:

Calories: 150   Carb: 31

* If your carb budget allows, you can substitute 2 teaspoons of brown sugar (8 grams carb and 22 calories).

LET'S TALK ABOUT FIBER

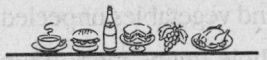

Fiber is the part of carbohydrates that you can't digest, and it has no calories. There is no need to count fiber, but you should try to include more high-fiber foods in your meals and snacks. The easiest switch is from white bread to whole wheat bread—more fiber, same amount of carb per portion. It's easy.

The main sources of fiber are fruits, vegetables, beans, and whole grains—all good-for-you foods. Eating more high-fiber foods will help normalize blood sugar, reduce cholesterol, help prevent colon cancer, prevent constipation, and even slightly lower blood pressure. Not bad for something that has no calories!

Slowly start eating fiber-rich foods—beans, berries, bran, fruits, oatmeal, vegetables, popcorn, and whole grains. Don't go overboard, because it takes your body a little time to adjust to the extra bulk passing through your digestive tract. And drink plenty of fluids. Fiber soaks up fluids like a sponge. This not only helps you feel fuller longer, but helps form soft, easily passed stools.

Add a Little Fiber to Your Life

- Eat whole fruits and vegetables instead of drinking juices

- Eat fruits and vegetables unpeeled

- Choose whole grains more often—whole wheat, cornmeal, barley, cracked wheat, and rye

- Eat whole grain or high-fiber cereals—oatmeal, oat flakes, bran, and shredded wheat

- Eat whole wheat bread, bagels, pasta, pretzels, crackers, and rolls

- Add beans, lentils, and peas to meals

- Try soybeans—edamame, soy nuts, tofu, or tempeh

- Snack on dried fruits, graham crackers, and popcorn

- Experiment with new versions of old favorites, like brown rice, buckwheat noodles, or baked sweet potatoes

---

Mash It, Smash It, Break It Apart

Fiber is fiber, no matter what you do in processing or cooking. Canned, pureed pumpkin is a rich source of fiber, as is split pea soup, mashed sweet potatoes, cream of broccoli soup, or a fruit smoothie.

MONITORING DIABETES

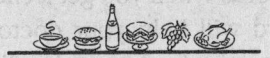

Many diabetes experts believe that self-monitoring is the key to successfully managing diabetes, reducing risks, and minimizing complications. Your diabetes educator, doctor, and dietitian will help you learn how to best monitor your condition.

Counting carbs and keeping a record of what you eat is one self-monitoring tool.

Checking Blood Sugar

Blood sugar is checked 2 ways: self-monitoring and the A1C test.

Your diabetes educator will tell you how often to check your blood sugar at home using a glucose monitor. At first you may do it more often, to be sure your medication and your diet are working together. Some people test 4 times a day, before each meal and at bedtime. If you have type 2 diabetes and your blood sugar is stable, you may test less frequently: 3 to 7 days a week before breakfast and randomly at other times during the day. At least 1 to 3 times a month, you should test before each meal and at bedtime to be sure your levels are within range.

You may be asked to keep a blood sugar log and to bring these records when you get a checkup. The numbers you record will help your doctor decide which type and how much of a drug or insulin you should be taking. They also give your diabetes educator information to help you adjust your daily carb budget.

YOU SHOULD KNOW

Target blood sugar values for people with diabetes

Time to Check	Target Blood Sugar Values
Upon waking, before eating	*90 to 130*
Before meals (at least 3 hours since your last meal)	*90 to 130*
2 hours after eating	*less than 160*
Bedtime (if it's lower, have a bedtime snack)	*110 to 150*

A1C is a blood test measuring a compound in your blood called *glycosylated hemoglobin*. The amount of this compound tells the average blood sugar level over the last 6 to 12 weeks. The A1C number is higher if blood sugar has been too high. For good control, the A1C value should be below 7%; a value of 6.5% means your average blood sugar is less than 155, which is very good. A1C tests should be done periodically throughout the year and are an excellent tool for monitoring long-term management of diabetes.

YOU SHOULD KNOW

- *Blood sugar below 70 is too low and above 240 is too high.*
- *Blood sugar equal to or over 200 increases your risk for infection and slows down wound healing.*

Low Blood Sugar: Hypoglycemia

If you ever think that your blood sugar is too low, test yourself with your glucose monitor. If the level is 70 or lower, have one of these "quick fix" foods immediately to raise your blood sugar. Each of the following equals 15 grams of carbohydrate or 1 carb choice.

- glucose gel packet or glucose tablets equaling 15 grams of carb
- ½ cup fruit juice
- 1 cup milk
- 1 to 2 teaspoons sugar or honey
- ½ cup regular soda
- 5 to 6 pieces of hard candy

Test your blood again in 15 minutes. If the level is still below 70, eat another 15 gram carb choice. Wait 15 minutes and test your blood again. If it will be an hour or more before your next meal, have a snack that contains both a carb and a protein. Good examples are:

- Peanut butter and crackers
- Cheese and crackers

- Half a ham or turkey sandwich
- Milk and cereal
- Hard or soft cooked egg and toast

It's a good idea to keep some of these "quick fix" choices in your house, desk drawer, or in the car when you drive long distances.

You Should Get a Round of Applause

Good diabetes control takes discipline, effort, and commitment. You need to monitor your diet, exercise, blood glucose, and drugs. Keep up the good work!

A WORD ABOUT THE GLYCEMIC INDEX

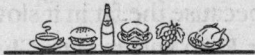

Decades ago, researcher David Jenkins at the University of Toronto coined the term *glycemic index* (GI). This index ranks carbohydrate foods by the amount they raise blood sugar after eating. Foods with a high glycemic index raise blood sugar levels quickly. Foods with a low GI produce a much smaller rise in blood sugar levels.

The theory behind the glycemic index is correct. Some foods do raise blood sugar quickly; others do not. But in practice, it's not that simple.

The glycemic index was devised based on eating one food at a time. Straight glucose was given a rating of 100 and individual foods were measured against it. White bread has a very high glycemic index. But if you add peanut butter, the glycemic response goes down because peanut butter, a high fat food, has a low glycemic index. The same goes for a baked potato, another high glycemic food; top it with cheese sauce and broccoli, and the glycemic index plunges.

It gets even more complicated. Ripe fruits have a lower glycemic index than unripe fruits. That's right, a hard peach will raise your blood sugar faster than a ripe, juicy one. Cooking pasta al dente is fine; overcook it, and its glycemic value goes up. Regular ice cream has a low glycemic index, because the fat in it slows down the absorption of sugar. Even sugars vary. Glucose is high on the index, but fructose (fruit sugar) is low.

GLYCEMIC INDEX OF COMMON FOODS

High (greater than 70)

White rice	*126*
Baked potato	*121*
Cornflakes	*119*
Rice cakes	*117*
Jellybeans	*114*
Carrots	*101*
White bread	*101*
Glucose	**100**
Wheat bread	*99*
Soda	*97*
Sucrose	*92*
Cheese pizza	*86*
Spaghetti	*83*
Popcorn	*79*
Corn	*78*
Banana	*76*
Orange juice	*74*

(continued)

Moderate (between 56 and 69)

Peas	68
Orange	62
Bran cereal	60
Apple juice	58
Pumpernickel bread	58

Low (55 and below)

Apple	52
Nonfat milk	46
Kidney beans	42
Fructose (fruit sugar)	32

Source: *Dietary Reference Intakes for Energy, Carbohydrate, Fiber, Fat, Fatty Acids, Cholesterol, Protein and Amino Acids, Part 1,* Institute of Medicine of the National Academies, The National Academies Press, 2002.

Bottom Line

Research into the health effects of the glycemic index is in its infancy. Most experts agree that the core concept is good: eat more high-fiber foods and fewer processed foods. Low GI foods include nonstarchy vegetables, most fruits, and dairy products, all good choices for someone with diabetes. Using the index might help you fine tune some of your carb choices, but exclusively eating-by-the-numbers could steer you away from otherwise healthy foods.

If you want to incorporate glycemic index choices into your carb budget for the day, that's fine. Some research has shown that this approach can give you a better blood sugar response.

YOU SHOULD KNOW

If you are considering using the glycemic index to help manage your diabetes, discuss the benefits with your diabetes educator, who can help you individualize this approach to your treatment goals.

WHEN YOU WANT
TO KNOW MORE

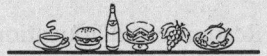

There are many resources available to help you learn more about diabetes, its treatment, and the newest research findings. Even food companies and pharmaceutical firms offer publications, newsletters, and recipes. Take advantage of all these resources because they provide interesting and worthwhile information. You can start with the following well-known and reliable resources.

American Diabetes Association
National Service Center
1701 North Beauregard Street
Alexandria, VA 22311
1-800-DIABETES (1-800-342-2383)
www.diabetes.org

National Diabetes Information Clearing House (NDIC)
1 Information Way
Bethesda, MD 20892-3560
1-800-860-8747
www.diabetes.niddk.nih.gov

National Diabetes Education Program (NDEP)
1 Diabetes Way
Bethesda, MD 20814-9692
1-800-438-5383
www.ndep.nih.gov

Diabetes Action Resource and Education Foundation
426 C Street, NE
Washington, DC 20002
202-333-4520
www.diabetesaction.org

Diabetes Exercise and Sports Association (DESA)
8001 Montcastle Drive
Nashville, TN 37221
1-800-898-4322
www.diabetes-exercise.org

Indian Health Service National Diabetes Program
5300 Homestead Road, NE
Albuquerque, NM 87110
505-246-4182
www.ihs.gov/MedicalPrograms/Diabetes/index.asp

Canadian Diabetes Association (CDA)
National Life Building
1400-522 University Avenue
Toronto, ON M5G 2R5
Canada
1-800-226-8464
www.diabetes.ca

International Diabetes Institute (IDI)
250 Kooyoung Road
Caulfield, Victoria 3162
Australia
061-03-9258-5050
www.diabetes.com.au *or* www.diabetes.org.au

USING YOUR DIABETES CARBOHYDRATE AND CALORIE COUNTER

The Diabetes Carbohydrate and Calorie Counter lists the portion size, calories, fat, carbohydrate, and sugar content for more than 11,000 foods. Now you can compare the values in your favorite foods and, when necessary, choose substitutes before you go out to shop or eat. This will save time and help you decide what to buy.

The carbohydrate and calorie values will help you stay within your carb and calorie budget for the day. Fat values have been included to help you plan lower fat meals to reduce your risk for heart disease. Sugar values were included to make you aware of which foods are high in sugar. Sugar is not counted separately, but is part of your total carb budget for the day.

The counter section of the book is divided into two parts: Part One: Brand Name, Nonbranded (Generic), and Take-Out Foods (page 67); and Part Two: Restaurant Chains (page 399). Each part lists foods or restaurant chains alphabetically.

In Part One, for each category, you will find non-branded (generic) foods listed first, in alphabetical order, followed by an alphabetical listing of brand name foods. The nonbranded listings will help you estimate calorie and carb values when you don't see your favorite. They can also help you to evaluate store brands. Large categories are divided into subcategories, such as canned, fresh, frozen, and ready-to-eat, to make it easier to find what you're looking for.

Because we eat out so often, more than 600 take-out foods are listed in Part One. These are found in the take-out subcategory in many categories throughout this section. Look there for foods you take out or order in, since they are not nutrition labeled.

Most foods are listed alphabetically, but in some cases, foods are grouped by category. For example, a tuna sandwich is found in the SANDWICH category. Other group categories include:

Asian Food   Page 73
    includes all types of Asian foods except
    egg rolls and sushi, which are found in
    separate categories

Deli Meats/Cold Cuts   Page 182
    includes all sandwich meats except
    chicken, ham, and turkey, which are
    found in separate categories

Dinner   Page 184
    includes all by brand name except
    pasta dinners, which are found in a
    separate category

Liquor/Liqueur   Page 252
includes all alcoholic beverages and
mixed drinks except beer, champagne,
and wine, which are found in separate
categories

Nutrition Supplements   Page 271
includes all dieting aids, meal
replacements, and drinks, except
energy bars and energy drinks, which
are found in separate categories

Sandwiches   Page 333
includes popular sandwich, calzone,
and panini choices

Snacks   Page 345
includes a variety of miscellaneous
snack items such as trail mix, pork
rinds, and cheese puffs

Spanish Food   Page 362
includes all types of Spanish and
Mexican foods except salsa and
tortillas, which are found in separate
categories

Part Two, Restaurant Chains, beginning on page 399, lists 89 national and regional restaurant, candy, coffee, doughnut, ice cream, pizza, sandwich, and sushi chains. Brand name foods are required by federal law to have nutrition information on their labels, but restaurants provide this information voluntarily.

With *The Diabetes Carbohydrate and Calorie Counter* as your guide, it will be easy for you to count carbs and manage your diabetes.

DEFINITIONS

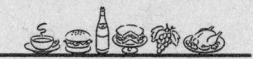

as prep (as prepared): refers to food that has been prepared according to package directions

lean and fat: describes meat with some fat on its edges that is not cut away before cooking, or poultry prepared with skin and fat as purchased

lean only: refers to lean meat that is trimmed of all visible fat, or poultry without skin

shelf stable: refers to prepared products found on the supermarket shelf that are ready-to-eat or are ready to be heated and do not require refrigeration

take-out: describes prepared dishes that you purchase ready-to-eat; those included serve as a guide to the calories in products you may purchase.

ABBREVIATIONS

avg	=	average
diam	=	diameter
fl	=	fluid
frzn	=	frozen
g	=	gram
in	=	inch
lb	=	pound
lg	=	large
med	=	medium
mg	=	milligram
oz	=	ounce
pkg	=	package
pt	=	pint
prep	=	prepared
qt	=	quart
reg	=	regular
sec	=	second
serv	=	serving
sm	=	small
sq	=	square
tbsp	=	tablespoon
tr	=	trace
tsp	=	teaspoon
w/	=	with
w/o	=	without
<	=	less than

NOTES

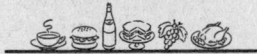

Cals = Calories
Carb = Carbohydrate
— (dash) indicates that values are not available
tr (trace) = less than 1 gram of fat, carbohydrate,
    or sugar
0 (zero) indicates there are no calories, fat,
    carbohydrate, or sugar

Discrepancies in figures are due to rounding, product reformulation, and reevaluation. Labeling law allows rounding of values. Some data listed is analysis data, obtained directly from manufacturers, not from labels. Therefore, some values may differ from those on labels because they have not been rounded.

PART ONE

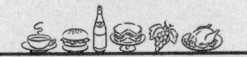

Brand Name, Nonbranded (Generic), and Take-Out Foods

YOU SHOULD KNOW

Naturally occurring compounds in certain healthy foods may help you manage your diabetes.

Green and black tea help to boost insulin activity and protect the eyes from damage.

Cinnamon lowers blood sugar.

Buckwheat lowers blood sugar.

Cherries lower blood sugar and help increase insulin production.

Foods high in vitamin C—citrus fruits, strawberries, watermelon, orange juice—help to prevent some complications from diabetes.

FOOD	PORTION	CALS	FAT	CARB	SUGAR
ABALONE					
breaded & fried	1 serv (3 oz)	162	6	9	tr
steamed	1 serv (3 oz)	127	3	6	tr
ACAI JUICE					
Zola Acai					
Juice	1 box (11 oz)	170	2	36	29
ACEROLA					
fresh	1 (5 g)	2	tr	tr	—
ACEROLA JUICE					
juice	1 cup	56	1	12	11
ADZUKI BEANS					
canned sweetened	½ cup	351	tr	81	—
AKEE					
fresh	3.5 oz	223	20	5	—
ALFALFA					
sprouts	½ cup	40	tr	1	tr
ALLIGATOR					
cooked	3 oz	126	2	0	0
ALLSPICE					
ground	1 tsp	5	tr	1	—
ALMONDS					
almond butter w/ salt	2 tbsp	203	19	7	2
almond paste	¼ cup	260	16	27	21
chocolate covered	6 pieces (0.6 oz)	102	8	6	3
dry roasted w/ salt	¼ cup	206	18	7	2
jordan almonds	6 pieces (0.7 oz)	99	4	14	13
praline	17 pieces (1.4 oz)	210	12	21	17
yogurt covered	6 pieces (0.8 oz)	122	8	10	8

FOOD	PORTION	CALS	FAT	CARB	SUGAR
American Almond					
Almond Paste	2 tbsp	140	9	13	11
Marzipan	2 tbsp	130	5	19	17
Blue Diamond					
Jalapeno Smokehouse	28 pieces (1 oz)	170	15	5	1
Milk Chocolate Covered	9 pieces (1.4 oz)	230	14	19	16
Smokehouse	28 pieces (1.3 oz)	170	16	5	1
Wasabi & Soy Sauce	28 pieces (1 oz)	170	15	6	2
Good Sense					
Raw Whole	¼ cup	180	15	6	0
Judy's					
Sugar Free Coconut Almond Brittle	¼ piece (1 oz)	90	5	2	0
Keto					
Chocolatey Covered	1 oz	169	13	7	0
Low Carb Creations					
Soft Almond Brittle	2 pieces (1 oz)	170	12	17	2
Mama Mellace's					
Butter Rum	1 oz	150	10	13	11
Cinnamon Roasted	1 oz	140	9	14	11
Sweet Delights					
Almond Roasters	⅓ pkg (1 oz)	190	14	6	3
AMARANTH					
leaves cooked	½ cup	14	tr	3	—
ANCHOVY					
boneless	1 oz	60	3	0	0
canned in oil drained	1 can (2 oz)	94	4	0	0
fresh	1 (4 g)	8	tr	0	0
ANISE					
seed	1 tsp	7	tr	1	—

FOOD	PORTION	CALS	FAT	CARB	SUGAR
ANTELOPE					
roasted	4 oz	215	4	0	0
APPLE					
CANNED					
sliced sweetened	½ cup	68	1	17	15
DRIED					
chopped	½ cup	104	tr	28	24
cooked w/o sugar	½ cup	73	tr	20	17
rings	5	78	tr	21	18
Crispy Green					
Crispy Apples	1 pkg (0.36 oz)	35	0	8	7
Del Monte					
Dried Apples	¼ cup	110	0	26	18
FRESH					
apple	1 sm	55	tr	15	11
apple	1 lg	110	tr	29	22
apple	1 med	72	tr	19	14
candied	1 sm (4.9 oz)	179	3	40	32
w/ skin sliced	1 cup	57	tr	15	11
w/o skin sliced	1 cup	53	tr	14	11
TreeTop					
Slices Red or Green	1 pkg (2 oz)	35	0	8	7
TAKE-OUT					
baked	1 (6 oz)	128	tr	42	37
baked no sugar	1 (5.6 oz)	136	tr	24	18
fried apple rings	1 serv (2.7 oz)	91	4	15	12
APPLE JUICE					
cider	1 cup	117	tr	29	27
mulled cider	1 serv	265	1	42	–
Hansen's					
100% Juice	8 oz	120	0	28	23

FOOD	PORTION	CALS	FAT	CARB	SUGAR
Hood					
100% Juice	1 cup	120	0	31	31
Kedem					
100% Juice	8 oz	110	0	28	28
Langers					
100% Cider	8 oz	120	0	28	26
100% Juice	8 oz	120	0	28	26
Diet Cocktail	8 oz	60	0	14	13
Low Carb Creations					
Apple Cider as prep	1 serv	10	0	2	tr
Minute Maid					
100% Juice	8 oz	100	0	28	26
Naked Juice					
Just Apple	8 oz	120	0	30	18
Ocean Spray					
100% Juice	8 oz	110	0	28	28
Odwalla					
Spiced Harvest Cider	8 fl oz	130	0	30	28
Red Cheek					
100% Juice	8 oz	120	0	29	23
Robert & James					
100% Juice	8 oz	110	0	28	28
Seneca					
100% Juice	8 oz	110	0	28	26
Snapple					
Diet	8 oz	15	0	4	3
TreeTop					
100% Juice	8 oz	120	0	29	26
Cider 100% Juice No Sugar Added	8 oz	120	0	29	26
APPLESAUCE					
sweetened	½ cup	97	tr	25	21
unsweetened	½ cup	52	tr	14	12

FOOD	PORTION	CALS	FAT	CARB	SUGAR
Jok'n'Al					
Low Carb	1 tbsp	10	0	2	1
Mott's					
Single-Serve Cinnamon	1 pkg (4 oz)	100	0	25	23
White House					
Apple Sauce	1 pkg (4 oz)	90	0	20	15
APRICOT JUICE					
nectar	6 oz	106	tr	27	26
APRICOTS					
CANNED					
heavy syrup	½ cup	91	tr	23	20
juice pack	½ cup	59	tr	15	13
light syrup	½ cup	80	tr	21	19
water pack	½ cup	33	tr	8	6
Del Monte					
Halves In Heavy Syrup	½ cup	100	0	26	25
Orchard Select Halves	½ cup	80	0	21	20
DRIED					
halves	6	51	tr	13	11
halves cooked w/o sugar	½ cup	106	tr	28	24
Crispy Green					
Crispy Apricots	1 pkg (0.36 oz)	40	0	9	7
FRESH					
apricots	1	17	tr	4	3
sliced	½ cup	40	tr	9	8
ARTICHOKE					
CANNED					
hearts in oil	1 serv (3 oz)	100	7	9	1
FRESH					
cooked	1 med	60	tr	13	1
hearts cooked	½ cup	42	tr	9	1

FOOD	PORTION	CALS	FAT	CARB	SUGAR
TAKE-OUT					
stuffed	1 (8.8 oz)	397	14	54	6
ARUGULA					
fresh	1 cup	3	tr	1	tr
ASIAN FOOD					
FRESH					
Azumaya					
Wrappers Large Square	8	160	1	31	1
Frieda's					
Won Ton Wrappers	4 (1 oz)	80	0	17	1
Nasoya					
Won Ton Wrappers	8	160	1	31	1
FROZEN					
Lean Cuisine					
Cafe Classics Asian Style Beef w/ Ginger & Soy	1 pkg (9.25 oz)	210	4	31	8
Cafe Classics Bowl Chicken Fried Rice	1 pkg (10 oz)	310	7	45	6
Cafe Classics Bowl Chicken Teriyaki	1 pkg (11 oz)	320	3	58	11
Cafe Classics Bowl Teriyaki Steak	1 pkg (10.5 oz)	340	7	47	10
Cafe Classics Chicken Teriyaki Stir Fry	1 pkg (10 oz)	300	5	49	11
Cafe Classics Hunan Beef & Broccoli	1 pkg (8.5 oz)	230	4	36	9
Cafe Classics Thai-Style Chicken	1 pkg (9 oz)	230	4	30	8
One Dish Favorites Asian Style Pot Stickers	1 pkg (9 oz)	320	6	55	11
One Dish Favorites Chicken Chow Mein	1 pkg (9 oz)	200	3	31	3

FOOD	PORTION	CALS	FAT	CARB	SUGAR
Skillet Asian Style Chicken & Vegetables	1 serv	160	3	22	5
MIX					
Annie Chun's					
Meal Kit Black Bean	1 serv	230	3	42	8
Meal Kit Garlic Scallion	1 serv	230	5	39	6
Meal Kit Soy Ginger	1 serv	220	2	42	9
TAKE-OUT					
buddha's delight w/ cellophane noodles fat choi jai	1 serv (7.6 oz)	211	4	44	3
cha siu bao steamed buns w/ chicken filling	1 (2.3 oz)	160	3	26	4
chop suey w/ beef & pork	1 cup	300	17	13	—
chop suey w/ pork	1 cup	375	29	29	—
chow mein chicken	1 cup	255	10	10	—
chow mein pork	1 cup	425	24	21	—
chow mein shrimp	1 cup	221	10	21	—
chow mein vegetable	1 serv (8 oz)	90	3	15	2
dim sum meat filled	3 pieces (4 oz)	124	3	11	1
egg foo yung beef	1 patty (6 oz)	243	16	7	3
egg foo yung chicken	1 patty (3 oz)	121	8	4	2
egg foo yung pork	1 patty (3 oz)	125	8	4	2
egg foo yung shrimp	1 patty (3 oz)	153	12	3	2
filipino chicken adobo	1 serv (15 oz)	555	26	45	tr
fried rice vegetable	1 cup	210	9	30	3
fried rice w/ egg	1 serv (6.7 oz)	395	20	49	—
kung pao chicken w/ rice	1 serv (1.75 cups)	240	3	42	3
phad thai	1 serv (9.2 oz)	232	9	30	2
sesame seed paste bun	1 (2.5 oz)	220	6	39	12
shrimp chips	1¼ cups (1 oz)	140	6	19	1

FOOD	PORTION	CALS	FAT	CARB	SUGAR
shu mai chicken & vegetable dumplings	6 (3.6 oz)	160	5	18	6
spring roll	1 (3.5 oz)	112	2	37	–
sweet & sour pork	1 serv (8 oz)	250	8	37	30
sweet red bean bun	1 (2.5 oz)	130	1	38	17
szechuan chicken w/ lo mein	1 cup (5.3 oz)	190	1	35	3
tempura vegetables	5 pieces (4 oz)	270	15	31	3
teriyaki chicken plain	¾ cup	399	27	7	–
teriyaki chicken w/ rice	1 serv (11 oz)	430	6	77	10
wonton fried	½ cup (1 oz)	111	8	8	–

ASPARAGUS
CANNED
spears	1 cup	46	2	6	3
Del Monte					
Cuts & Tips	½ cup	20	0	3	0
Tips	½ cup	20	0	3	0
FRESH					
cooked	4 spears	13	tr	2	1
Frieda's					
White	⅔ cup	20	0	4	2

AVOCADO
california mashed	¼ cup	96	9	5	tr
california peeled & pitted	1	289	27	15	1
florida mashed	¼ cup	69	6	5	0
florida peeled & pitted	1	365	31	24	7
Brooks Tropical					
Lite SlimCado	1 tbsp	35	3	3	0
Calavo					
Fresh	⅕ med (1 oz)	55	5	3	0
Frieda's					
Fresh Cocktail	1 (1.4 oz)	60	6	3	0

FOOD	PORTION	CALS	FAT	CARB	SUGAR
TAKE-OUT					
guacamole	1 serv (2.2 oz)	105	10	5	1
BACON					
bacon grease	1 tbsp	116	13	0	0
beef breakfast strips cooked	3 strips	153	12	tr	0
pan fried	3 strips	109	9	tr	—
BACON SUBSTITUTES					
bacon bits meatless	1 tbsp	33	2	2	0
meatless	1 strip	16	1	tr	0
Lightlife					
Organic Tempeh Smokey Strips	3 slices (2 oz)	80	3	6	1
Smart Bacon	2 strips (0.8 oz)	45	2	1	1
BAGEL					
cinnamon raisin	1 mini	71	tr	14	2
cinnamon raisin	1 lg (4 in)	244	2	49	5
egg	1 lg (4.5 in)	364	3	69	—
low carb	1 (4 oz)	216	0	42	0
mini onion	1 (1.4 oz)	100	0	20	1
oat bran	1 lg (4 in)	227	1	47	1
plain	1 lg (4.5 in)	360	2	70	—
plain	1 med (3.5 in)	289	2	56	—
plain	1 sm (3 in)	190	1	37	—
Alvarado Street Bakery					
Sprouted Wheat Cinnamon Raisin	1 (3.3 oz)	280	1	59	28
Pepperidge Farm					
100% Whole Wheat	1	250	2	49	9
Mini 100% Whole Wheat	1	100	1	20	3

FOOD	PORTION	CALS	FAT	CARB	SUGAR
Sara Lee					
Heart Healthy 100% Whole Wheat	1 (3.3 oz)	220	2	47	8
Heart Healthy Cinnamon Raisin	1 (3.3 oz)	250	2	50	13
Whole Grain Plain	1 (3.3 oz)	240	1	50	6
Thomas'					
Carb Consider Plain	1	150	3	24	tr
Carb Consider Whole Wheat	1	140	3	23	tr
Weight Watchers					
Original	1 (2.8 oz)	190	2	44	3

BAKING POWDER

FOOD	PORTION	CALS	FAT	CARB	SUGAR
baking powder	1 tsp	2	0	1	—

BAKING SODA

FOOD	PORTION	CALS	FAT	CARB	SUGAR
baking soda	1 tsp	0	0	0	0

BALSAM PEAR (BITTER GOURD)

FOOD	PORTION	CALS	FAT	CARB	SUGAR
leafy tips cooked w/o salt	1 cup	20	tr	4	1
pods sliced cooked w/ salt	1 cup	24	tr	5	2

BAMBOO SHOOTS

FOOD	PORTION	CALS	FAT	CARB	SUGAR
canned sliced	½ cup	12	tr	2	1
raw sliced	½ cup	20	tr	4	2

BANANA

FOOD	PORTION	CALS	FAT	CARB	SUGAR
banana chips	1 oz	147	10	17	—
fresh	1 med (7 in)	105	tr	27	14
fresh	1 lg (8 in)	121	tr	31	17
fresh	1 sm (6 in)	90	tr	23	12
fresh baby	1 extra sm (<6 in)	72	tr	19	10
fresh mashed	½ cup	100	tr	26	14
fresh sliced	1 cup	134	1	34	18

FOOD	PORTION	CALS	FAT	CARB	SUGAR
powder	1 tbsp	21	tr	5	3
whole dried	1 piece (1.2 oz)	130	1	33	22
Frieda's					
Burro	1 (3 oz)	80	0	20	13
Goodniks					
Nutty Bananas Crunchy Snack	⅔ cup	230	16	21	3

BARBECUE SAUCE
Carb Options

Original	2 tbsp	10	0	3	0
Consorzio					
Organic Original	1 tbsp	50	0	11	10
Organic Spicy	1 tbsp	50	0	11	10
Hunt's					
Hickory	2 tbsp	45	0	11	9
Hickory & Brown Sugar	2 tbsp	70	0	16	15
Honey Hickory	2 tbsp	50	0	12	11
Honey Mustard	2 tbsp	50	0	12	10
Hot & Spicy	2 tbsp	45	0	11	8
Mesquite	2 tbsp	40	0	9	6
Original	2 tbsp	50	0	13	10
Nando's					
Barbecue	1 tbsp	7	0	2	1
Steel's					
Sugar Free	2 tbsp	15	0	2	0

BARLEY

flour	1 cup	511	2	110	1
pearled cooked	1 cup (5.5 oz)	193	1	44	tr

BARRACUDA

broiled	4 oz	239	14	tr	tr
cooked flaked	1 cup	287	16	1	tr

FOOD	PORTION	CALS	FAT	CARB	SUGAR
TAKE-OUT					
breaded & fried	4 oz	282	17	5	tr
BASIL					
fresh chopped	1 tbsp	1	tr	tr	tr
ground	1 tsp	4	tr	1	–
BASS					
freshwater raw	3 oz	97	3	0	0
sea cooked	3 oz	105	2	0	0
striped baked	3 oz	105	3	0	0
BAY LEAF					
crumbled	1 tsp	2	tr	tr	–
BEANS					
CANNED					
baked beans w/ pork & tomato sauce	½ cup	119	1	24	7
Bush's					
Barbecue	½ cup	150	1	32	13
Homestyle	½ cup	140	1	29	12
Onion 98% Fat Free	½ cup	140	1	29	12
Vegetarian Fat Free	½ cup (4.6 oz)	130	0	24	4
Heinz					
Vegetarian	1 cup	250	1	48	24
Old El Paso					
Refried Fat Free	½ cup	100	0	18	1
Ranch Style					
Original Texas	½ cup	138	3	20	2
Read					
3 Bean Salad	½ cup	60	0	13	8
Van Camp's					
Pork And Beans	½ cup	110	1	23	7

FOOD	PORTION	CALS	FAT	CARB	SUGAR
FROZEN					
Lean Cuisine					
Cafe Classics Sante Fe Style Rice & Beans	1 pkg (10.4 oz)	290	5	50	10
TAKE-OUT					
refried beans	½ cup	43	2	5	–
three bean salad	¾ cup	230	11	31	–
BEAR					
simmered	3 oz	220	11	0	0
BEAVER					
roasted	3 oz	140	6	0	0
BEEF					
FRESH					
arm pot roast trim 0 fat braised	3.5 oz	297	19	0	0
arm pot roast trim ⅛ in fat braised	3.5 oz	302	19	0	0
beef crumbles 70% lean pan browned	3 oz	230	15	0	0
bottom round roast trim 0 in fat braised	4 oz	253	10	0	0
bottom round roast trim 0 in fat roasted	3.5 oz	187	8	0	0
bottom round roast trim ½ in fat braised	4 oz	337	22	0	0
bottom round roast trim ⅛ in fat braised	4 oz	280	13	0	0
bottom round roast trim ⅛ in fat roasted	4 oz	247	13	0	0
bottom sirloin butt roast trim 0 in roasted	3.5 oz	182	8	0	0

FOOD	PORTION	CALS	FAT	CARB	SUGAR
brisket flat half trim ⅛ in fat braised	3.5 oz	298	19	0	0
brisket flat trim 0 fat braised	3.5 oz	221	9	0	0
brisket point half trim 0 fat braised	3.5 oz	358	29	0	0
brisket point half trim ¼ in fat braised	3.5 oz	404	22	0	0
brisket point half trim ⅛ in fat braised	3.5 oz	349	27	0	0
chuck boston cut roast trim 0 fat roasted	3.5 oz	207	11	0	0
chuck boston cut roast trim ¼ in fat roasted	3.5 oz	242	15	0	0
chuck bottom roast trim 0 fat braised	3.5 oz	334	24	0	0
chuck bottom roast trim ¼ in fat braised	3.5 oz	345	26	0	0
chuck fillet steak trim 0 fat broiled	4 oz	181	6	0	0
chuck top roast trim 0 fat broiled	4 oz	245	13	0	0
club steak trim ½ in fat broiled	4 oz	384	29	0	0
corned beef brisket cooked	3 oz	213	16	tr	0
crosscut shank trim ¼ in fat stewed	1 serv (6.8 oz)	510	28	0	0
delmonico steak trim ¼ in fat broiled	4 oz	409	33	0	0
entrecote steak trim ½ in fat broiled	4 oz	413	33	0	0

FOOD	PORTION	CALS	FAT	CARB	SUGAR
eye round roast trim 0 in fat roasted	4 oz	190	5	0	0
eye round roast trim ¼ in fat roasted	4 oz	283	17	0	0
eye round roast trim ⅛ in fat roasted	4 oz	236	11	0	0
filet mignon roast trim ¼ in fat roasted	4 oz	376	29	0	0
filet mignon roast trim ⅛ in fat roasted	4 oz	367	28	0	0
filet mignon trim 0 in fat broiled	4 oz	247	13	0	0
filet mignon trim ⅛ in fat broiled	4 oz	303	19	0	0
ground 70% lean broiled	3.5 oz	273	18	0	0
ground 75% lean broiled	2.5 oz	195	13	0	0
ground 80% lean broiled	3 oz	234	15	0	0
ground 85% lean pan fried	3 oz	197	12	0	0
ground 90% lean pan fried	3 oz	173	9	0	0
ground 95% lean pan fried	3 oz	139	5	0	0
ground 97% fat free irradiated	4 oz	160	8	0	0
london broil trim 0 fat broiled	3.5 oz	188	8	0	0
london broil trim ¼ in fat broiled	4 oz	260	12	0	0
new york strip steak trim 0 fat broiled	4 oz	219	9	0	0
porterhouse steak trim 0 in fat broiled	1 lb	1252	87	0	0

FOOD	PORTION	CALS	FAT	CARB	SUGAR
porterhouse steak trim ¼ in fat broiled	1 lb	1284	117	0	0
porterhouse steak trim ⅛ in fat broiled	4 oz	337	25	0	0
porterhouse steak trim ⅛ in fat broiled	1 lb	1346	99	0	0
rib eye roast trim ¼ in fat roasted	3.5 oz	365	30	0	0
rib eye steak trim ⅛ in fat broiled	4 oz	221	9	0	0
rib roast trim ¼ in fat roasted	4 oz	406	33	0	0
rib steak trim ¼ in fat broiled	4 oz	388	31	0	0
round tip roast trim 0 in fat roasted	4 oz	213	9	0	0
sandwich steaks thinly sliced	1 serv (2 oz)	173	15	0	0
shell steak trim ¼ in fat broiled	4 oz	366	27	0	0
shortribs lean & fat braised	1 serv (7.8 oz)	1060	94	0	0
skirt steak trim 0 fat broiled	4 oz	289	19	0	0
t-bone steak trim 0 fat broiled	4 oz	280	18	0	0
t-bone steak trim ¼ in fat broiled	1 lb	1388	103	0	0
t-bone steak trim ⅛ in fat broiled	1 lb	804	56	0	0
tip round roast trim ⅛ in fat roasted	4 oz	248	13	0	0

FOOD	PORTION	CALS	FAT	CARB	SUGAR
top loin steak boneless trim ⅛ in fat broiled	4 oz	299	19	0	0
top round roast trim 0 fat braised	4 oz	237	7	0	0
top round roast trim ¼ in fat braised	4 oz	281	13	0	0
top round roast trim ¼ in fat roasted	4 oz	265	15	0	0
top round steak trim ¼ in fat pan fried	4 oz	314	17	0	0
top sirloin steak trim ⅛ in fat broiled	4 oz	275	16	0	0
top sirloin steak trim ⅛ in fat pan fried	4 oz	355	24	0	0
tri-tip roast trim 0 fat roasted	3.5 oz	218	12	0	0
tri-tip steak trim 0 fat broiled	4 oz	300	17	0	0
READY-TO-EAT					
roast beef spread	¼ cup	127	9	2	tr

BEEF DISHES

CANNED

Hormel

FOOD	PORTION	CALS	FAT	CARB	SUGAR
Corned Beef Hash 50% Reduced Fat	1 cup	290	12	24	2
Libby's					
Hash Corned Beef	1 cup	420	24	33	1
REFRIGERATED					
Hormel					
Beef Roast Au Jus	1 serv (5 oz)	200	9	3	3
Beef Tips w/ Gravy	½ cup	160	7	5	3
Huxtable's					
Shepherds Pie Beef	1 pkg (10 oz)	270	11	27	1

FOOD	PORTION	CALS	FAT	CARB	SUGAR
Morton's Of Omaha					
Beef Pot Roast w/ Gravy	1 serv (3 oz)	160	5	2	0
TAKE-OUT					
beef bouriguignon	1 serv (7 oz)	254	16	3	—
beef curry	1 cup	432	31	14	6
bool kogi korean marinated beef ribs	4 oz	190	10	6	4
bubble & squeak	5 oz	186	13	16	—
bulgoghi korean grilled beef	1 serv (5.2 oz)	256	15	5	3
cornish pasty	1 (8 oz)	847	52	79	—
greek moussaka	1 serv (8.5 oz)	450	33	12	4
irish stew	1 cup (7 oz)	280	16	10	—
kebab indian	1 (5.4 oz)	553	40	2	—
kheena	6.7 oz	781	71	1	—
koftas	5	280	22	3	—
pot roast w/ gravy	1 serv (6 oz)	320	10	4	0
samosa	2 (4 oz)	652	62	20	—
shepherds pie	1 serv (7 oz)	282	16	20	—
steak & kidney pie w/ top crust	1 slice (5 oz)	400	26	23	—
stew w/ vegetables	1 serv (8 oz)	218	12	16	2
stroganoff	¾ cup	260	19	43	—
swiss steak	4.6 oz	214	9	10	—
toad in the hole	1 (4.7 oz)	383	29	23	—
BEEFALO					
roasted	4 oz	213	7	0	0
BEER AND ALE					
alcohol free beer	7 fl oz	50	tr	11	5
ale brown	10 oz	77	0	8	—
ale pale	10 oz	88	0	12	—
beer light	12 oz can	103	0	5	tr

FOOD	PORTION	CALS	FAT	CARB	SUGAR
beer regular	12 oz can	139	0	11	0
black & tan	1 serv (12 oz)	146	0	13	—
boilermaker	1 serv	216	0	13	—
lager	10 oz	80	0	4	—
mead	1 serv	250	0	13	—
pilsener lager	7 oz	85	tr	13	2
shandy	1 serv	125	0	12	—
stout	10 oz	102	0	6	—
Coors					
Nonalcoholic	1 bottle (12 oz)	73	0	14	—
Original	1 bottle (12 oz)	148	0	11	—
Corona					
Light	1 bottle (12 oz)	109	0	7	—
Edison					
Light	1 bottle	109	0	7	—
Genessee					
Genny Light	1 bottle (12 oz)	96	0	6	—
Guiness					
Draught	1 bottle (12 oz)	125	0	10	—
Foreign Extra Stout	1 bottle (12 oz)	176	0	14	—
Michelob					
Ultra Low Carbohydrate	1 bottle (12 oz)	95	0	3	—
BEETS					
CANNED					
harvard	½ cup	90	tr	22	—
pickled	½ cup	74	tr	18	—
sliced	½ cup	37	tr	9	8
Del Monte					
Pickled Sliced	½ cup	35	0	8	5
Sliced	½ cup	35	0	8	5
FRESH					
greens cooked w/o salt	½ cup	19	tr	4	tr

FOOD	PORTION	CALS	FAT	CARB	SUGAR
sliced cooked	½ cup	37	tr	8	7
whole cooked	2 med (3.5 oz)	44	tr	10	8
Frieda's					
Beets	½ cup	35	0	8	5

BISCUIT
MIX
Bisquick

Reduced Fat	⅓ cup	150	3	27	3
Jiffy					
Buttermilk as prep	1	170	4	29	2
MiniCarb					
Buttery as prep	1	255	21	3	0

REFRIGERATED

plain baked	1 (1 oz)	93	4	13	tr

TAKE-OUT

buttermilk	1 lg (2.7 oz)	280	13	37	1
plain	1 sm (1.2 oz)	127	6	17	tr
tea biscuit	1 (3 oz)	210	3	30	12
w/ egg	1 (4.8 oz)	373	22	32	—
w/ egg & bacon	1 (5.3 oz)	458	31	29	1
w/ egg & ham	1 (6.7 oz)	442	27	30	2
w/ egg & sausage	1 (6.3 oz)	581	39	11	1
w/ ham	1 (4 oz)	386	18	44	1
w/ sausage	1 (4.4 oz)	485	32	40	1

BISON

roasted	3 oz	122	2	0	0

BITTERMELON
Frieda's

Foo Qua	1 cup	15	0	3	0

BLACK BEANS

dried cooked	1 cup	227	1	41	—

FOOD	PORTION	CALS	FAT	CARB	SUGAR
BLACKBERRIES					
canned in heavy syrup	½ cup	118	tr	30	25
fresh	½ cup	31	tr	7	4
unsweetened frzn	½ cup	48	tr	12	8
BLACKBERRY JUICE					
canned	6 oz	65	1	13	13
BLACKEYE PEAS					
DRIED					
cooked	1 cup	198	1	36	–
BLINTZE					
Cohen's & Wilton					
Cheese	1	80	3	10	5
Golden					
Cheese	1 (2.1 oz)	80	2	13	5
Potato	1	90	4	15	2
Vegetable	1	110	5	15	0
Ratner's					
Cheese	1 (2.2 oz)	90	2	14	5
TAKE-OUT					
cheese	1 (2.7 oz)	160	9	15	4
BLUEBERRIES					
canned in heavy syrup	½ cup	113	tr	28	26
fresh	½ cup	41	tr	11	7
fresh	1 pt	229	1	58	40
frzn unsweetened	½ cup	40	1	9	7
A&L Farms					
Bleuets Fresh	1 pt	80	0	19	9
Frieda's					
Dried	¼ cup (1.4 oz)	140	0	33	17

FOOD	PORTION	CALS	FAT	CARB	SUGAR
BLUEBERRY JUICE					
Hi-C					
Blazin' Blueberry	1 box	100	0	26	26
Van Dyk's					
100% Juice	6 oz	74	0	18	15
BLUEFIN					
fillet baked	4.1 oz	186	6	0	0
BLUEFISH					
fresh baked	3 oz	135	5	0	0
BOAR					
wild roasted	3 oz	136	4	0	–
BONITO					
fresh	3 oz	117	4	0	0
BOYSENBERRIES					
frzn unsweetened	½ cup	33	tr	8	5
BRAINS					
beef pan-fried	3 oz	167	13	0	0
beef simmered	3 oz	123	9	0	0
lamb braised	3 oz	123	9	0	0
lamb fried	3 oz	232	19	0	0
pork braised	3 oz	117	8	0	0
veal braised	3 oz	116	8	0	0
veal fried	3 oz	181	14	0	0
BRAN					
oat	½ cup (1.6 oz)	116	3	31	–
wheat	½ cup (2 oz)	63	1	19	–
Hodgson Mill					
Oat	¼ cup	120	3	23	0
Wheat Unprocessed	¼ cup	30	0	10	0

FOOD	PORTION	CALS	FAT	CARB	SUGAR
BREAD					
CANNED					
boston brown	1 slice (1.6 oz)	88	1	19	5
FROZEN					
Pepperidge Farm					
Whole Grain Garlic	1 serv (2.5 inch)	170	8	20	1
Whole Grain Garlic Texas Toast	1 slice	150	8	14	1
MIX					
Buitoni					
Focaccia Rosemary & Garlic	1 piece (1 oz)	110	1	22	2
Foccacia Italian Herb & Cheese	1 slice	110	2	21	3
MiniCarb					
Country White as prep	1 slice	80	3	7	0
Sassafras					
12 Grain & Sunflower	1 slice (1.4 oz)	150	2	28	4
READY-TO-EAT					
anadama	1 (1.1 oz)	87	1	16	3
baguette parisian	2 oz	120	0	26	0
baguette whole wheat	2 oz	140	0	29	tr
challah	1 slice (1.4 oz)	115	2	19	1
cinnamon	1 slice (0.9 oz)	69	1	13	1
cuban bread	1 slice (1.1 oz)	83	1	16	1
french	1 slice (1.1 oz)	88	1	17	tr
navajo fry	1 piece	281	10	41	2
oat bran	1 slice (1.1 oz)	71	1	12	2
oatmeal	1 slice (0.9 oz)	73	1	13	2
pan criollo	1 piece (0.9 oz)	69	1	13	tr
pannetone	1 slice (0.9 oz)	86	2	15	5
pita	1 lg (2 oz)	165	1	33	1
pita	1 sm (1 oz)	77	tr	16	tr

FOOD	PORTION	CALS	FAT	CARB	SUGAR
pita whole wheat	1 sm (1 oz)	74	1	15	tr
pita whole wheat	1 lg (2.2 oz)	170	2	35	1
potato scallion	1 slice (2 oz)	120	1	24	1
pumpernickel	1 slice (0.9 oz)	65	1	12	tr
raisin	1 slice (1.1 oz)	88	1	17	2
rye	1 slice (1.1 oz)	83	1	15	tr
seven grain	1 slice (1.1 oz)	80	1	15	3
wheat berry	1 slice (0.9 oz)	65	1	12	1
wheat bran	1 slice (1.3 oz)	89	1	17	3
wheat germ	1 slice (1 oz)	73	1	14	1
white cubed	1 cup	93	1	18	2
whole wheat	1 slice (1 oz)	69	1	13	6
Alvarado Street Bakery					
Diabetic Lifestyle	1 (1.2 oz)	80	0	15	2
Arnold					
Bakery Light 100% Whole Wheat	1 slice	80	1	18	3
Country Classics Buttermilk	1 slice	110	2	19	4
Country Classics Wheat	1 slice	100	2	19	4
Raisin Cinnamon	1 slice (1 oz)	80	2	15	6
Smart & Healthy Omega-3 100% Whole Wheat	1 slice	80	1	16	2
Smart & Healthy Sugar Free 100% Whole Wheat	1 slice	80	1	15	0
Beefsteak					
Rye Soft	1 slice	70	1	14	1
Cedar's					
Wraps Whole Wheat	1 (2 oz)	180	4	34	tr
Damascus					
Roll-Up Flax	1 (2 oz)	110	3	15	1
Roll-Up Whole Wheat	1 (2 oz)	110	3	17	1

FOOD	PORTION	CALS	FAT	CARB	SUGAR
Wraps Honey Wheat	½ wrap (2 oz)	130	0	28	0
Wraps Spinach	1 (4 oz)	280	0	52	tr
Ecce Panis					
Country Wheat	1 slice (2 oz)	150	0	32	tr
European Baguette	2 oz	150	0	34	tr
Enjoy Life					
Rye-Less Rye	1 slice	80	1	18	2
Food For Life					
Brown Rice Bread Yeast Free	1 slice	100	1	20	1
Rice Bread Fruit & Seed Yeast Free	1 slice	140	1	35	3
Rice Bread Multi Seed Yeast Free	1 slice	120	1	26	1
White Rice Bread Yeast Free	1 slice	100	0	23	0
Freihofer's					
100% Whole Wheat	1 slice	90	2	17	3
Whole Wheat Light	2 slices	80	1	19	3
French Meadow Bakery					
Health Seed	1 slice	110	4	18	0
Healthy Hemp	1 slice	92	2	12	1
Men's Bread	1 slice	89	3	9	0
Woman's Bread	1 slice	81	2	11	0
Kangaroo					
Bread Wraps	1 (2.6 oz)	140	3	30	0
Greek Pita Flat	1 (2.6 oz)	200	2	38	2
Greek Pita Flat Wheat	1 (2.4 oz)	145	2	30	1
Pita Pockets Onion	½ (1.2 oz)	90	0	18	1
Pita Pockets Wheat N'Honey	½ (1.2 oz)	90	0	16	1
Pita Pockets White	½ (1.2 oz)	90	0	18	1
Salad Pockets	1 (1.2 oz)	90	0	16	1

FOOD	PORTION	CALS	FAT	CARB	SUGAR
Sandwich Pockets Whole Grain	1 (1.2 oz)	80	1	16	1
Matthew's					
All Natural Cinnamon Raisin	1 slice	80	1	17	6
Natural Ovens					
100% Whole Grain	1 slice	60	1	14	1
7 Grain Herb	1 slice	70	1	16	1
Better White	1 slice	80	1	19	1
Cracked Wheat	1 slice	80	1	16	1
English Muffin Bread	1 slice	80	1	16	1
Glorious Cinnamon Raisin	1 slice	70	1	15	3
Happiness Raisin Pecan	1 slice	70	1	15	3
Health Max	1 slice	80	1	16	2
Hunger Filler	1 slice	60	1	13	1
Lo Carb Golden Crunch	1 slice	70	4	7	2
Lo Carb Original	1 slice	60	2	8	2
Mild Rye	1 slice	70	1	13	0
Multi-Grain Stay Slim	1 slice	60	1	14	1
Nutty Natural	1 slice	70	1	16	1
Right Wheat	1 slice	60	1	13	1
Soft Wheat	1 slice	70	1	15	1
Sunny Millet	1 slice	60	1	14	1
Nature's Path					
Manna Carrot Raisin	1 slice	130	0	27	10
Manna Millet Rice	1 slice	130	0	28	9
Manna SunSeed	1 slice	160	2	29	11
Pepperidge Farm					
Deli Rye Seedless	1 slice	80	1	14	tr
Farmhouse Soft 100% Whole Wheat	1 slice	110	2	19	3
Farmhouse Soft Oatmeal	1 slice	120	2	21	3
Hearty 100% Whole Wheat	1 slice	110	2	20	4

FOOD	PORTION	CALS	FAT	CARB	SUGAR
Hearty 15 Grain	1 slice	120	2	20	3
Jewish Rye Seeded	1 slice	80	1	15	tr
Natural Whole Grain 100% Whole Wheat	1 slice	110	2	20	3
Natural Whole Grain 9 Grain	1 slice	110	2	20	3
Natural Whole Grain German Dark Wheat	1 slice	110	2	20	3
Natural Whole Grain Multi Grain	1 slice	120	2	20	3
Soft Honey Whole Wheat	1 slice	110	2	20	4
Stoneground 100% Whole Wheat	1 slice	70	1	12	1
Swirl French Vanilla	1 slice	140	4	23	7
Whole Grain Cinnamon Raisin Swirl	1 slice	110	3	19	6
Whole Grain Cinnamon Swirl	1 slice	110	3	18	5
Whole Grain Honey Oat	1 slice	110	2	20	4
Sara Lee					
Blueberry Crumble	1 slice	180	3	33	10
Brown Sugar Cinnamon	1 slice	200	6	31	11
Cinnamon Raisin	1 slice	190	4	32	16
Delightful 100% Whole Wheat	1 slice	90	1	18	2
Delightful 100% Whole Wheat w/ Honey	1 slice	90	1	18	2
Delightful White	1 slice	90	1	15	1
Earth Grains Buttermilk	1 slice	220	3	40	7
Earth Grains Honey Whole Grain	1 slice	220	3	37	6
Earth Grains Oat & Nut	1 slice	230	5	40	8
Earth Grains Potato	1 slice	210	2	40	7

FOOD	PORTION	CALS	FAT	CARB	SUGAR
Earth Grains Wheat Berry	1 slice	200	2	40	4
Multigrain	1 slice	100	2	19	4
White Whole Grain	1 slice	150	2	28	5
Stroehmann					
Family Grains Twisted Bread	1 slice	70	1	14	2
Honey Cracked Wheat	1 slice	90	1	16	2
New York Rye	1 slice (1 oz)	80	1	15	1
Super Bakery					
Athlete's Formula	1 slice (1.5 oz)	100	4	12	1
Fitness Formula	1 slice (1.5 oz)	90	3	12	1
Wrap Organic	1 (4 oz)	340	8	56	0
Thomas'					
Toasting Cinnamon	1 slice	130	5	20	6
Toasting Cinnamon Raisin	1 slice	120	3	22	10
Toasting Corn	1 slice	110	2	19	3
Whole Grain Swirl Cinnamon Raisin	1 slice (1.3 oz)	110	3	20	8
Whole Grain Swirl Oatmeal Raisin	1 slice	110	2	20	6
Toufayan					
Wraps Sundried Tomato Basil	1 (2 oz)	183	5	30	1
Wraps Wheat	1 (2 oz)	183	5	29	1
TAKE-OUT					
chapatis as prep w/ fat	1 bread (1.6 oz)	95	2	18	1
cornbread	1 piece (2.3 oz)	183	6	27	4
cornstick	1 (1.4 oz)	118	4	18	3
focaccia onion	1 piece (4.6 oz)	282	10	43	2
focaccia rosemary	1 piece (3.5 oz)	251	7	40	1
focaccia tomato olive	1 piece (4.7 oz)	270	8	42	1
garlic bread	1 slice (1 oz)	96	4	13	tr
italian garlic	1 loaf (11 oz)	990	38	137	1

FOOD	PORTION	CALS	FAT	CARB	SUGAR
naan	1 bread (3.5 oz)	286	9	43	3
papadums fried	2 (1.5 oz)	81	4	9	–
paratha	1 bread (2.1 oz)	201	10	23	1
poori indian puffed bread	1 piece (1.3 oz)	112	4	16	tr
zucchini	1 slice (1.4 oz)	150	7	19	10

BREAD COATING
Fryin' Magic
Cornmeal	1 tbsp	30	0	6	0

BREADCRUMBS
dry seasoned	¼ cup	115	2	21	2
fresh	¼ cup	30	tr	6	tr
plain	¼ cup	107	1	19	2

4C
Carb Careful Seasoned	⅓ cup	110	1	9	2

Arnold
Italian	¼ cup	110	2	19	1

Progresso
Italian Style	¼ cup	110	2	20	2

Rienzi
Italian Style	¼ cup	120	2	20	2

Ronzoni
Italian Flavored	¼ cup	120	2	21	2

BREADFRUIT
fresh	1 small (13.5 oz)	396	1	104	42
fried	1 cup	379	21	52	21
raw	1 cup	227	1	60	24

BREAD MACHINE MIX
Carbsense
Harvest Wheat as prep	1 slice	60	0	4	0

Keto
Cinnamon Raisin as prep	1 slice	79	0	6	tr

FOOD	PORTION	CALS	FAT	CARB	SUGAR
French Loaf as prep	1 slice	79	0	5	tr
Sourdough Rye as prep	1 slice	79	1	5	tr
Ketogenics					
Low Carb Honey Wheat as prep	1 slice	80	1	7	1
Low Carb Pumpernickel Rye as prep	1 slice	80	2	7	1
BREADSTICKS					
plain	1 sm	21	tr	3	tr
plain	1 lg	41	1	7	tr
Angonoa					
Deli Style Sesame	3 (0.5 oz)	730	3	10	tr
John Wm Macy's					
CheeseSticks Original Cheddar	3 (1 oz)	130	6	14	0
Pepperidge Farm					
Snack Sticks Wheat	9 (1 oz)	130	4	22	4
Stella D'Oro					
Mini Cracked Pepper	4 (0.5 oz)	70	2	11	tr
Original	1 (0.4 oz)	40	1	6	0
Roasted Garlic	1	45	1	7	0
Sesame	1 (0.4 oz)	50	2	7	0
BREAKFAST DRINKS					
Carnation					
Instant Breakfast Chocolate Malt as prep w/ fat free milk	1 serv	220	1	39	19
Instant Breakfast Classic French Vanilla as prep w/ fat free milk	1 serv	220	1	39	18

FOOD	PORTION	CALS	FAT	CARB	SUGAR
Instant Breakfast Milk Chocolate as prep w/ fat free milk	1 serv	220	1	39	20
Instant Breakfast Ready-To-Drink Carb Conscious French Vanilla	1 pkg	150	5	13	12
Instant Breakfast Ready-To-Drink Carb Conscious Milk Chocolate	1 pkg	150	5	15	12
Instant Breakfast Ready-To-Drink Creamy Milk Chocolate	1 pkg	250	5	40	38
Instant Breakfast Ready-To-Drink French Vanilla	1 pkg	240	5	34	30
Instant Breakfast Ready-To-Drink Strawberry Creme	1 pkg	250	5	37	36
Instant Breakfast Strawberry as prep w/ fat free milk	1 serv	220	6	39	19
Instant Breakfast Junior Vanilla	1 box (8.8 oz)	250	12	27	12
Instant Breakfast No Sugar Added Vanilla as prep w/ fat free milk	1 serv	150	1	24	8
BROAD BEANS					
fava fresh cooked	½ cup	94	tr	17	2
BROCCOFLOWER					
fresh raw	½ cup (1.8 oz)	16	tr	3	–

FOOD	PORTION	CALS	FAT	CARB	SUGAR
BROCCOLI					
FRESH					
chinese broccoli (gai lan) cooked	½ cup	10	tr	2	tr
raab cooked	½ cup	28	tr	3	1
raw	1 bunch (1.3 lbs)	207	2	40	10
raw flower	1 piece	3	tr	1	—
raw flowers	1 cup	20	tr	4	—
River Ranch					
Broccoli Slaw	1 cup	25	0	5	2
Florets	1¼ cups	25	0	4	2
FROZEN					
chopped cooked	½ cup	26	tr	5	1
spears cooked	1 pkg (10 oz)	70	tr	13	4
spears cooked	½ cup	26	tr	5	1
TAKE-OUT					
batter dipped & fried	4 pieces	77	5	6	1
w/ cheese sauce	1 cup	242	15	16	5
BROWNIE					
MIX					
Aunt Paula's					
Low Carb Chef Fudge Brownie as prep	1 (2.5 inch)	89	5	9	0
Big Train					
Low Carb Chocolate Chip as prep	1 (2 inch)	140	9	15	4
Jiffy					
Fudge as prep	1	160	5	28	18
Keto					
Chocolate Fudge as prep	1	59	3	2	0
MiniCarb					
Chocolate Brownie as prep	1	220	17	10	1

FOOD	PORTION	CALS	FAT	CARB	SUGAR
Nature's Path					
Organic Double Fudge	¹⁄₁₀ pkg	150	3	31	21
Organic HempPlus	¹⁄₁₀ pkg	140	2	31	20
No Pudge!					
All Flavors	1	100	0	21	13
READY-TO-EAT					
Laura's Wholesome Junk Food					
Gluten Free Better Brownie	2	120	6	16	8
TAKE-OUT					
plain	1 (2.1 oz)	243	10	39	—
BRUSSELS SPROUTS					
FRESH					
cooked	6 pieces	45	1	9	2
FROZEN					
cooked	1 cup	65	1	13	3
BUCKWHEAT					
groats roasted cooked	½ cup	323	1	17	1
BUFFALO					
burger	4 oz	150	5	1	0
water buffalo roasted	3 oz	111	2	0	0
BULGUR					
cooked	½ cup	76	tr	17	tr
TAKE-OUT					
tabbouleh	1 cup	198	15	16	2
BURBOT (FISH)					
fresh baked	3 oz	98	1	0	0
BURDOCK ROOT					
cooked w/o salt	1 cup	110	tr	26	4
cooked w/o salt	1 root (5.8 oz)	146	tr	35	6

FOOD	PORTION	CALS	FAT	CARB	SUGAR
Frieda's					
Gobo Root	¾ cup	60	0	15	0
BUTTER					
clarified butter	3.5 oz	876	99	0	0
stick	1 stick (4 oz)	813	92	tr	—
stick	1 pat (5 g)	36	4	tr	—
whipped	1 pat (4 g)	27	3	tr	—
whipped	1 tbsp	70	7	0	0
Cabot					
Salted	1 tbsp	100	11	0	0
Unsalted	1 tbsp	100	11	0	0
Land O Lakes					
Unsalted	1 tbsp	100	11	0	0
BUTTER SUBSTITUTES					
Butter Buds					
Granules	1 pkg (2 g)	5	0	2	—
Keto					
Butta	1 tsp	43	5	0	0
Molly McButter					
Natural Butter	1 tsp	5	0	1	—
Natural Cheese	1 tsp	5	0	1	—
Roasted Garlic	1 tsp	5	0	1	—
CABBAGE					
chinese bok choy shredded cooked	½ cup	10	tr	2	—
green raw shredded	½ cup (1.2 oz)	9	tr	2	—
green shredded cooked	½ cup (2.6 oz)	17	tr	3	—
red shredded cooked	½ cup	16	tr	3	—
savoy shredded cooked	½ cup	18	tr	4	—
Frieda's					
Baby Bok Choy	⅔ cup	10	0	2	1
Bok Choy	1 cup	10	0	2	1

FOOD	PORTION	CALS	FAT	CARB	SUGAR
Gai Choy	1 cup (3 oz)	20	0	4	1
Napa	1 cup (3 oz)	15	0	3	1
Salad Savoy	⅔ cup (3 oz)	25	0	5	2
Tuscan	⅔ cup (3 oz)	20	0	5	3
Lohmann					
Red Cabbage Sweet & Sour	¼ cup	40	0	10	8
River Ranch					
Angel Hair	1 ½ cups	20	0	5	3
TAKE-OUT					
korean kimchee	½ cup	22	tr	4	—
stuffed cabbage	1 (6 oz)	373	22	18	—
sweet & sour red cabbage	4 oz	61	3	8	—
CACTUS					
napoles fresh sliced	½ cup (1.5 oz)	7	tr	1	—
prickly pear fresh	1 cup (5.3 oz)	56	1	13	—
Frieda's					
Cactus Pads	¾ cup (3 oz)	20	0	4	0
CAKE					
sponge	1 piece (1.3 oz)	110	1	23	14
sponge cake dessert shell	1 (0.8 oz)	70	2	12	7
Arnold					
Date Nut Loaf	1 inch slice (2 oz)	190	5	32	18
Boboli					
Mini Eclairs Custard Filled	4 (2.3 oz)	224	12	22	18
Drake's					
Coffee Cakes	1 (1.2 oz)	140	6	20	11

FOOD	PORTION	CALS	FAT	CARB	SUGAR
Entenmann's					
Coffee Cake Cheese Filled Crumb	1 serv (1.9 oz)	200	10	25	11
Coffee Cake Crumb	1 serv (2 oz)	260	12	34	13
Danish Twist Raspberry	⅛ cake	220	11	28	15
Fudge Iced Golden Cake	⅛ cake	290	13	41	30
Light Loaf Cake Fat Free	⅛ cake (1.7 oz)	120	0	27	16
Loaf All Butter	⅙ cake (2.4 oz)	220	9	31	19
Louisiana Crunch	⅑ cake (2.9 oz)	330	14	49	35
Marble Loaf	⅛ cake	190	8	28	16
Mini's Carrot Cake	1 (1.4 oz)	160	7	22	15
Ultimate Crumb Cake	⅒ cake	250	13	32	15
Goody Man					
Happy Birthday Cupcake Chocolate	1 (1.75 oz)	200	6	34	24
Happy Birthday Cupcake White	1 (1.75 oz)	190	5	37	26
Hostess					
Shortcake Dessert Cups	1 (1.1 oz)	100	1	22	13
Low Carb Creations					
Cheesecake Blueberry Swirl	1 slice (3 oz)	220	16	21	2
Cheesecake Chocolate	1 slice (3 oz)	250	20	19	2
Cheesecake Key Lime	1 slice (3 oz)	250	20	19	2
Cheesecake New York	1 slice (3 oz)	250	15	19	1
Cheesecake Pumpkin Swirl	1 slice (3 oz)	220	16	22	2
Nature's Path					
Organic Toaster Pastry Apple Cinnamon	1 (2 oz)	210	5	40	18
Organic Toaster Pastry Blueberry	1 (2 oz)	210	5	40	18

FOOD	PORTION	CALS	FAT	CARB	SUGAR
Organic Toaster Pastry Frosted Apple Cinnamon	1 (2 oz)	210	5	39	21
Organic Toaster Pastry Frosted Blueberry	1 (2 oz)	200	4	38	20
Organic Toaster Pastry Frosted Strawberry	1 (2 oz)	210	4	40	19
Philadelphia					
Snack Bars Classic Cheesecake	1 bar (1.5 oz)	190	11	22	12
Snack Bars Strawberry Cheesecake	1 bar (1.5 oz)	190	9	22	13
Snack & Smile					
Mini Loaf Apple Cinnamon	1 loaf (2 oz)	190	8	29	16
Mini Loaf Banana	1 loaf (2 oz)	200	8	30	17
Mini Loaf Blueberry	1 loaf (2 oz)	190	8	29	16
Mini Loaf Carrot	1 loaf (2 oz)	200	8	30	16
Tastykake					
Koffee Kakes	1 (2 oz)	210	7	34	18
Krimpets Butterscotch Iced	2 (2 oz)	210	5	38	24
TAKE-OUT					
angelfood	1 slice (2 oz)	141	tr	32	16
apple crisp	1 serv (8.6 oz)	384	8	76	49
baklava	1 piece (2.7 oz)	334	23	29	10
basbousa namoura	1 piece (1 oz)	60	3	10	10
bean cake	1 cake (1.1 oz)	130	7	16	7
black forest chocolate cherry	1 piece (2.5 oz)	187	9	27	23
boston cream pie	1 slice (3.2 oz)	232	8	39	33
cannoli w/ cannoli cream	1	369	21	42	28
carrot w/ icing	1 slice (4.7 oz)	543	28	70	52
cheesecake	1 slice (4.5 oz)	410	25	37	28

FOOD	PORTION	CALS	FAT	CARB	SUGAR
cheesecake chocolate	1 slice (4.5 oz)	489	32	49	29
chinese moon cake	1 (4.8 oz)	458	6	92	49
coconut mochiko filipino cake	1 piece (2.7 oz)	252	12	35	11
coffeecake iced	1 piece (1.6 oz)	175	8	24	15
cream puff custard filled chocolate frosted	1 (3.9 oz)	293	18	27	7
dutch honey cake	1 slice (0.8 oz)	70	0	17	8
eclair	1 (3.5 oz)	262	16	24	7
french apple tart	1 (3.5 oz)	302	15	37	15
fruitcake	1 slice (1.5 oz)	139	4	26	13
funnel cake	1 (3.2 oz)	276	14	29	4
gingerbread	1 piece (2.4 oz)	213	7	35	22
jelly roll	1 slice (1.8 oz)	146	2	28	20
jelly roll lemon filled	1 slice (3 oz)	210	2	48	29
napoleon	1 mini (1 oz)	123	9	9	1
napoleon	1 (3 oz)	348	25	25	4
panettone	½ cake (2.9 oz)	300	12	43	21
petit fours	2 (0.9 oz)	120	7	15	12
pineapple upside down	1 piece (4.2 oz)	387	15	61	41
pound fat free	1 slice (2 oz)	160	1	35	19
sacher torte	1 slice (2.2 oz)	240	11	30	11
strawberry shortcake	1 serv (4.1 oz)	211	5	40	35
strudel apple	1 piece (2.2 oz)	175	7	26	16
strudel cheese	1 piece (2.2 oz)	195	8	24	14
strudel cherry	1 piece (2.2 oz)	179	6	29	18
tiramisu	1 piece (5.1 oz)	409	30	31	17
torte chocolate ganache	1 slice (3.5 oz)	400	26	40	24
white w/ coconut icing	1 slice (3.9 oz)	399	12	71	64

CAKE ICING

FOOD	PORTION	CALS	FAT	CARB	SUGAR
chocolate	¼ cup	269	7	53	51
vanilla	¼ cup	322	8	64	62

FOOD	PORTION	CALS	FAT	CARB	SUGAR
Jiffy					
Fudge Frosting	¼ cup	150	4	28	27
White Frosting	¼ cup	150	5	27	29
CAKE MIX					
Bob's Red Mills					
Gluten Free Chocolate as prep	⅙ cake	170	7	24	12
Carbsense					
Zero Carb Baking Mix	1 oz	110	1	4	0
Jiffy					
Devil's Food as prep	⅕ cake	220	6	40	23
Golden Yellow as prep	⅕ cake	220	5	39	24
White Cake as prep	⅕ cake	210	5	39	32
MiniCarb					
Carrot as prep	1 slice	280	20	10	0
Chocolate as prep	1 slice	230	18	16	0
Zero Carb Baking Mix not prep	½ cup	55	1	2	2
CALABAZA					
fresh	½ cup	32	tr	8	–
CANADIAN BACON					
Jones					
Slices	3	70	3	0	0
CANDY					
crisped rice bar chocolate chip	1 bar (1 oz)	115	4	21	9
fudge chocolate marshmallow	1 piece (0.7 oz)	84	3	14	–
fudge chocolate w/ nuts	1 piece (0.7 oz)	81	3	14	–
gumdrops	10 sm (0.4 oz)	135	0	35	–
jelly beans	10 sm (0.4 oz)	40	tr	10	–
lollipop	1 (6 g)	22	0	6	–

FOOD	PORTION	CALS	FAT	CARB	SUGAR
marzipan	1 oz	128	7	15	—
milk chocolate w/ almonds	1 bar (1.45 oz)	215	14	22	20
peanut brittle	1 oz	128	5	20	—
peanuts chocolate covered	10 (1.4 oz)	208	13	20	—
pretzels chocolate covered	1 (0.4 oz)	50	2	8	—
3 Musketeers					
Bar	1 (2.1 oz)	260	8	46	40
Fun Size	2 (1.2 oz)	140	5	25	22
Minatures	7 (1.4 oz)	180	5	31	27
Almond Joy					
Bar	1 (0.68 oz)	90	5	11	9
Altoids					
All Flavors	3 pieces	10	0	2	2
Anastasia					
Coco Rhum Bites	2 pieces (1 oz)	110	5	16	9
At Last!					
Chocolate Almond	1 bar	120	10	13	0
Chocolate Crisp	1 bar	110	9	14	0
Chocolate Mint	1 bar	110	10	15	0
Chocolate Peanut Butter	1 bar	120	11	14	0
Baby Ruth					
Fun Size	1 bar (0.7 oz)	100	5	14	11
Brach's					
Bridge Mix	16 pieces	190	8	26	22
Candy Corn	26 pieces	140	0	35	28
Caramel Clusters	3 pieces	210	13	23	19
Circus Peanuts	6 pieces	160	0	39	34
Fruit Rippers Berry Punch	1 pkg (0.5 oz)	60	0	11	8
Fruit Slices	3 pieces	150	0	38	29

FOOD	PORTION	CALS	FAT	CARB	SUGAR
Malts	15 pieces	190	7	30	21
Mellowcreme Pumpkins	6 pieces	130	0	33	26
Milk Maid Caramels	4 pieces	160	5	30	18
Mint Patties	3 pieces	140	3	29	26
Orange Slices	2 pieces	130	0	32	23
Peanut Butter Meltaways	3 pieces	200	13	19	17
Root Beer Barrels	3 pieces	70	0	17	11
Spearmint Leaves	5 pieces	130	0	34	23
Spice Drops	12 pieces	130	0	33	23
Sprinkles	17 pieces	200	9	29	26
Star Brites Butterscotch	3 pieces	60	0	16	10
Stars	10 pieces	200	11	24	23
Wild'N Fruity Gummi Bears	14 pieces	140	0	32	22
Breath Savers					
Sugar Free Peppermint	1 piece	5	0	2	0
Butterfinger					
Bar	1 (2.1 oz)	270	11	43	29
Crisps	1 bar (1.8 oz)	250	13	33	24
Crisps Minis	4 (1.5 oz)	220	11	29	22
Minis	4 (1.4 oz)	180	7	29	20
Cadbury					
Milk Chocolate Roast Almond	10 blocks (1.4 oz)	220	13	21	18
Royal Dark	10 blocks (1.4 oz)	220	13	24	20
Carbolite					
Caramel	1 bar	100	5	18	0
CarbAway	1 bar	100	5	17	0
CarboSnack	1 bar	110	6	20	0
Chocolate Truffle	1 bar (1 oz)	122	8	17	0
Chocolate Almond	1 bar (1.75 oz)	298	21	3	tr
Chocolate Crisp	1 bar (1.75 oz)	256	14	3	0

FOOD	PORTION	CALS	FAT	CARB	SUGAR
Chocolate Peanut Butter	1 bar (1.75 oz)	256	21	3	0
Crisy Caramel	1 bar (1 oz)	130	9	17	0
Milk Chocolate	1 bar (1.75 oz)	263	18	1	0
Peanut Butter Cup	1	170	14	17	0
Pecan Cluster	1 bar	120	8	15	0
CarbSlim					
Crunch Bites Chocolate Caramel	1 pkg	122	14	21	0
Crunch Bites Peanut Butter	1 pkg	171	14	21	0
Cary's Of Oregon					
English Toffee Milk Chocolate Almond	1 piece (0.75 oz)	110	8	12	10
ChocoSoy					
Soy Milk Chocolate	1 piece (0.4 oz)	50	3	6	5
CocoaVia					
Blueberry & Almond Chocolate	1 bar	100	6	12	9
Chocolate	1 bar	80	2	13	6
Chocolate Almond	1 bar	80	2	13	8
Chocolate Blueberry	1 bar	80	2	13	8
Chocolate Cherry	1 bar	80	2	13	7
Chocolate Covered Almonds	1 bar	140	11	12	8
Crispy Chocolate	1 bar	90	5	11	7
Original Chocolate	1 bar	100	6	12	9
Coffee Rio					
Coffee Candy All Flavors	4 pieces	60	2	10	10
Daboga					
Organic Milk Chocolate	1 bar (2 oz)	318	20	30	28
Doctor's CarbRite					
Sugar Free Dark Chocolate	1 oz	124	8	2	0

FOOD	PORTION	CALS	FAT	CARB	SUGAR
Sugar Free Dark Chocolate With Almonds	4 sq (1 oz)	132	10	16	0
Sugar Free Milk Chocolate	1 oz	128	9	0	0
Sugar Free Milk Chocolate With Peanuts	4 sq (1 oz)	132	10	12	0
Sugar Free Milk Chocolate With Soy Crisps	4 sq (1 oz)	120	8	12	0
Sugar Free Mint Chocolate	1 oz	128	9	0	0
Dove					
Dark Chocolate	1 bar (1.3 oz)	200	12	22	19
Dark Chocolate Miniatures	5 (1.4 oz)	210	13	24	20
Milk Chocolate	1 bar (1.3 oz)	200	12	22	20
Milk Chocolate Miniatures	5 (1.4 oz)	220	13	24	22
Eclipse					
Mints Sugarless All Flavors	3 pieces	5	0	2	0
Estee					
Fructose Sweetened Peanut Butter Cups	5	200	12	19	13
Fructose Sweetened Dark Chocolate	½ bar (1.4 oz)	200	14	23	15
Fructose Sweetened Milk Chocolate	½ bar (1.4 oz)	230	17	17	15
Fructose Sweetened Milk Chocolate w/ Almonds	½ bar (1.4 oz)	230	17	16	14
Fructose Sweetened Milk Chocolate w/ Crisp Rice	½ bar (1.2 oz)	370	26	29	24
Peanut Brittle	⅓ box (1.3 oz)	210	9	28	1
Sugar Free Assorted Fruit	3	15	0	16	0
Sugar Free Butterscotch	4	15	0	16	0
Sugar Free Gourmet Jelly Beans	26	70	0	24	0
Sugar Free Gum Drops Assorted Fruit	11	110	0	34	0

FOOD	PORTION	CALS	FAT	CARB	SUGAR
Sugar Free Gummy Bears Assorted Fruit	17	70	0	30	0
Sugar Free Peppermint	3	15	0	14	0
Sugar Free Sour Citrus Slices	9	60	0	30	0
Sugar Free Toffee	4	15	0	16	0
Sugar Free Tropical Fruit	3	15	0	16	0
Fauchon					
Assortment Truffles	3 pieces (1.3 oz)	160	11	19	16
Chocolate Assortment	3 pieces (1.1 oz)	170	11	19	15
Ferrero Rocher					
Candy	3 pieces (1.3 oz)	220	15	17	16
Fruitzels					
Assorted	7 pieces	120	0	29	19
Godiva					
Chocolatier Dark Chocolate w/ Raspberry	1 bar (1.5 oz)	220	11	28	22
Chocolatier Milk Chocolate	1 bar (1.5 oz)	230	13	26	25
Chocolatier Milk Chocolate w/ Almonds	1 bar (1.5 oz)	230	15	20	18
Sugar Free Chocolate	1 bar (1.5 oz)	190	15	24	0
Sugar Free Chocolate w/ Almonds	1 bar (1.5 oz)	200	15	23	0
Sugar Free Dark Chocolate	1 bar (1.5 oz)	190	14	25	0
Goetze's					
Caramel Creams	3 pieces	130	3	23	13
Gol D Lite					
Milk Chocolate Crisp	1 bar	125	9	15	0
Seashell Truffle	1 piece	54	3	6	0
Goldenberg's					
Peanut Chews	3 pieces	180	8	22	14

FOOD	PORTION	CALS	FAT	CARB	SUGAR
Golightly					
Sugar Free Caramels	5 pieces	150	6	31	0
Sugar Free Doublers Chews Peach & Creme	7 pieces	150	7	31	0
Sugar Free Fudgie Rolls	6 pieces	130	5	28	0
Sugar Free Hard Candy	4 pieces	45	0	15	0
Hershey's					
Chocolate Miniatures Sugar Free	5 pieces (1.4 oz)	170	13	25	0
Chocolate w/ Almonds Miniatures Sugar Free	5 pieces (1.4 oz)	180	14	23	0
Dark Chocolate Miniatures Sugar Free	5 pieces (1.4 oz)	190	15	23	0
Hugs	1 piece	25	2	3	–
Kisses	1	25	2	3	–
Milk Chocolate	1 bar (1.4 oz)	210	12	23	20
Milk Chocolate w/ Almonds	1 bar (1.4 oz)	230	14	21	17
Nuggets Cookies 'N' Creme	4	190	10	22	19
Nuggets Dark Chocolate w/ Almonds	4	220	14	20	16
Nuggets Milk Chocolate	4	230	13	24	21
Pot Of Gold	3 pieces	130	5	21	18
Take 5	2 pkg (1.5 oz)	220	11	25	18
Hint Mint					
All Flavors	2 pieces	10	0	2	2
Jelly Belly					
Jelly Beans Sugar Free	35	80	0	37	0
Jolly Rancher					
All Flavors	4 pieces	60	0	15	9
Lollipops All Flavors	1 (0.6 oz)	60	0	16	12
Sugar Free	4 pieces (0.6 oz)	35	0	13	0

FOOD	PORTION	CALS	FAT	CARB	SUGAR
Joyva					
Halvah Chocolate Covered	1 serv (2 oz)	380	25	20	19
Halvah Marble	1 serv (2 oz)	390	25	18	10
Judy's					
Sugar Free Almond Caramel Cluster	1 piece (1.5 oz)	200	15	10	0
Sugar Free Cashew Caramel Cluster	1 piece (1.5 oz)	190	14	12	1
Sugar Free English Toffee	1 piece (1.5 oz)	220	17	9	0
Sugar Free Macadamia Caramel Cluster	1 piece (1.5 oz)	220	20	9	tr
Sugar Free Peanut Brittle	¾ cup	100	6	2	0
Sugar Free Pecan Almond Cluster	1 piece (1.5 oz)	220	19	9	0
Junior Mints					
Snack Size	1 box (0.7 oz)	80	2	16	14
Klein					
Sugar Free Hard Candy All Flavors	3 pieces	12	0	5	0
Lambertz					
Petits Soleils Chocolate Coated Gingerbread	1 piece (0.4 oz)	47	2	7	5
Landies Candies					
Sugar Free Almond Clusters	2 pieces (1.5 oz)	240	17	17	tr
Sugar Free Bon Bons Peanut Butter	2 (1.5 oz)	240	17	17	0
Sugar Free Coconut Clusters	2 pieces (1.5 oz)	250	18	18	tr
Sugar Free Cookies & Cream	2 pieces (1.5 oz)	240	15	23	0
Sugar Free Dark Almond Bark	1 piece (1.5 oz)	230	15	23	0

FOOD	PORTION	CALS	FAT	CARB	SUGAR
Sugar Free Dark Miniature Bars	7 pieces (1.5 oz)	230	14	26	0
Sugar Free Milk Miniature Bars	7 pieces (1.5 oz)	240	15	21	0
Sugar Free Mint Discs	7 pieces (1.5 oz)	240	15	21	0
Sugar Free Peanut Clusters	2 (1.5 oz)	240	17	17	0
Sugar Free White Almond Bark	1 piece (1.5 oz)	230	15	21	0
Sugar Free White Caps	6 pieces (1.5 oz)	230	15	24	0
Lean Protein Bites					
Milk Chocolate	1 pkg (1 oz)	120	6	1	0
Peanut Butter	1 pkg (1 oz)	120	5	1	1
White Chocolate	1 pkg (1 oz)	120	4	2	2
Legacy Chocolates					
Truffles Assorted	1 piece (0.5 oz)	90	6	6	4
Lindt					
Dark Chocolate 70% Cocoa	4 blocks (1.4 oz)	220	17	13	11
Lindor Truffles Dark Chocolate	3 pieces	220	18	15	13
Lindor Truffles Milk Chocolate	3 pieces	220	17	16	15
Low Carb Chef					
Gummi Bears	14 pieces	138	0	30	0
Jelly Beans	37 pieces	120	0	36	0
Sugar Free Caramel Marshmallow Treats	3 pieces	140	7	28	0
Sugar Free Cherry Cordials	3 pieces	250	8	28	0
Sugar Free Coconut Clusters	4 pieces	210	18	19	0

FOOD	PORTION	CALS	FAT	CARB	SUGAR
Sugar Free Milk Chocolate Covered Vanilla Caramels	3 pieces	160	8	27	0
Sugar Free Peanut Butter Cups	1 piece	200	16	19	0
Sugar Free Peanut Butter Truffes	2 pieces	200	16	19	0
Sugar Free Peanut Clusters	4 pieces	210	17	16	0
Sugar Free Pecan Turtles	1 piece	120	13	20	0
Sugar Free Peppermint Patties	3 pieces	150	9	28	0
M&M's					
Almond	1 pkg (1.3 oz)	200	11	21	18
Chewlicious	1 bar (0.8 oz)	100	3	18	15
Crispy	1 pkg (1.5 oz)	200	8	31	25
Crispy Fun Size	3 pkg (1.5 oz)	200	8	30	25
Crunchy M-Azing	1 bar (1.52 oz)	220	12	29	26
Mega	27 pieces	200	9	28	25
Mega Peanut	12 pieces	210	11	24	21
Minis	1 pkg (1.1 oz)	150	7	21	19
Peanut	1 pkg (1.7 oz)	250	15	30	25
Peanut Butter	1 pkg (1.6 oz)	240	14	26	22
Plain	1 pkg (1.7 oz)	240	10	34	31
Plain Fun Size	1 pkg (0.7 oz)	100	5	15	13
Maple Grove Farms					
Maple Sugar Candy	5 pieces (1.3 oz)	140	0	36	32
Mauna Loa					
Kona Coffee Crunch Chocolate	1 bar (1.8 oz)	270	16	29	24
Macadamia Crisp Milk Chocolate	1 bar (1.8 oz)	270	17	29	25
Macadamia Milk Chocolate	1 bar (1.8 oz)	280	18	27	25

FOOD	PORTION	CALS	FAT	CARB	SUGAR
Mentos					
Sugar Free Mixed Berries	1 piece	5	0	3	0
Milky Way					
Bar	2 fun size (1.4 oz)	180	7	28	24
Bar	1 (2 oz)	270	10	41	35
Caramel Dark Chocolate	5 pieces	200	9	29	24
Caramels Milk Chocolate	5 pieces	200	8	30	26
Midnight	2 fun size (1.4 oz)	170	7	28	23
Midnight	1 bar (1.8 oz)	220	8	36	30
Midnight Miniatures	5 (1.4 oz)	180	7	29	24
Miniature	5 (1.5 oz)	190	7	30	25
Mon Cheri					
Hazelnut	4 pieces	260	18	20	20
Mounds					
Bar	1 (0.7 oz)	90	5	11	9
Mr. Goodbar					
Bar	1 (1.75 oz)	270	16	27	23
Mrs. Fields					
Decadent Chocolates	3 pieces (1.8 oz)	240	12	29	22
Munch					
Nut Bar	1 (1.42 oz)	220	15	18	12
Nestle					
Toll House Brownie Bar	2 pieces (2 oz)	250	12	36	23
Toll House Cookie Bar	1 piece (1 oz)	130	6	18	11
Turtles Original	3 pieces	240	14	30	23
Odense					
Marzipan	2 tbsp (1.4 oz)	170	4	29	24
Pearson's					
Mint Patties	1	30	1	6	5

FOOD	PORTION	CALS	FAT	CARB	SUGAR
Perlege					
Sugar Free Belgium Chocolate All Flavors	1 bar (3.5 oz)	532	42	14	0
Sugar Free Cream Filled Belgian Chocolate All Flavors	1 bar (1.5 oz)	226	16	22	0
Planters					
CarbWell Peanut Butter Crunch	1 bar (1.25 oz)	160	12	16	1
Pure De-Lite					
Caramel	1 bar	120	5	19	0
Caramel Crisp	1 bar	120	6	18	0
Caramel Nougat	1 bar	110	5	20	0
Caramel Peanut Butter	1 bar	120	6	17	0
Caramel Pecan	1 bar	130	7	17	0
Sugar Free Dark Chocolate	1 bar	173	14	1	0
Sugar Free Milk Chocolate	1 bar	187	14	3	0
Sugar Free Milk Chocolate w/ Almonds	1 bar	190	14	4	0
Sugar Free Milk Chocolate w/ Coconut	1 bar	190	14	4	0
Sugar Free Milk Chocolate w/ Mint	1 bar	187	14	3	0
Sugar Free Milk Chocolate w/ Orange	1 bar	187	14	3	0
Sugar Free Milk Chocolate w/ Peanuts	1 bar	190	14	4	0
Sugar Free White Chocolate	1 bar	187	14	3	0
Truffle Bar Caramel	1 bar	140	8	16	0
Truffle Bar Dark Mint	1 bar	160	12	13	0
Truffle Bar Hazelnut	1 bar	160	12	12	0
Truffle Bar Peanut Butter	1 bar	160	11	13	0

FOOD	PORTION	CALS	FAT	CARB	SUGAR
Reese's					
Bites	16 pieces	220	12	23	20
FastBreak	1 bar (0.7 oz)	90	5	11	10
Miniatures Peanut Butter Cups Sugar Free	5 pieces (1.4 oz)	170	12	24	0
Nutrageous	1 bar (0.6 oz)	95	6	9	8
Peanut Butter Cups	1 piece (1.4 oz)	210	12	22	19
Peanut Butter Cups Miniatures	5 (1.4 oz)	210	12	22	19
Peanut Butter Cups Sugar Free	1 piece (1.5 oz)	180	13	26	0
Pieces	25	90	5	11	–
White Miniatures Peanut Butter Cups	4 pieces (1.4 oz)	210	12	21	19
White Miniatures Peanut Butter Cups Sugar Free	5 pieces (1.4 oz)	180	13	21	0
Ritter Sport					
Dark Chocolate Whole Hazelnuts	6 pieces (1.3 oz)	210	15	16	14
Russell Stover					
Assorted	3 pieces (1.4 oz)	170	7	27	23
Low Carb Pecan Delights	1 piece (1 oz)	130	9	15	0
Pecan Delights	1 pkg (2 oz)	280	18	27	20
Smucker's					
Jelly Beans	25	150	0	37	31
Snickers					
Bar	1 bar (2.07 oz)	280	14	35	30
Cruncher	1 bar (1.6 oz)	230	13	25	17
Cruncher	3 fun size (1.4 oz)	230	13	25	18
Fun Size	2 bars (1.4 oz)	190	10	24	20
Miniatures	4 (1.3 oz)	170	9	22	18

FOOD	PORTION	CALS	FAT	CARB	SUGAR
Sour Patch					
Connectors	1.5 oz	150	0	37	26
Kids	1.5 oz	140	0	36	29
Starburst					
Fruit Chew Pop	1	50	0	13	10
Fruit Chews	1 pkg (2.07 oz)	240	5	48	34
Hard Candies	3 pieces	50	0	13	12
Jellybeans	¼ cup	150	0	38	30
Swedish Fish					
Aqua Life	1.5 oz	140	0	36	29
Original	20 pieces (1.5 oz)	140	0	36	28
Take 5					
Snack Size	2 pieces	220	11	25	18
The Chocolate Traveler					
Carb Controlled Wedges Bittersweet	4 pieces	120	9	12	0
Carb Controlled Wedges Dark Chocolate Coffee	4 pieces	110	8	15	0
Carb Controlled Wedges Dark Chocolate Mint	4 pieces	110	8	15	0
Carb Controlled Wedges Milk Chocolate	4 pieces	120	8	15	0
Wedges Bittersweet	4 pieces	130	10	10	7
Wedges Dark Chocolate Coffee	4 pieces	130	8	15	12
Wedges Dark Chocolate Mint	4 pieces	130	8	15	12
Wedges Milk Chocolate	4 pieces	130	8	15	14
Toblerone					
Bittersweet Chocolate w/ Honey & Almond Nugget	⅓ bar (1.2 oz)	170	9	20	16

FOOD	PORTION	CALS	FAT	CARB	SUGAR
Torras					
Sugar Free Dark Chocolate	1 oz	136	10	15	0
Sugar Free Milk Chocolate	1 oz	140	10	17	0
Sugar Free Milk Chocolate w/ Almonds	1 oz	146	10	15	0
Sugar Free Milk Chocolate w/ Hazelnuts	1 oz	148	11	15	0
Sugar Free White Chocolate	1 oz	138	10	17	0
Twix					
Caramel	1 bar	280	14	37	27
Peanut Butter	1 bar	280	17	28	19
Twizzlers					
Strawberry Snack Size	3 pkgs	130	1	30	19
Sugar Free	4 pieces (1.5 oz)	130	1	33	0
Unique Origin					
Guaranda Dark Chocolate	1 piece (0.3 oz)	54	4	4	3
Weight Watchers					
English Toffee Squares	3 pieces	160	10	23	7
Mint Patties	2	100	6	15	5
Peanut Butter Crunch	4 pieces	180	8	31	9
Pecan Crowns	3 pieces	150	9	21	7
Whitman's					
Sampler	3 pieces (1.4 oz)	220	10	31	26
Whoppers					
Malted Milk Balls	18 pieces	190	7	31	25
Yamate Chocolatier					
No Sugar Almonds & Caramel	1 piece (0.6 oz)	70	6	9	1
York					
Peppermint Patty	3 (1.4 oz)	150	3	29	24

FOOD	PORTION	CALS	FAT	CARB	SUGAR
Peppermint Patty Sugar Free	3 (1.3 oz)	110	4	28	0

CANTALOUPE
fresh cubed	1 cup	57	tr	13	–
fresh half	½	94	1	22	–

CARAWAY
seed	1 tsp	7	tr	1	–

CARDAMOM
ground	1 tsp	6	tr	1	–

CARDOON
Frieda's
Cardoon	1 cup	15	0	4	1

CARIBOU
roasted	3 oz	142	4	0	0

CARP
fresh	3 oz	108	5	0	0
fresh cooked	3 oz	138	6	0	0
roe salted in olive oil	2 tbsp (1 oz)	40	–	6	–

CARROT JUICE
Bolthouse Farms
Carrot Juice	8 oz	70	0	14	14

Luvli Juices
Zingy Carrot	1 bottle (10 oz)	145	0	35	31

Naked Juice
Just Carrot	8 oz	80	0	13	13

CARROTS
CANNED
slices	½ cup	17	tr	4	–

FOOD	PORTION	CALS	FAT	CARB	SUGAR
Del Monte					
Savory Sides Honey Glazed	½ cup	70	0	18	12
Sliced	½ cup	35	0	8	5
Glory					
Seasoned Honey	½ cup	50	0	12	9
FRESH					
baby raw	1 (½ oz)	6	tr	1	–
raw	1 (2.5 oz)	31	tr	7	–
raw shredded	½ cup	24	tr	6	–
slices cooked	½ cup	35	tr	8	–
Bolthouse Farms					
Baby	1 pkg (2.25 oz)	25	0	7	4
Matchstix	3 oz	35	0	9	6
Earthbound Farms					
Organic Mini Peeled	½ cup	30	0	7	4
Frieda's					
Gold	⅔ cup (3 oz)	35	0	9	6
Nature's Gold					
Fresh	1 med (2.7 oz)	40	0	9	5
River Ranch					
Shredded	¾ cup	35	0	9	6
CASABA					
cubed	1 cup	45	tr	11	–
CASHEWS					
dry roasted w/ salt	18 nuts (1 oz)	160	13	9	–
Bowlby's					
Bits Cashew	½ cup	200	19	5	1
Frito Lay					
Salted	3 tbsp	160	13	7	2
Good Sense					
Jumbo Honey Roasted	¼ cup	170	11	13	4

FOOD	PORTION	CALS	FAT	CARB	SUGAR
Jumbo Roasted & Salted	¼ cup	190	16	9	2
Sweet Delights					
Cashew Roasters	⅓ pkg (1 oz)	170	14	10	1

CASSAVA

fresh	3.5 oz	120	tr	27	–

CATFISH

channel breaded & fried	3 oz	194	11	7	–
wolffish atlantic baked	3 oz	105	3	0	0

CAULIFLOWER
FRESH

cooked	½ cup (2.2 oz)	14	tr	3	–
flowerets cooked	3 (2 oz)	12	tr	2	–
flowerets raw	3 (2 oz)	14	tr	3	–
green raw floweret	1 (0.9 oz)	8	tr	2	–
raw	½ cup (1.8 oz)	13	tr	3	–
River Ranch					
Florets	1 cup	20	0	4	2

CAVIAR

black or red	2 tbsp	81	6	1	0

CELERY

diced cooked	½ cup	13	tr	3	–
fresh	1 stalk (1.3 oz)	6	tr	1	–
seed	1 tsp	8	tr	1	–
Dole					
Stalks	2 med (3 oz)	15	0	3	0
Frieda's					
Celery Root	¾ cup	35	0	8	2
River Ranch					
Sticks Fresh	4 (3 oz)	15	0	3	2

FOOD	PORTION	CALS	FAT	CARB	SUGAR
CEREAL					
Alti Plano					
Hot Cereal Chai Almond	1 pkg	210	7	33	15
Hot Cereal Oaxacan Chocolate	1 pkg	170	3	30	9
Hot Cereal Orange Date	1 pkg	180	3	36	20
Hot Cereal Regular	1 pkg	190	3	32	1
Hot Cereal Spiced Apple Raisin	1 pkg	160	2	35	12
Alvarado Street Bakery					
Plain Grinola	½ cup	220	5	38	7
Aunt Paula's					
Hot Flax Cereal	1 serv (1½ oz)	100	5	8	0
Back To Nature					
Banana Nut Multibran	¾ cup	140	3	37	9
Flax & Fiber Crunch	1 cup	200	3	41	9
Granola Apple Blueberry	½ cup	200	3	39	6
Granola Apple Cinnamon	½ cup	180	3	36	11
Granola Classic	½ cup	180	3	36	5
Granola French Vanilla	½ cup	220	6	35	12
Hi Protein Crunch	½ cup	150	1	27	10
Hi-Fiber Multibran	½ cup	70	1	22	5
Muesli	¾ cup	230	4	48	12
Multigrain Harvest	1 cup	210	3	46	10
Oat & Soy Crisp	¾ cup	180	3	33	8
Strawberry & Seven Grains	1 cup	210	1	50	15
Barbara's Bakery					
Shredded Spoonfuls	¾ cup	120	2	24	5
Bear Naked					
Apple Cinnamon	¼ cup	140	7	17	5
Banana Nut	¼ cup	140	7	17	5
Fruit And Nut	¼ cup	140	7	16	5
Peak Protein	½ cup	200	8	24	11

FOOD	PORTION	CALS	FAT	CARB	SUGAR
Carbsense					
Hot Cereal Country Spice not prep	½ cup	130	6	15	0
Hot Cereal Roasted Hazelnut not prep	½ cup	140	9	15	0
CoCo Wheats					
Hot Cereal	⅓ cup	200	1	41	2
Country Choice Naturals					
Instant Oatmeal Apples 'N' Cinnamon	1 pkg	140	2	27	11
Instant Oatmeal Maple Syrup	1 pkg	170	2	32	9
Instant Oatmeal Organic Plus French Vanilla	1 pkg	180	3	32	12
Instant Oatmeal Organic Plus Golden Brown Sugar	1 pkg	180	3	32	12
Instant Oatmeal Regular	1 pkg	110	2	19	tr
Oatmeal Steel Cut not prep	½ cup	150	3	27	0
Oats Old Fashioned not prep	½ cup	150	3	27	1
Oats Quick not prep	½ cup	150	3	27	1
Organic Multi Grain Hot Cereal not prep	½ cup	130	2	29	2
Deliciously Slim					
Granola Cranberry Cashew	¾ cup	230	13	29	2
Granola Strawberry Almond	¾ cup	230	13	29	2
Enjoy Life					
Cinnamon Crunch Nut & Gluten Free	¾ cup	160	5	26	5

FOOD	PORTION	CALS	FAT	CARB	SUGAR
EnviroKidz					
Organic Orangutan O's	¾ cup	120	1	26	9
Erewhon					
Apple Stroodles	¾ cup	110	1	25	4
Aztec	1 cup	110	0	26	1
Banana O's	¾ cup	110	0	26	7
Brown Rice Cream	¼ cup	170	1	36	0
Corn Flakes	1¼ cups	210	3	45	tr
Crispy Brown Rice	1 cup	110	0	25	1
Crispy Brown Rice No Salt Added	1 cup	110	0	25	1
Fruit'n Wheat	¾ cup	170	2	39	12
Kamut Flakes	⅔ cup	110	0	25	1
Raisin Bran	1 cup	170	1	40	10
Rice Twice	¾ cup	120	0	28	8
Whole Wheat Flakes	1 cup	180	1	42	tr
General Mills					
Cheerios	1 cup	110	2	22	1
Cheerios Apple Cinnamon	¾ cup	120	2	25	13
Fiber One	½ cup (1 oz)	60	1	25	0
Fiber One Honey Clusters	1¼ cup	170	1	47	5
Total Honey Clusters	¾ cup	170	2	39	13
Total Protein	¾ cup	120	4	11	2
Total Raisin Bran	1 cup	170	1	41	20
Total Whole Grain	¾ cup (1 oz)	100	1	23	5
Gram's Gourmet					
Cream Of Flax not prep	½ cup	142	5	11	1
Crunch Granolas All Flavors	½ cup	349	30	10	1
Grandy Oats					
Organic Granola Classic	½ cup	252	14	27	6
Organic Granola Low Fat Cranberry Chew	½ cup	191	1	41	17

FOOD	PORTION	CALS	FAT	CARB	SUGAR
Organic Granola Mainely Maple	½ cup	204	7	31	9
Hi-Lo					
Low Carb Cereal	½ cup	90	2	11	1
Hodgson Mill					
Bulgur Wheat w/ Soy Grits	¼ cup	116	1	22	0
Cracked Wheat	¼ cup	110	1	26	0
Multi Grain w/ Flaxseed & Soy	⅓ cup	160	3	25	1
Kashi					
GoLean	1 cup	140	1	30	6
GoLean Crunch!	1 cup (1.9 oz)	190	3	36	13
Good Friends	1 cup	170	2	43	9
Heart To Heart	¾ cup	110	2	25	5
Mighty Bites All Flavors	1 cup	120	2	23	5
Organic Promise Cranberry Sunshine	1 cup	110	1	26	9
Kellogg's					
Raisin Bran	1 cup	190	2	45	19
Smart Start Antioxidants	1 cup	180	1	43	14
Smart Start Healthy Heart	1¼ cups	230	2	49	17
Special K Vanilla Almond	1 cup (1.1 oz)	110	2	24	12
Keto					
Cocoa Crisp	½ cup	110	2	4	0
Frosted Flakes All Flavors	¾ cup	110	1	9	tr
Hot Cereal Apple Cinnamon	2 scoops	150	4	12	tr
Hot Cereal Strawberry & Creme	2 scoops	150	4	12	tr
Low Carb Crispy Soy	¾ cup	110	2	2	0
Oatmeal Old Fashioned	2 scoops	150	4	12	tr
Liquid Cereal					
Apple & Cinnamon	1 can (11 oz)	160	1	32	21

FOOD	PORTION	CALS	FAT	CARB	SUGAR
Chocolate	1 can (11 oz)	170	1	33	21
Fruit	1 can (11 oz)	150	0	31	31
Peanut Butter	1 can (11 oz)	170	2	32	21
MiniCarb					
Milk Chocolate Hot Cereal not prep	½ cup	140	6	17	2
Mother's					
Cinnamon Oat Crunch	1 cup	230	3	48	15
Cocoa Bumpers	1 cup	120	1	29	15
Groovy Grahams	¾ cup	100	1	24	13
Honey Round-Ups	¾ cups	110	1	25	10
Multigrain Hot Cereal	½ cup	130	1	29	0
Oat Bran Hot Cereal	½ cup	150	3	25	1
Oatmeal Instant	½ cup	150	3	27	1
Peanut Butter Bumpers	1 cup	130	3	26	10
Rolled Oats	½ cup	150	3	27	1
Toasted Oat Bran	¾ cup	120	2	24	5
Whole Wheat Hot Cereal	½ cup	130	1	30	0
Natural Ovens					
Great Granola	¼ cup	110	4	18	3
Paul's Oatmeal not prep	⅓ cup	120	3	22	3
Nature's Path					
Optimum Organic ReBound	¾ cup	190	6	35	9
Organic Zen Instant Oatmeal Cranberry Ginger	1 pkg	150	3	30	11
Perky's					
Nutty Flax	¾ cup	230	5	41	41
PerkyO's Original	¾ cup	120	1	28	2
Post					
Grape-Nuts	½ cup	200	1	47	5

FOOD	PORTION	CALS	FAT	CARB	SUGAR
Great Grains Raisins Dates Pecans	½ cup	210	5	40	14
Raisin Bran	1 cup (2 oz)	190	1	46	19
Shredded Wheat Spoon Size	1 cup	170	1	40	0
Quaker					
Instant Oatmeal Apples & Cinnamon	1 pkg	130	2	27	12
Instant Oatmeal Cinnamon & Spice	1 pkg	170	2	35	15
Instant Oatmeal Cinnamon Roll	1 pkg	160	2	33	13
Instant Oatmeal Lower Sugar Apples & Cinnamon	1 pkg	110	2	22	6
Instant Oatmeal Lower Sugar Maple & Brown Sugar	1 pkg	120	2	24	4
Instant Oatmeal Maple & Brown Sugar	1 pkg	160	2	33	13
Instant Oatmeal Nutrition For Women Golden Brown Sugar	1 pkg	170	2	32	12
Instant Oatmeal Nutrition For Women Vanilla Cinnamon	½ pkg	160	2	32	13
Instant Oatmeal Peaches & Cream	1 pkg	130	3	25	6
Instant Oatmeal Raisin & Spice	1 pkg	150	2	33	16
Instant Oatmeal Regular	1 pkg	100	2	19	0
Instant Oatmeal Strawberries & Cream	1 pkg	130	3	25	6

FOOD	PORTION	CALS	FAT	CARB	SUGAR
Instant Oatmeal Take Heart Blueberry	1 pkg	160	2	33	9
Instant Oatmeal Take Heart Golden Maple	1 pkg	160	2	34	9
Instant Oatmeal Weight Control Banana Bread	1 pkg	160	3	29	1
Instant Oatmeal Weight Control Cinnamon	1 pkg	160	3	29	1
Life	¾ cup	120	2	25	6
Life Cinnamon	¾ cup	120	2	25	8
Life Honey Graham	¾ cup	120	2	25	7
Life Vanilla Yogurt Crunch	1¼ cup	210	3	43	12
Old Fashioned Oats not prep	½ cup	150	3	27	1
Ralston					
100% Hot Wheat	⅓ cup	150	1	31	0
Apple Dapples	1 cup	120	1	30	16
Cocoa Crumbles	1 cup	120	1	26	14
Confruity Crisp	¾ cup	110	1	25	12
Corn Biscuits	1 cup	110	0	26	3
Corn Flakes	1 cup	100	0	24	2
Crisp Crunch	¾ cup	120	1	27	14
Crisp Crunch Berry Treats	1 cup	120	1	27	13
Crisp Rice	1¼ cups	120	0	29	3
Enriched Bran Flakes	¾ cup	90	1	23	5
Farina	3 tbsp	120	0	25	0
Freaky Fruits	1 cup	120	1	27	13
Frosted Flakes	¾ cup	120	0	28	12
Fruit Rings	1 cup	120	1	28	15
Grits	¼ cup	140	1	32	0
Instant Oats Bananas & Cream	1 pkg	130	4	27	10
Magic Stars	¾ cup	120	1	27	13

FOOD	PORTION	CALS	FAT	CARB	SUGAR
Oats & More W/ Almonds	¾ cup	130	2	27	6
Oats Instant	1 pkg	100	2	19	0
Oats Instant Apples & Cinnamon	1 pkg	130	2	26	12
Oats Instant Blueberries & Cream	1 pkg	130	3	26	11
Oats Instant Cinnamon & Spice	1 pkg	170	2	34	16
Oats Instant For Kids Cinnawow	1 pkg	140	2	30	10
Oats Instant For Kids Maplicious & Brown Sugar	1 pkg	150	2	31	9
Oats Instant For Kids Roarin' Raspberry	1 pkg	150	3	29	11
Oats Instant For Kids Strawberries & Stars	1 pkg	140	2	30	13
Oats Instant Maple Brown Sugar	1 pkg	160	2	32	13
Oats Instant Peaches & Cream	1 pkg	130	3	36	12
Oats Instant Raisins & Spice	1 pkg	150	2	32	16
Oats Instant Strawberries & Cream	1 pkg	140	3	26	11
Oats Old Fashioned	½ cup	150	3	27	0
Oats Quick	½ cup	140	3	26	0
Raisin Bran	1 cup	200	2	47	18
Rice Biscuits	1¼ cups	120	0	27	2
Shredded Wheat Frosted Bite Size	1¼ cups	200	1	47	11
Silly Spheres	1½ cups	110	1	25	3
Tasteeos	1 cup	110	2	22	1

FOOD	PORTION	CALS	FAT	CARB	SUGAR
Tasteeos Apple Cinnamon	¾ cup	120	2	26	13
Tasteeos Honey Nut	1 cup	120	2	24	11
South Beach Diet					
Toasted Wheats	1¼ cups	210	1	48	3
Whole Grain Crunch	¾ cup	110	3	21	4

CEREAL BARS

All Bran

Brown Sugar Cinnamon	1	130	3	27	11
Honey Oat	1	130	3	27	11
Oatmeal Raisin	1	130	3	26	13

Enjoy Life

Caramel Apple Nut & Gluten Free	1 (1 oz)	110	3	21	7

Entenmann's

Multi-Grain Chocolate Chip	1	140	3	28	16
Multi-Grain Rainbow Chip	1	180	8	26	15
Multi-Grain Real Raspberry	1	140	3	26	16

EnviroKidz

Crispy Rice Panda Peanut Butter	1 (1 oz)	110	3	20	7

Estee

Rice Crunchy Chocolate	1	60	1	14	0
Rice Crunchy Chocolate Chip	1	70	1	15	0
Rice Crunchy Peanut Butter	1	60	1	14	0
Rice Crunchy Vanilla	1	70	0	15	0

General Mills

Team Cheerios Strawberry	1	160	4	30	11
Trix	1	160	4	30	11

FOOD	PORTION	CALS	FAT	CARB	SUGAR
Glenny's					
Slim Carb Bars Peanut Caramel	1	140	4	19	1
Kashi					
Chewy Granola Honey Almond Flax	1 (1.2 oz)	140	5	21	6
Chewy Granola Peanut Peanut Butter	1 (1.2 oz)	130	5	20	5
Chewy Granola Trail Mix	1 (1.2 oz)	130	5	20	6
Kudos					
Granola Chocolate Chip	1	130	5	20	13
Granola Peanut Butter	1	130	6	18	13
Granola w/ M&M's	1	100	3	17	10
Granola w/ Snickers	1	100	4	16	10
Natural Ovens					
Great Granola Chocolate Almond	1	150	6	23	14
Great Granola Fruit & Lemon	1	130	3	24	8
Great Granola Mixed Fruit	1	130	3	24	8
Nature Valley					
Chewy Trail Mix Fruit & Nut	1	140	4	25	13
Healthy Heart Honey Nut	1	160	4	28	13
Nutri-Grain					
Apple Cinnamon	1	140	3	26	13
Banana Muffin	1	170	4	30	16
Blueberry	1	140	3	26	13
Blueberry Muffin	1	170	4	31	7
Cherry	1	140	3	26	14
Chewy Granola Chocolatey Chunk	1	110	4	18	8

FOOD	PORTION	CALS	FAT	CARB	SUGAR
Chewy Granola Honey Oat & Raisin	1	110	3	18	9
Cinnamon Raisin Muffin	1	170	4	32	18
Mixed Berry	1	140	3	26	13
Raspberry	1	140	3	26	13
Strawberry	1	140	3	26	13
Strawberry Yogurt	1	140	3	26	14
Vanilla Yogurt	1	140	3	26	14
Quaker					
Breakfast Squares Brown Sugar Cinnamon	1 (2.1 oz)	220	4	43	21
Chewy Chocolate Chip	1 (1 oz)	120	4	21	9
Chewy Peanut Butter Chocolate Chunk	1 (1 oz)	120	4	20	9
Chewy Low Fat Maple Brown Sugar	1 (1 oz)	110	2	22	9
Chewy Low Fat S'mores	1 (1 oz)	110	2	22	10
Oatmeal To Go Brown Sugar Cinnamon	1 (2.1 oz)	220	4	43	20
Rice Krispies					
Treats Original	1 (0.8 oz)	90	2	18	8
Skippy					
Peanut Butter	1	180	11	18	11
Peanut Butter & Fudge	1	190	12	18	11
Peanut Butter & Marshmallow	1	140	12	14	11
Peanut Butter & Strawberry	1	170	12	14	11
South Beach Diet					
Chocolate	1	140	5	15	7
Cinnamon Raisin	1	140	5	15	7
Cranberry Almond	1	140	5	15	7

FOOD	PORTION	CALS	FAT	CARB	SUGAR
Maple Nut	1	140	5	15	7
Peanut Butter	1	140	5	15	6
Special K					
Blueberry	1	90	2	18	9
Chocolatey Drizzle	1	90	2	17	8
Cranberry Apple	1	90	2	18	9
Peach Berry	1	90	2	18	9
Strawberry	1	90	2	18	9
Vanilla Crisp	1	90	2	17	7

CHAMPAGNE

FOOD	PORTION	CALS	FAT	CARB	SUGAR
mimosa	1 serv	117	tr	12	–
punch	1 serv	113	0	5	–
sekt german champagne	3.5 fl oz	84	0	5	–

CHAYOTE

FOOD	PORTION	CALS	FAT	CARB	SUGAR
fresh cooked	1 cup	38	1	8	–

CHEESE

FOOD	PORTION	CALS	FAT	CARB	SUGAR
beaufort	1 oz	115	9	tr	tr
blue	1 oz	100	8	1	–
brie	1 oz	95	8	tr	–
cacio di roma sheep's milk cheese	1 oz	130	10	0	0
camembert	1 oz	85	7	tr	–
cantal	1 oz	105	9	tr	tr
cheddar	1 oz	114	9	tr	–
cheddar low fat	1 oz	49	2	1	–
edam	1 oz	101	8	tr	–
feta	1 oz	75	6	1	–
goat fresh	1 oz	23	2	tr	tr
gouda	1 oz	101	8	1	–
grana padano parmesan shaved	1 tbsp	20	2	0	0
limburger	1 oz	93	8	tr	–

FOOD	PORTION	CALS	FAT	CARB	SUGAR
mozzarella	1 oz	80	6	1	–
mozzarella fresh	1 oz	80	6	tr	0
muenster	1 oz	104	9	tr	–
parmesan grated	1 tbsp (5 g)	23	2	tr	–
provolone	1 oz	100	8	1	–
queso anego	1 oz	106	9	1	–
queso asadero	1 oz	101	8	1	–
queso chichuahua	1 oz	106	8	2	–
queso fresco	1 oz	41	2	1	–
queso manchego	1 oz	107	8	tr	–
queso panela	1 oz	74	5	1	–
raclette	1 oz	102	8	tr	tr
ricotta part skim	½ cup (4.4 oz)	171	10	6	–
ricotta whole milk	½ cup (4.4 oz)	216	16	4	–
romano	1 oz	110	8	1	–
roquefort	1 oz	105	9	1	–
saint marcellin	1 oz	94	8	tr	tr
swiss	1 oz	107	8	1	–
triple creme	1 oz	113	11	tr	tr
whey cheese	1 oz	126	8	9	0
yogurt cheese	1 oz	80	7	0	0
Athenos					
Blue	1 oz	100	8	tr	0
Feta	1 oz (1 in cube)	80	6	tr	0
Feta Crumbled	¼ cup	90	7	2	0
Gorgonzola Crumbled	3 tbsp	110	9	2	0
Back To Nature					
Organic American Slices	1 slice (0.7 oz)	80	7	tr	0
Organic Cheddar Cubes	8 pieces (1.1 oz)	130	11	0	0
Organic Cheddar Shredded	¼ cup	110	10	tr	0
Organic Cream Cheese	⅛ pkg (1 oz)	100	10	tr	tr

FOOD	PORTION	CALS	FAT	CARB	SUGAR
Organic Mozzarella Shredded	¼ cup	80	5	tr	0
Organic White Cheddar Slices Reduced Fat	1 slice (0.7 oz)	60	4	0	0
Boar's Head					
Feta	1 oz	60	4	1	0
Cabot					
American	1 slice (0.7 oz)	80	7	1	0
Cheddar	1 oz	110	9	tr	0
Cheddar Smoked	1 oz	110	9	tr	0
Cheddar Light 50% Reduced Fat	1 oz	70	5	1	0
Cheddar Light 50% Reduced Fat Jalapeno	1 oz	70	5	1	0
Cheddar Light 75% Reduced Fat	1 oz	60	3	tr	0
Cheddar Shake	2 tsp	25	2	1	1
Colby Jack	1 oz	110	9	7	0
Fancy Blend Shredded	¼ cup	100	7	1	0
Monterey Jack	1 oz	110	9	tr	0
Mozzarella Shredded	¼ cup	80	6	1	0
Pepper Jack	1 oz	110	9	tr	0
Swiss Slices	1 slice (1 oz)	110	8	1	0
Cantare					
Baked Brie En Croute	1 oz	100	7	4	0
Chavrie					
Goat's Milk	2 tbsp	50	4	1	1
Connoisseur					
Asiago Spread	1 tbsp	90	7	2	2
Cracker Barrel					
Sharp Cheddar 2% Milk	1 oz	90	6	tr	0
Fage					
Feta	1 oz	80	7	0	0

FOOD	PORTION	CALS	FAT	CARB	SUGAR
Finlandia					
Muenster	1 slice (1.1 oz)	120	10	tr	0
Formaggio					
Fresh Mozzarella	1 oz	90	6	1	1
Heluva Good Cheese					
Cheddar Extra Sharp	1 oz	110	9	1	0
Jordan's					
Provolone	1 slice (1 oz)	100	8	0	0
Kraft					
Cheddar Extra Sharp	1 oz	120	10	0	0
Laughing Cow					
Cheese Bites Light	6 pieces (0.8 oz)	35	2	1	1
Creamy French Onion Light	1 wedge	35	2	1	1
Creamy Garlic & Herb Light	1 wedge (0.7 oz)	35	2	1	1
Creamy Swiss Light Original	1 wedge (0.7 oz)	35	2	1	1
Creamy Swiss Original	1 wedge (0.7 oz)	50	4	1	1
Mini Babybel Bonbel	1 piece (0.7 oz)	70	6	0	0
Mini Babybel Gouda	1 piece (0.7 oz)	80	6	0	0
Mini Babybel Light Original	1 piece (0.7 oz)	50	3.	0	0
Mini Babybel Mild Cheddar	1 piece (0.7 oz)	70	5	1	0
Mini Babybel Original	1 piece (0.7 oz)	70	6	0	0
Meza					
Baked Brie In Pastry w/ Cranberries & Spiced Almonds	1 oz	110	7	8	2
Miller's					
Mozzarella	1 slice (1 oz)	81	5	0	0

FOOD	PORTION	CALS	FAT	CARB	SUGAR
Mont Chevre					
Assorted Crottins	1 oz	70	6	1	tr
Polly-O					
Mozzarella Part Skim	1 oz	70	5	tr	tr
Mozzarella Shredded	¼ cup	90	7	tr	0
Ricotta Part Skim	¼ cup	90	6	2	2
Ricotta Lite	¼ cup	70	3	3	2
String-Ums	1 stick (1 oz)	80	6	tr	0
President					
Feta	1 inch cube (1 oz)	90	7	2	0
Sargento					
Cheddar Extra Sharp	1 oz	110	9	1	0
Muenster Deli Style	1 slice (0.7 oz)	80	6	0	0
Reduced Fat 4 Cheese Mexican Shredded	¼ cup (1 oz)	80	6	tr	0
String	1 piece (0.8 oz)	70	5	tr	0
Sorrento					
Mozzarella Fresh	1 oz	90	6	0	0
Mozzarella w/ Tomato & Basil Shredded	¼ cup	80	5	1	1
Pizza Cheese Shredded	¼ cup	90	7	1	0
Stringsters	1 stick (1 oz)	80	5	1	0
Suisse Delicat					
Healthy Swiss	1 oz	90	6	0	0
CHEESE DISHES					
TAKE-OUT					
fondue	½ cup (3.8 oz)	247	15	4	—
fried mozzarella sticks	3 (4.6 oz)	503	32	20	2
souffle	1 serv (7 oz)	504	38	18	5
CHERIMOYA					
fresh	1	515	2	131	—

FOOD	PORTION	CALS	FAT	CARB	SUGAR
CHERRIES					
CANNED					
Del Monte					
Sweet Dark Pitted In Heavy Syrup	½ cup	100	0	24	24
DRIED					
bing unsulfured	¼ cup	130	0	31	21
montmorency tart pitted	⅓ cup	160	1	36	24
rainier unsulfured	⅓ cup	140	1	32	30
yogurt covered	¼ cup	170	6	29	22
Frieda's					
Bing	¼ cup (1.4 oz)	120	0	26	17
Tart	⅓ cup (1.4 oz)	150	0	33	22
Good Sense					
Cherries	⅓ cup	145	0	33	22
FRESH					
sour	1 cup	51	tr	13	–
sweet	10	49	1	11	–
Super Cherry					
Rainier	21	90	0	19	14
FROZEN					
dark sweet unsweetened	1 cup	110	1	25	20
CHERRY JUICE					
Hi-C					
Sour Blast Wild Cherry	1 pkg	110	0	29	28
Wild Cherry	1 box	100	0	28	27
Minute Maid					
Coolers Clear Cherry	1 pouch (7 oz)	100	0	28	27
Ocean Spray					
Black Cherry	8 oz	140	0	33	33
CHERVIL					
seed	1 tsp	1	tr	tr	–

FOOD	PORTION	CALS	FAT	CARB	SUGAR
CHESTNUTS					
chinese steamed	3 (1 oz)	43	tr	10	–
creme de marrons	1 oz	73	tr	18	10
japanese roasted	1 oz	57	tr	13	–
ready-to-eat vacuum packed	5 (1 oz)	40	0	8	0
roasted	3 (1 oz)	70	1	15	3
CHEWING GUM					
Bazooka					
Bubble Gum	1 piece (4 g)	15	0	4	3
Big Red					
Gum	1 piece	10	0	2	2
Brach's					
Abra Cabubble	1 piece	45	0	10	7
CareFree					
Koolerz Lemonaide	1 piece	5	0	2	0
Doublemint					
Gum	1 piece	10	0	2	2
Eclipse					
Sugarless All Flavors	2 pieces	5	0	2	0
Extra					
Sugar Free All Flavors	1 piece	5	0	2	0
Sugar Free Bubble Gum	1 piece	5	0	1	0
Glee Gum					
Peppermint	2 pieces (2.5 g)	5	0	2	2
Juicy Fruit					
Gum	2 pieces	10	0	2	2
Orbit					
All Flavors	1 piece	5	0	2	0
Sugarless All Flavors	2 pieces	5	0	2	0
SteviaDent					
Gum	2 pieces	3	0	1	0

FOOD	PORTION	CALS	FAT	CARB	SUGAR
Winterfresh					
Gum	1 stick	10	0	2	2
Wrigley's					
Spearmint	1 stick	10	0	2	2
Xylichew					
Licorice	2 pieces	4	0	2	0
CHICKEN					
CANNED					
breast meat in water	2 oz	70	1	0	0
w/ broth	½ can (2.5 oz)	117	6	0	0
FRESH					
broiler/fryer breast w/ skin batter dipped & fried	½ breast (4.9 oz)	364	18	13	—
broiler/fryer breast w/ skin roasted	½ breast (3.4 oz)	193	8	0	0
broiler/fryer breast w/ skin stewed	½ breast (3.9 oz)	202	8	0	0
broiler/fryer breast w/o skin fried	½ breast (3 oz)	161	4	tr	—
broiler/fryer breast w/o skin roasted	½ breast (3 oz)	142	3	0	0
broiler/fryer drumstick w/ skin batter dipped & fried	1 (2.6 oz)	193	11	6	—
broiler/fryer drumstick w/ skin floured & fried	1 (1.7 oz)	120	7	1	—
broiler/fryer drumstick w/ skin roasted	1 (1.8 oz)	112	6	0	0
broiler/fryer drumstick w/ skin stewed	1 (2 oz)	116	6	0	0
broiler/fryer drumstick w/o skin fried	1 (1.5 oz)	82	3	0	0
broiler/fryer drumstick w/o skin roasted	1 (1.5 oz)	76	2	0	0

FOOD	PORTION	CALS	FAT	CARB	SUGAR
broiler/fryer drumstick w/o skin stewed	1 (1.6 oz)	78	3	0	0
broiler/fryer leg w/ skin batter dipped & fried	1 (5.5 oz)	431	26	14	—
broiler/fryer leg w/ skin floured & fried	1 (3.9 oz)	285	16	3	—
broiler/fryer leg w/ skin roasted	1 (4 oz)	265	15	0	0
broiler/fryer leg w/ skin stewed	1 (4.4 oz)	275	16	0	0
broiler/fryer leg w/o skin fried	1 (3.3 oz)	195	9	1	—
broiler/fryer leg w/o skin roasted	1 (3.3 oz)	182	8	0	0
broiler/fryer leg w/o skin stewed	1 (3.5 oz)	187	8	0	0
broiler/fryer neck w/ skin stewed	1 (1.3 oz)	94	7	0	0
broiler/fryer neck w/o skin stewed	1 (.6 oz)	32	1	0	0
broiler/fryer skin floured & fried	from ½ chicken (2 oz)	281	24	5	—
broiler/fryer skin roasted	from ½ chicken (2 oz)	254	23	0	0
broiler/fryer skin stewed	from ½ chicken (2.5 oz)	261	24	0	0
broiler/fryer thigh w/ skin batter dipped & fried	1 (3 oz)	238	14	8	—
broiler/fryer thigh w/ skin floured & fried	1 (2.2 oz)	162	9	2	—
broiler/fryer thigh w/ skin roasted	1 (2.2 oz)	153	10	0	0

FOOD	PORTION	CALS	FAT	CARB	SUGAR
broiler/fryer thigh w/ skin stewed	1 (2.4 oz)	158	10	0	0
broiler/fryer thigh w/o skin fried	1 (1.8 oz)	113	5	1	—
broiler/fryer thigh w/o skin roasted	1 (1.8 oz)	109	6	0	0
broiler/fryer thigh w/o skin stewed	1 (1.9 oz)	107	5	0	0
broiler/fryer w/ skin floured & fried	½ chicken (11 oz)	844	47	10	—
broiler/fryer w/ skin fried	½ chicken (16.4 oz)	1347	81	44	—
broiler/fryer w/ skin roasted	½ chicken (10.5 oz)	715	41	0	0
broiler/fryer w/ skin stewed	½ chicken (11.7 oz)	730	42	0	0
broiler/fryer w/ skin neck & giblets batter dipped & fried	1 chicken (2.3 lbs)	2987	180	93	—
broiler/fryer w/ skin neck & giblets roasted	1 chicken (1.5 lbs)	1598	90	tr	—
broiler/fryer w/ skin neck & giblets stewed	1 chicken (1.6 lbs)	1625	93	tr	—
broiler/fryer w/o skin fried	1 cup	307	13	2	—
broiler/fryer w/o skin roasted	1 cup (5 oz)	266	10	0	0
broiler/fryer w/o skin stewed	1 cup (5 oz)	248	9	0	0
broiler/fryer wing w/ skin batter dipped & fried	1 (1.7 oz)	159	11	5	—
broiler/fryer wing w/ skin floured & fried	1 (1.1 oz)	103	7	1	—

FOOD	PORTION	CALS	FAT	CARB	SUGAR
broiler/fryer wing w/ skin roasted	1 (1.2 oz)	99	7	0	0
broiler/fryer wing w/ skin stewed	1 (1.4 oz)	100	7	0	0
capon w/ skin neck & giblets roasted	1 chicken (3.1 lbs)	3211	165	1	—
cornish hen w/skin roasted	½ hen (4 oz)	296	21	0	—
cornish hen w/ skin roasted	1 hen (8 oz)	595	42	0	0
cornish hen w/o skin & bone roasted	1 hen (3.8 oz)	144	4	0	—
cornish hen w/o skin & bone roasted	½ hen (2 oz)	72	2	0	—
roaster dark meat w/o skin roasted	1 cup (5 oz)	250	12	0	—
roaster light meat w/o skin roasted	1 cup (5 oz)	214	6	0	—
roaster w/ skin neck & giblets roasted	1 chicken (2.4 lbs)	2363	140	1	—
roaster w/ skin roasted	½ chicken (1.1 lbs)	1071	64	0	0
roaster w/o skin roasted	1 cup (5 oz)	469	28	0	0
stewing dark meat w/o skin stewed	1 cup (5 oz)	361	21	0	—
stewing w/ skin neck & giblets stewed	1 chicken (1.3 lbs)	1636	107	tr	—
stewing w/ skin stewed	½ chicken (9.2 oz)	744	49	0	0
Amish Select					
Boneless Skinless Breast w/ Honey Dijon Mustard	1 serv (4 oz)	130	2	4	3

FOOD	PORTION	CALS	FAT	CARB	SUGAR
Murray's					
Breast Boneless & Skinless	4 oz	110	1	0	0
Ground	3 oz	130	7	0	0
Whole Lean	4 oz	170	9	0	0
FROZEN					
Bell & Evans					
Breaded Breast Nuggets	1 serv (4 oz)	190	6	13	1
Breaded Whole Breast Tenders	1 (4 oz)	190	6	13	1
Burgers	1 (3 oz)	120	6	tr	0
Chicken Sandwich Steaks	1 serv (2 oz)	60	1	tr	0
Weaver					
Breast Strips	3 pieces	230	14	14	1
Breast Tenders	5 pieces	240	15	15	0
Buffalo Popcorn Chicken	7 pieces	230	14	13	1
Crispy Breast Strips	2 pieces	220	14	13	1
Crispy Mini Drums	5 pieces	250	16	14	2
Croquettes	2 + gravy	230	14	15	2
Honey Batter Breast Tenders	5 pieces	220	13	13	3
Hot Wings Buffalo Style	3 pieces	190	13	0	0
Nuggets	4 pieces	210	15	9	0
Patties Italian	1	210	14	12	1
Patties Breast	1	170	10	10	1
Patties Original	1	180	11	10	1
Wings Honey BBQ BB	3	200	11	7	2
READY-TO-EAT					
chicken salad sandwich spread	¼ cup	104	7	4	0
Hillshire Farm					
Smoked Breast	6 slices (2 oz)	60	1	2	1
Perdue					
Short Cuts Grilled Italian	½ cup	80	1	4	1

FOOD	PORTION	CALS	FAT	CARB	SUGAR
Short Cuts Grilled Lemon Pepper	½ cup (2.5 oz)	80	1	3	–
Tyson					
Roasted Whole Chicken w/ Skin	1 serv (3 oz)	160	11	1	1

CHICKEN DISHES
FROZEN
Maple Leaf Farms

FOOD	PORTION	CALS	FAT	CARB	SUGAR
Chicken Breast Stuffed Broccoli & Cheese	1 serv (6 oz)	340	19	20	2

REFRIGERATED
Lloyd's

FOOD	PORTION	CALS	FAT	CARB	SUGAR
Barbecue Shredded Chicken	¼ cup (2 oz)	90	2	11	9

Old El Paso

FOOD	PORTION	CALS	FAT	CARB	SUGAR
For Tacos Shredded Chicken	¼ cup	60	2	4	1

Oscar Mayer

FOOD	PORTION	CALS	FAT	CARB	SUGAR
Lunchables Chicken Wraps	1 pkg	440	13	64	25

Tyson

FOOD	PORTION	CALS	FAT	CARB	SUGAR
Chicken Breast Medallions In Tomato & Herb Sauce	1 serv (5 oz)	120	4	5	2

TAKE-OUT

FOOD	PORTION	CALS	FAT	CARB	SUGAR
boneless breast w/ apple stuffing	1 serv (5 oz)	260	9	10	2
breast & wing breaded & fried	2 pieces (5.7 oz)	494	30	20	–
chicken & dumplings	¾ cup	256	12	12	–
chicken & noodles	1 cup	365	18	26	–
chicken a la king	1 cup	470	34	12	–
chicken cacciatore	¾ cup	394	24	9	–
chicken pie w/ top crust	1 slice (5.6 oz)	472	31	32	–

FOOD	PORTION	CALS	FAT	CARB	SUGAR
chicken cordon bleu	1 serv (5 oz)	280	13	10	0
chicken curry ½ breast	1 serv	160	9	6	3
chicken curry boneless	1 serv (6.2 oz)	219	12	8	4
chicken curry leg & thigh	1 serv	180	10	7	3
drumstick breaded & fried	2 pieces (5.2 oz)	430	27	16	–
grilled breast strips	4 strips (3 oz)	100	2	0	0
groundnut stew hkatenkwan	1 serv (15.7 oz)	576	40	18	3
jamaican jerk wings	4 wings (9.9 oz)	709	51	3	tr
sancocho de pollo dominican chicken stew	1 serv	702	30	34	4
tandoori chicken breast	1 serv	260	13	5	–
tandoori chicken leg & thigh	1 serv	300	17	6	–
thigh breaded & fried	2 pieces (5.2 oz)	430	27	16	–

CHICKEN SUBSTITUTES
Lightlife

FOOD	PORTION	CALS	FAT	CARB	SUGAR
Smart Cutlet Seasoned Chicken	1 (4 oz)	180	4	11	3
Smart Menu Chick'n Nuggets	4 pieces	220	11	16	1
Smart Menu Chick'n Patties	1 patty	160	7	14	0
Smart Menu Chick'n Strips	1 serv (3 oz)	80	0	5	0
Quorn					
Cutlets	1 (3.5 oz)	200	8	20	2
Gruyere Cutlet	1 (4 oz)	260	15	23	3
Naked Cutlet	1 (2.4 oz)	80	3	5	0
Nuggets	3–4 pieces (3 oz)	180	8	18	2
Patties	1 patty (2.6 oz)	160	7	12	2
Tenders	1 cup (3 oz)	90	2	8	1

FOOD	PORTION	CALS	FAT	CARB	SUGAR
CHICKPEAS					
DRIED					
cooked	1 cup	269	4	45	—
CHICORY					
endive fresh chopped	½ cup	4	tr	1	—
Frieda's					
Belgian Endive	2 cups	115	0	3	1
CHILI					
powder	1 tsp	8	tr	1	—
Bush's					
ChiliMagic Chili Starter as prep	1 cup	250	11	17	5
Original No Beans	1 cup	240	14	16	5
Del Monte					
Sauce	1 tbsp	20	0	5	4
Frieda's					
California Dried	2 tbsp	15	0	2	1
Peppadew	⅓ cup	40	0	32	29
Gringo Billy's					
Chili Mix	1 tbsp	24	1	2	0
Hunt's					
Family Favorites Chili	¼ cup (2.2 oz)	25	0	9	3
Lean Cuisine					
Cafe Classics Three Bean Chili	1 pkg (10 oz)	260	7	40	8
Lightlife					
Smart Chili	1 pkg	200	0	34	8
McCormick					
Mexican Style Chili Powder	¼ tsp	0	0	0	0
Pacific Foods					
Beef Steak w/ Beans	1 cup	250	7	29	5

FOOD	PORTION	CALS	FAT	CARB	SUGAR
Ro-Tel					
Chili Fixin's	½ cup	35	1	8	5
Stagg					
Classic w/ Beans	1 cup	310	17	24	7
Country Blend	1 cup	330	17	30	7
Country Blend w/ Beans	1 cup	33	17	30	7
CHINESE PRESERVING MELON					
cooked	½ cup	11	tr	3	–
CHIPS					
apple chips	10	101	5	16	14
Bachman					
Potato Golden Crips	1 pkg (1 oz)	150	9	16	0
Cape Cod					
Potato 40% Reduced Fat	19	130	6	18	tr
Potato Beachside BBQ	19	150	8	17	tr
Potato Classic	19	150	8	17	tr
Potato Fresh Garden Herb Reduced Fat	19	130	6	19	tr
Potato Jalapeno & Cheddar	19	140	8	16	tr
Potato No Salt	19	150	10	14	tr
Potato Robust Russet	19	150	8	16	tr
Potato Salt & Vinegar	19	150	8	17	tr
Potato Sea Salt & Cracked Pepper	19	140	7	16	tr
Tortilla Reduced Carb	10	140	6	11	0
Tortilla Veggie	12	140	6	18	0
Deliciously Slim					
Tortilla Black Bean & Sour Cream	1 oz	140	9	13	1
Tortilla Lightly Salted	1 oz	140	8	13	0
Tortilla Ranch	1 oz	140	9	13	1

FOOD	PORTION	CALS	FAT	CARB	SUGAR
Doritos					
Baked Cooler Ranch	15 (1 oz)	120	4	21	1
Baked Nacho Cheesier	15	120	4	21	1
Cooler Ranch	12	140	7	18	tr
Four Cheese	12	140	8	17	0
Guacamole	12	150	8	16	0
Light Nacho Cheesier	11	90	1	18	1
Natural White Nacho Cheese	11	150	8	17	tr
Ranchero	12	150	1	17	0
Rollitos Cooler Ranch	17	140	8	17	tr
Rollitos Zesty Taco	17	150	8	17	tr
Toasted Corn	13	140	7	18	0
Fritos					
Corn Chips King Size	12	160	10	16	0
Original	32	160	10	15	tr
Scoops	10	160	10	16	0
Twists	23	150	9	17	tr
Glenny's					
Soy Crisps Low Fat Lightly Salted	1 pkg (1.3 oz)	140	2	18	2
Soy Crispy Wispys Sour Cream & Onion	⅕ bag (0.5 oz)	60	2	7	0
Spud Delites Sea Salt	1 pkg (1.1 oz)	100	1	21	0
Veggie Fries	1 pkg (1.3 oz)	140	2	26	0
Guiltless Gourmet					
Guiltless Carbs Salsa Verde	1 oz	110	3	9	0
Guiltless Carbs Southwest Ranch	1 oz	110	3	9	0
Guiltless Carbs Three Pepper	1 oz	110	3	9	0
Tortilla Blue Corn	18 (1 oz)	110	2	22	0
Tortilla Chili Lime	18 (1 oz)	110	2	22	0

FOOD	PORTION	CALS	FAT	CARB	SUGAR
Tortilla Chili Verde	18 (1 oz)	120	2	22	1
Tortilla Chipotle	18 (1 oz)	120	2	22	1
Tortilla Mucho Nacho	18 (1 oz)	110	2	20	1
Tortilla Organic Red Corn	18 (1 oz)	110	2	22	0
Tortilla Spicy Black Bean	18 (1 oz)	110	2	22	0
Tortilla Sweet White Corn	18 (1 oz)	110	2	22	0
Tortilla Yellow Corn	18 (1 oz)	110	2	22	0
Tortilla Yellow Corn Unsalted	18 (1 oz)	110	1	22	0
Herr's					
Potato	1 oz	140	8	16	0
Keto					
Low Carb Tortilla All Flavors	1 oz	150	8	8	0
Lay's					
Baked KC Masterpiece	11 (1 oz)	120	3	22	2
Baked Sour Cream & Onion	12 (1 oz)	120	3	21	3
Chile Limon	1 oz	150	10	14	0
Classic	1 pkg (1 oz)	150	10	15	0
Deli Style Original	17 (1 oz)	150	10	16	0
Dill Pickle	20 (1 oz)	160	10	13	1
Flamin' Hot	17 (1 oz)	160	10	15	1
KC Masterpiece BBQ	15 (1 oz)	150	10	15	2
Kettle Cooked Jalapeno	15 (1 oz)	140	8	16	0
Kettle Cooked Mesquite BBQ	18 (1 oz)	140	8	16	1
Kettle Cooked Original	22 (1 oz)	150	8	16	0
Kettle Cooked Sea Salt & Vinegar	18 (1 oz)	140	7	17	tr
Light Fat Free KC Masterpiece	20 (1 oz)	75	0	17	1
Light Fat Free Original	20 (1 oz)	75	0	18	0

FOOD	PORTION	CALS	FAT	CARB	SUGAR
Limon	17 (1 oz)	150	10	15	0
Natural Country BBQ	14 (1 oz)	150	9	16	1
Natural Sea Salt & Vinegar	16 (1 oz)	150	9	15	tr
Natural Sea Salted	16 (1 oz)	150	9	15	0
Original Baked	11 (1 oz)	110	2	23	2
Salt & Vinegar	17 (1 oz)	150	10	15	1
Sour Cream & Onion	17 (1 oz)	160	11	12	tr
Stax	13 (1 oz)	160	10	15	1
Wavy	11 (1 oz)	150	10	15	0
Wavy Au Gratin	13 (1 oz)	150	10	14	tr
Wavy Hickory Barbecue	13 (1 oz)	150	9	16	tr
Wavy Ranch	12 (1 oz)	150	10	16	tr
Manny's					
Organic Tortilla Blues	1 oz	150	7	20	0
Tortilla No Salt Added	1 oz	150	7	20	0
Maui					
Shrimp Chips	17	140	8	19	0
Met-Rx					
Pro Chips Bar-B-Que	1 pkg (2 oz)	260	9	8	4
Pro Chips Nacho	1 pkg (2 oz)	260	10	6	2
Pringles					
Sour Cream & Onion	14 (1 oz)	160	10	15	1
Racquet					
Wheat Chips All Flavors	6 chips	30	1	4	0
Revival					
Baked Soy Pasta Chips Lightly Salted Sunshine	1 bag (0.9 oz)	100	2	13	0
Baked Soy Pasta Chips Naturally Nice	1 bag (0.9 oz)	80	1	12	0
Baked Soy Pasta Chips Rev It Up Ranch	1 bag (0.9 oz)	105	3	12	1
Ruffles					
Baked Original	10	120	3	21	2

FOOD	PORTION	CALS	FAT	CARB	SUGAR
Cheddar & Sour Cream	11	160	10	14	0
KC Masterpiece Mesquite BBQ	11	150	10	15	tr
Light Cheddar & Sour Cream	15	75	0	16	tr
Light Original	17	70	0	17	0
Original	12	160	10	14	0
Potato Crisps	16	160	10	16	0
Reduced Fat Sea Salted	15	140	7	17	0
Sour Cream & Onion	11	160	10	14	1
Santitas					
White Corn	9	130	6	19	0
Yellow Corn	9	130	6	19	0
Snyder's Of Hanover					
Veggie Crisps	1 pkg (1.5 oz)	190	9	26	0
Stacy's					
Twisted Pasta Low Fat	1 oz	110	2	21	1
Sunchips					
French Onion	10	140	6	18	3
Harvest Cheddar	10	140	6	19	2
Tastee					
Potato Yukon Gold	1 oz	130	5	19	2
Terra Chips					
Spiced Sweet Potato	1 pkg (½ oz)	190	13	17	3
Tostitos					
Blue Corn	6	140	6	19	0
Crispy Rounds	13	140	7	18	0
Gold	6	140	7	19	0
Light Restaurant Style	6	90	1	20	0
Original Bite Size	20	110	1	24	0
Restaurant Style	6	130	6	19	0
Santa Fe	7	140	6	19	0
Scoops	13	140	7	18	0

FOOD	PORTION	CALS	FAT	CARB	SUGAR
Yellow Corn	6	140	6	19	0
Utz					
No Salt Added	20 (1 oz)	150	9	14	0

CHITTERLINGS
pork cooked	3 oz	258	24	0	0

CHIVES
fresh chopped	1 tbsp	1	tr	tr	—

CHOCOLATE
BAKING
grated unsweetened	¼ cup	165	17	10	tr
liquid unsweetened	1 oz	134	14	10	0
mexican	1 sq (0.7 oz)	85	3	15	14
squares unsweetened	1 square (1 oz)	145	15	9	tr

CHIPS
Baker's
Chocolate Chunks	13 pieces (0.5 oz)	70	5	9	8
Ghirardelli					
Semi-Sweet	33 pieces (0.5 oz)	70	4	9	7

CHOCOLATE SPREAD
Twist
Sugar Free Chocolate Spread	2 tbsp	170	12	2	0

CHOCOLATE SYRUP
syrup	2 tbsp	82	tr	22	—
Colac					
Chocolate Topping	1 tbsp	37	1	15	0
DaVinci Gourmet					
Sugar Free	2 tbsp	15	0	5	0

FOOD	PORTION	CALS	FAT	CARB	SUGAR
Hershey's					
Syrup	2 tbsp	100	0	25	20
Nesquik					
Calcium Fortified	2 tbsp	100	0	27	25
Smucker's					
Sundae Syrup Chocolate	2 tbsp	110	0	26	21
Walden Farms					
Sugar Free	2 tbsp	0	0	0	0
CINNAMON					
cinnamon sugar	1 tsp	16	tr	4	4
ground	1 tsp	6	tr	2	—
sticks	0.5 oz	39	tr	8	0
Gringo Billy's					
Cinnamon Sweetener	½ tsp	0	0	0	0
CISCO					
smoked	1 oz	50	3	0	0
CLAMS					
CANNED					
meat only	1 cup	236	3	8	—
Brunswick					
Baby	2 oz	50	1	0	0
Bumble Bee					
Baby	¼ cup	50	1	2	0
Chopped or Minced	¼ cup	25	0	2	0
Smoked	¼ cup	130	9	1	0
Chicken Of The Sea					
Chopped	¼ cup	30	0	2	0
Minced	¼ cup	30	0	2	1
Whole Baby	¼ cup	30	0	1	0
Orleans					
Clam Juice	1 tbsp	0	0	0	0

FOOD	PORTION	CALS	FAT	CARB	SUGAR
FRESH					
cooked	20 sm	133	2	5	–
raw	20 sm (6.3 oz)	133	2	5	–
TAKE-OUT					
breaded & fried	20 sm	379	21	19	–
CLEMENTINES					
Haddon House					
In Light Syrup	½ cup	80	0	19	18
Sunkist					
Fresh	2	80	0	17	13
Tina					
Fresh	1	50	1	15	12
CLOVES					
ground	1 tsp	7	tr	1	–
COCOA					
powder unsweetened	1 tbsp (5 g)	11	1	3	–
COCONUT					
fresh	1 piece (1.5 oz)	159	15	7	–
fresh shredded	1 cup	283	27	12	–
Frieda's					
White	¼ cup (1.4 oz)	140	13	6	1
COCONUT JUICE					
coconut water	1 cup	46	tr	9	–
cream canned	1 tbsp	36	3	2	–
milk canned	1 tbsp	30	3	tr	–
A Taste Of Thai					
Coconut Milk	⅓ cup	140	15	3	0
Lite Coconut Milk	⅓ cup	45	4	3	0
Amy & Brian					
Juice	8 oz	76	0	19	10

FOOD	PORTION	CALS	FAT	CARB	SUGAR
Thai Kitchen					
Milk	2 oz	124	12	3	1
Vita Coco					
Coconut Water	1 box (11 oz)	65	0	17	17
Coconut Water w/ Fruit Juice All Flavors	1 box (11 oz)	110	0	27	27
Zico					
Coconut Water Mango	11 oz	60	0	15	14
Coconut Water Natural	11 oz	60	0	15	14
Coconut Water Passion Fruit + Orange Peel	11 oz	60	0	15	14
COD					
atlantic canned	3 oz	89	1	0	0
atlantic dried	3 oz	246	2	0	0
atlantic fresh cooked	3 oz	89	1	0	0
pacific fresh baked	3 oz	95	1	0	0
roe canned	1 oz	34	1	tr	–
roe tarama	3.5 oz	547	55	6	tr
TAKE-OUT					
roe baked w/ butter & lemon juice	1 oz	36	1	tr	–
COFFEE					
INSTANT					
decaffeinated as prep	8 oz	2	0	0	0
decaffeinated powder	1 rounded tsp	4	0	1	0
powder	1 rounded tsp	4	tr	1	0
REGULAR					
brewed	8 oz	2	tr	0	0
roasted beans	1 oz	64	4	18	–
Soy Java					
All Flavors	1 tbsp	20	0	0	0

FOOD	PORTION	CALS	FAT	CARB	SUGAR
TAKE-OUT					
turkish	1 cup (4 oz)	50	1	12	12
COFFEE BEVERAGES					
AchievONE					
All Flavors	1 bottle (9.5 oz)	120	0	5	4
America's Best Brew					
Iced Coffee All Flavors	8 oz	110	2	25	22
Big Train					
Low Carb Blended Ice Mocha as prep	1 serv (16 oz)	90	5	14	2
Cinnabon					
Latte Caramel Nut	1 can (8 oz)	170	6	27	25
Latte Cinnamon Vanilla	1 can (8 oz)	170	6	27	25
Double Bean Elixir					
Coffee Soda All Flavors	8 oz	90	0	23	23
Double Hit					
Maximum Energy Coffee Drink	1 can (12 oz)	80	0	20	20
Flavour Creations					
Coffee Flavoring Tablets All Flavors	1 tablet	0	0	tr	tr
Frappio					
Iced Coffee Energy Drink	1 can (15 oz)	260	4	42	38
Jakada					
Latte Mocha	1 bottle (10.5 oz)	180	3.5	33	32
Latte Vanilla	1 bottle (10.5 oz)	180	4	32	31
Loco-Joe					
Iced Coffee	1 box (8.25 oz)	160	4	26	25
Low Carb Creations					
Cappuccino	1 cup	30	2	3	tr

FOOD	PORTION	CALS	FAT	CARB	SUGAR
Shock					
Latte	8 oz	150	3	28	24
Triple Mocha	1 can (8 oz)	125	2	27	27
Sipper Sweets					
Sugar Free Low Carb Cappuccino	1 serv	50	3	3	0
Starbucks					
Frappuccino	1 bottle (9.5 oz)	190	3	39	30
Frappuccino Mocha	1 bottle (9.5 oz)	190	3	39	30
Frappuccino Vanilla	1 bottle (9.5 oz)	190	3	39	30
Wolfgang Puck					
Gourmet Heated Lattes All Flavors	1 can (10 oz)	100	5	9	8
TAKE-OUT					
cafe amaretto w/ alcohol	1 serv	192	9	15	—
cafe au lait	1 cup (8 oz)	77	4	6	7
cafe brulot	1 cup	48	0	3	3
cafe brulot w/ alcohol	1 serv	130	tr	16	—
cappuccino	1 cup (8 oz)	77	4	6	7
coffee con leche	1 cup (6 oz)	104	4	16	17
espresso	1 cup (4 oz)	2	tr	0	0
irish coffee	1 serv (8 oz)	209	11	5	4
latte w/ skim milk	1 serv (13 oz)	88	tr	12	11
latte w/ whole milk	1 serv (14 oz)	143	6	15	14
mocha	1 serv (17 oz)	403	9	69	54

COFFEE SUBSTITUTES
Teeccino

FOOD	PORTION	CALS	FAT	CARB	SUGAR
Herbal Coffee All Flavors	1 cup	15	0	3	1

COFFEE WHITENERS
Coffee-Mate

FOOD	PORTION	CALS	FAT	CARB	SUGAR
Half & Half Original	2 tbsp	40	4	1	1
Half & Half Vanilla	2 tbsp	60	4	7	7

FOOD	PORTION	CALS	FAT	CARB	SUGAR
Latte Classic	2 tbsp	100	6	12	4
Latte Mocha	2 tbsp	90	4	14	9
Latte Vanilla	2 tbsp	90	4	14	9
Liquid All Flavors	1 tbsp	40	2	5	5
Sugar Free All Flavors	1 tbsp	15	1	1	0
Hood					
Country Creamer Non Dairy	1 tbsp	20	2	2	0

COLESLAW
Dole
Classic Cole Slaw no dressing	1½ cup (3 oz)	25	0	5	2

Fresh Express
3 Color Deli	1½ cups	20	0	5	3
Cole Slaw Kit as prep	2 cups	120	8	12	10

River Ranch
Country Homestyle Kit	1 cup	140	9	14	12
Honey Dijon Peppercorn Kit	1 cup	120	8	11	8
Mix	1¼ cups	25	0	5	3

TAKE-OUT
coleslaw w/ dressing	¾ cup	147	11	13	—

COLLARDS
fresh cooked	½ cup	17	tr	4	—

Allens
Seasoned Southern Style	½ cup	35	1	5	1

COOKIES
MIX
Aunt Paula's
Low Carb Chef Chocolate Chip as prep	1	66	4	4	0

FOOD	PORTION	CALS	FAT	CARB	SUGAR
Low Carb Chef Peanut Butter as prep	1	66	4	4	0
Big Train					
Low Carb Chocolate Chip as prep	2	140	9	11	5
Low Carb Peanut Butter as prep	2	140	9	9	2
Bob's Red Mill					
Gluten Free Chocolate Chip as prep	2	260	10	41	24
Keto					
Chocolate Chip as prep	1	47	2	2	1
Oatmeal Raisin as prep	2	59	3	2	0
MiniCarb					
All Flavors as prep	1	110	2	7	1
Nature's Path					
Organic Chocolate Chip	1/10 pkg	150	2	31	16
READY-TO-EAT					
cream cheese	1 (1.1 oz)	141	9	14	6
hermits	1 (1 oz)	117	5	18	10
jumbles coconut	1 (1 oz)	121	7	13	7
madeleines	1 (0.8 oz)	86	5	10	5
pinenut cookies	1 (1.1 oz)	134	9	11	8
spritz	1 (0.4 oz)	42	2	6	3
toll house original	1 (0.8 oz)	105	6	13	9
zeppole	1 (0.8 oz)	78	6	6	4
Alex & Dani's					
Original Hazelnut	3 (1 oz)	130	6	17	8
Annie's Homegrown					
Bunny Grahams All Flavors	26	130	4	20	6
Archway					
Fruit Filled Apricot	1 (0.8 oz)	90	3	15	7
Fruit Filled Raspberry	1 (0.8 oz)	90	3	15	7

FOOD	PORTION	CALS	FAT	CARB	SUGAR
Oatmeal Raisin	1	120	4	20	11
Windmill	1	90	4	14	7
Arico					
Gluten Free Casein Free	1 bar	150	5	25	14
Gluten Free Casein Free Almond Cranberry	1 bar	150	6	23	12
Gluten Free Casein Free Double Chocolate	1 bar	150	5	25	13
Back To Nature					
Chocolate Chunk	2	130	6	17	9
Crispy Oatmeal	2	120	5	18	8
Sandwich Chocolate & Mint Creme	2	130	6	18	11
Sandwich Classic Creme	2	130	6	18	11
Bahlsen					
Butter Leaves	7 (1 oz)	140	7	19	7
Hanover Waffelin	5 (1 oz)	160	10	16	8
Nuss Dessert	3 (1.1 oz)	170	11	17	8
Carbolite					
Chocolate Chip	1 (1 oz)	120	9	12	0
Peanut Butter	1 (1 oz)	120	9	12	0
Shortbread	1 (1 oz)	180	9	14	0
Country Choice Naturals					
Chocolate Chip Walnut	1	100	4	16	10
Double Fudge Brownie	1 (0.8 oz)	90	3	16	10
Ginger	1	90	2	17	10
Ginger Snaps	5	120	5	19	9
Lemon	1	90	3	17	10
Oatmeal Chocolate Chip	1 (0.8 oz)	100	4	15	8
Oatmeal Raisin	1 (0.8 oz)	100	3	16	9
Old Fashioned Oatmeal	1 (0.8 oz)	100	3	16	8
Peanut Butter	1	100	5	13	8

FOOD	PORTION	CALS	FAT	CARB	SUGAR
Sandwich Cremes Chocolate	1	130	5	19	11
Sandwich Cremes Duplex	2	130	5	19	11
Sandwich Cremes Ginger Lemon	2	130	5	19	11
Sandwich Cremes Mint Creme	2	130	5	19	11
Sandwich Cremes Vanilla	2	130	5	19	11
Vanilla Wafers	7	120	5	19	8
David's					
Hamantash Raspberry	1 (0.7 oz)	85	6	12	5
De Beukelaer					
Pirouline	8 (1 oz)	130	4	23	13
Doritos					
Barras De Coco	5	120	4	21	7
Dove					
Beyond Chocolate Chunk	1	110	6	13	7
Chocolate Walnut Oasis	1	110	6	13	6
Chocolate Walnut Rendezvous	1	110	8	13	7
Milk Chocolate Moment	3	150	9	20	12
Mint Chocolate Serenade	3	160	8	19	10
Toffee Chocolate Tango	3	160	8	20	12
Dunkaroos					
Chocolate Graham	1 pkg	120	5	20	14
Cinnamon Graham	1 pkg	130	5	21	14
Honey Graham	1 pkg	120	5	20	13
Elite					
Tea Biscuits Chocolate	4	80	2	14	4
Enjoy Life					
Gingerbread Spice Nut & Gluten Free	2 (1 oz)	100	4	16	9

FOOD	PORTION	CALS	FAT	CARB	SUGAR
No-Oat Oatmeal Nut & Gluten Free	2 (1 oz)	110	4	19	10
Snickerdoodle Nut & Gluten Free	2 (1 oz)	130	5	21	10
Entenmann's					
Original Chocolate Chip	3	140	7	20	11
Estee					
Fructose Sweetened Chocolate Chip	4	160	8	21	6
Fructose Sweetened Lemon	4	160	6	20	6
Fructose Sweetened Sandwich Chocolate	3	170	6	26	12
Fructose Sweetened Sandwich Original	3	170	6	26	13
Fructose Sweetened Sandwich Peanut Butter	3	190	8	25	11
Fructose Sweetened Vanilla	4	160	7	21	7
Fructose Sweetened Vanilla Sandwich	3	170	6	27	12
Sugar Free Chocolate Chip	3	110	4	22	0
Sugar Free Lemon	3	110	3	22	0
Sugar Free Wafer Chocolate Creme	4	150	8	20	9
Sugar Free Wafer Lemon Creme	4	150	9	21	0
Sugar Free Wafer Peanut Butter Creme	4	150	9	20	0
Sugar Free Wafer Strawberry Creme	4	150	9	21	0

FOOD	PORTION	CALS	FAT	CARB	SUGAR
Sugar Free Wafer Vanilla Creme	4	150	9	20	0
Frieda's					
Asian Almond	2 (1 oz)	170	10	19	6
Gamesa					
Animalitos	14	110	1	25	7
Arcoiris Marshmallow	6	220	4	44	20
Arcoiris Marshmallow	2	120	5	18	8
Arcoiris Merengue	6	200	3	43	22
Emperador Chocolate	2	120	4	19	10
Emperador Fresa	2	120	4	19	10
Emperador Limon	6	270	8	45	19
Emperador Vanilla	2	120	4	19	9
Hawaianas	3	130	4	22	9
Marias	8	120	2	24	7
Ricanelas	8	140	4	24	7
Roscas	3	130	4	22	8
Sugar Wafers Chocolate	3	160	7	23	15
Sugar Wafers Strawberry	3	160	6	24	16
Sugar Wafers Vanilla	3	160	7	25	17
Glenny's					
Soy Fudgies All Flavors	3	70	2	14	0
Gol D Lite					
Low Carb Pizzelle	1 (0.3 oz)	46	2	6	0
Golightly					
Fabulous Tastes Caramel Dulce De Leche	4	100	6	14	0
Grandma's					
Homestyle Big Chocolate Chip	1 (1.4 oz)	190	9	25	15
Homestyle Big Fudge Chocolate Chip	1 (1.4 oz)	170	7	27	10

FOOD	PORTION	CALS	FAT	CARB	SUGAR
Homestyle Big Oatmeal Raisin	1 (1.4 oz)	180	6	30	15
Homestyle Big Peanut Butter	1 (1.4 oz)	200	10	24	13
Mini Vanilla Creme	9	150	7	22	10
Peanut Butter Sandwich	5	210	10	28	13
Rich N'Chewy Chocolate Chip	1 pkg	270	12	38	23
Vanilla Creme Sandwich	5	210	10	30	15
Granny Oats					
Low Carb Oatmeal	4	98	6	10	0
Heavenly					
Meringues All Flavors Sugar Free Fat Free	1	0	0	1	0
Karen's					
Fabulous Tastes Heavenly Chocolate Chip	4	90	5	16	0
Fabulous Tastes Luscious Raspberry Almond	4	110	6	15	0
Fabulous Tastes Pecan Vanilla Pralines	4	120	8	15	0
Kedem					
Tea Biscuits Chocolate	2	32	1	6	2
Tea Biscuits Orange	2	32	1	6	2
Keebler					
Chips Deluxe	1 (0.5 oz)	80	5	9	5
Graham Honey	8 (1.1 oz)	140	4	23	7
Sandies Fruit Delights Lemon	1 (0.6 oz)	80	4	11	6
Sandies Strawberry Shortcake	1 (0.6 oz)	80	4	11	6
Soft Batch Chocolate Chip	1 (0.6 oz)	80	4	10	6

FOOD	PORTION	CALS	FAT	CARB	SUGAR
Keto					
Low Carb Biscotti Chocolate	1 (1.2 oz)	157	9	6	0
Low Carb Biscotti Lemon Nut	1 (1.2 oz)	157	9	6	0
Low Carb Biscotti Vanilla Almond	1 (1.2 oz)	157	9	6	0
Laura's Wholesome Junk Food					
Anna Banana Split	1	105	5	13	8
Gluten Free Charlotte's Chocolate Chip	2	120	6	16	8
Gluten Free Sally's Raisin	2	110	5	16	9
Lemon Vanilla	2	120	6	15	8
Oatmeal Chocolate Chip	2	110	5	14	8
Oatmeal Raisin	2	100	4	11	9
Wheat Free X-Treme Chocolate Fudge	2	110	5	13	7
Leibniz					
Butter Biscuits	6	130	3	23	7
Little Debbie					
Apple Flips	1 (1.2 oz)	150	5	24	13
Low Carb Creations					
Chocolate Chip	1 (1 oz)	140	10	11	tr
Coconut	1 (1 oz)	140	10	9	tr
Lemon	1 (1 oz)	140	11	9	tr
Snickerdoodle	1 (1 oz)	140	11	9	tr
LU					
Chocolatier	3 (1 oz)	150	9	17	12
Le Fondant	4 (1.1 oz)	170	10	19	9
Le Petit Fruit Strawberry	5 (1.2 oz)	110	1	26	19
Pim's Sensation Bar Chocolate	1	110	6	13	8

FOOD	PORTION	CALS	FAT	CARB	SUGAR
Pim's Sensation Bar Hazelnut	1	110	6	13	8
Shortbread	2	140	8	16	5
Mauna Loa					
Macadamia Nut Chocolate chip	2	130	6	18	14
Macadamia Nut Hawaiian Crunch	2	150	8	15	8
Macadamia Nut White Chocolate Chip	2	130	6	18	14
Nabisco					
Honey Maid Cinnamon Sticks	1 pkg (1 oz)	120	3	23	8
Mallomars	2	120	5	17	12
Oreo Mini	1 pkg (1.2 oz)	170	7	25	14
Natural Ovens					
Carob Chip	1	90	4	16	6
Chocolate Raspberry	1	120	5	19	6
Oatmeal Raisin	1	90	3	15	6
Nature's Path					
Organic Signature Lemon Poppyseed	4	130	4	23	8
Organic Animal Vanilla	9	120	4	20	8
Pepperidge Farm					
Brussels	2	100	5	13	7
Soft Baked Chocolate Chunk	1 (1.1 oz)	140	6	21	13
Whims Chocolate Cashew	9 (1 oz)	150	7	20	11
Pure De-Lite					
High Protein Chocolate Fudge	1 (2.2 oz)	210	8	29	0
High Protein Peanut Butter Crunch	1 (2.2 oz)	210	8	28	0

FOOD	PORTION	CALS	FAT	CARB	SUGAR
SnackWell's					
Creme Sandwich	1 pkg (1.7 oz)	210	5	38	18
Mint Creme	2	110	4	19	13
South Beach Diet					
Chocolate Chip	2	100	5	16	4
Peanut Butter	2	100	5	15	3
Soybite					
All Flavors	1	79	5	7	0
Stella D'Oro					
Lady Stella	3	130	5	20	9
Super Chip					
Chocolate Chip	2 (0.9 oz)	100	7	10	0
TAKE-OUT					
biscotti with nuts chocolate dipped	1 (1.3 oz)	117	6	16	11
black & white	1 lg (3 oz)	302	9	52	31
finikia	1 (1.2 oz)	171	5	16	5
koulourakia butter cookie twist	1 (0.9 oz)	113	6	14	5
linzer tart	1 (2.4 oz)	280	14	34	12
CORIANDER					
cilantro fresh	1 tsp (2 g)	tr	tr	tr	–
leaf dried	1 tsp	2	tr	tr	–
leaf fresh	¼ cup	1	tr	tr	–
seed	1 tsp	5	tr	1	–
CORN					
CANNED					
Del Monte					
Cream Style	½ cup	60	1	14	7
Fiesta	½ cup	50	1	12	5
Gold & White	½ cup	80	1	18	6

FOOD	PORTION	CALS	FAT	CARB	SUGAR
Savory Sides In Butter Sauce	½ cup	90	3	14	5
Savory Sides Santa Fe	½ cup	70	1	16	1
Summer Crisp	½ cup	70	1	13	4
White	½ cup	60	1	11	7
Green Giant					
Mexicorn	⅓ cup	70	1	14	4
Yellow & White	⅓ cup	60	1	12	3
FRESH					
yellow cooked	1 ear (2.7 oz)	83	1	19	—
FROZEN					
cooked	½ cup	67	tr	17	—
Birds Eye					
Baby Gold & White	⅔ cup	100	1	21	3
TAKE-OUT					
fritters	1 (1 oz)	62	2	9	—
on-the-cob w/ butter cooked	1 ear	155	3	32	—
scalloped	1 cup	257	11	34	11
CORNMEAL					
cornmeal mush as prep w/ water	1 cup	223	1	47	tr
cornmeal yellow	1 cup	505	2	107	1
harina de maize con leche	1 cup	295	7	51	32
Indian Head					
Stone Ground	¼ cup	100	1	20	0
Quaker					
Old Fashioned Grits not prep	¼ cup	140	1	32	0
Quick Grits not prep	¼ cup	130	1	29	0
TAKE-OUT					
corn pone	1 piece (2.1 oz)	128	3	23	tr
fritter puerto rican style	1 (1.4 oz)	109	7	8	tr

FOOD	PORTION	CALS	FAT	CARB	SUGAR
harina de maiz con coco	½ cup	383	27	36	21
hush puppies	1 (0.8 oz)	74	3	10	tr
johnnycake	1 piece (1.7 oz)	134	4	21	4

CORNSTARCH

cornstarch	1 cup (4.5 oz)	488	tr	117	–

COTTAGE CHEESE

Breakstone's
Fat Free	½ cup	80	0	8	6

Cabot
Cottage Cheese	½ cup	100	5	4	4
No Fat	½ cup	70	0	5	5

Hood
4% Fat w/ Pineapple	½ cup	130	4	15	13
Fat Free	½ cup	80	0	6	5
Low Fat	½ cup	90	1	5	4
Low Fat No Salt Added	½ cup	90	1	6	5
Low Fat w/ Peaches	½ cup	110	1	18	16

Light N'Lively
Lowfat	½ cup	80	2	6	5

COUSCOUS

cooked	1 cup (5.5 oz)	176	tr	36	–

Near East
Broccoli & Cheese as prep	1 cup	230	3	41	2
Curry as prep	1 cup	220	4	42	3
Herbed Chicken as prep	1 cup	220	3	42	2
Original as prep	1 cup	230	5	46	1
Parmesan as prep	1 cup	220	5	41	3
Roasted Garlic Olive Oil as prep	1 cup	230	5	41	1
Toasted Pine Nut as prep	1 cup	230	6	40	2
Tomato Lentil as prep	1 cup	220	3	42	3

FOOD	PORTION	CALS	FAT	CARB	SUGAR
Wild Mushroom Herb as prep	1 cup	230	4	42	2

CRAB
CANNED
blue	½ cup	67	1	0	0
blue drained	1 can (6.5 oz)	124	2	0	0
Brunswick					
Crabmeat 15% Leg	2 oz	40	1	1	1
Fancy Lump	2 oz	45	1	1	0
Bumble Bee					
Lump	¼ cup	40	1	0	0
Pink	¼ cup	35	1	0	0
White	¼ cup	40	1	0	0
Chicken Of The Sea					
Fancy	½ can (2 oz)	40	0	2	0
Lump	½ can (2 oz)	35	1	1	1
Madam					
Crab Meat	½ cup	40	1	12	0
Terry's					
Crabmeat	¼ cup	40	0	2	1
FRESH					
alaska king meat only steamed	3 oz	82	1	0	0
blue cooked flaked	1 cup (4 oz)	120	2	0	0
dungeness steamed	3 oz	94	1	1	–
queen steamed	3 oz	98	1	0	0
FROZEN					
Margaritaville					
Coral Reef Cakes + Sauce	1	200	10	4	4
Phillips Seafood					
Crab Cakes	1 (3 oz)	160	10	7	0
Crab Meat Stuffing	1 serv (3.5 oz)	170	4	15	3
Mini Cakes	4	160	10	7	0

FOOD	PORTION	CALS	FAT	CARB	SUGAR
Slammers	2	150	9	12	2
TAKE-OUT					
alaska king leg steamed	1 leg (4.7 oz)	130	2	0	0
baked	1 (3.8 oz)	160	2	4	—
cakes	2 (4.2 oz)	186	9	1	—
crab imperial	1 crab (6.8 oz)	289	15	6	3
crab salad	1 serv (5.5 oz)	285	21	3	1
crab thermidor	1 serv (6.4 oz)	456	37	8	tr
deviled	1 serv (4.5 oz)	254	13	17	6
dungeness steamed	1 crab (4.5 oz)	140	2	1	—
empanada de jueyes	1 (4.4 oz)	341	16	38	7
fried crab puffs	4 (3.2 oz)	323	18	30	tr
kenagi korean crab cooked	1 serv (3 oz)	71	tr	0	0
salmorejo de jueyes (in tomato sauce)	1 serv (4.5 oz)	215	14	3	1
soft-shell breaded & fried	1 med (2.3 oz)	216	13	11	1
taco de jueyes	1 (4.2 oz)	266	14	18	1
CRACKER CRUMBS					
cracker meal	1 cup	440	2	93	tr
graham cracker crumbs	1 cup	355	8	65	26
CRACKERS					
melba toast round	1	12	tr	2	tr
oyster cracker	¼ cup	48	1	8	tr
saltines	1	13	tr	2	tr
American Vintage					
Wine Biscuits All Flavors	5	140	7	17	5
Andre's					
CarboSave Crackerbread All Flavors	1 oz	140	8	8	2
Annie's Homegrown					
Cheddar Bunnies BBQ	50	130	6	18	1

FOOD	PORTION	CALS	FAT	CARB	SUGAR
Cheddar Bunnies Original	50	150	7	19	0
Cheddar Bunnies Ranch	50	130	6	17	1
Cheddar Bunnies Whole Wheat	50	130	6	17	1
Back To Nature					
Classic Rounds	5	70	2	11	1
Crispy Wheats	17	130	4	22	4
Rice Thin Sesame Ginger	16	120	3	23	0
Rice Thin White Cheddar	16	120	3	23	tr
Blue Diamond					
Nut-Thins Almond	16	130	3	23	0
Nut-Thins Hazelnut	16	130	3	23	0
Nut-Thins Pecan	16	130	4	23	0
Bran-A-Crisp					
Low Carb Wheat Bran	1	20	0	6	tr
Breton					
Cabaret	3 (5 g)	70	4	9	1
Garden Vegetable	3	60	3	8	1
Multi Grain	3	70	4	8	2
Original	3	60	3	8	2
Reduced Fat & Sodium	3	60	2	9	1
Sesame	3	60	3	7	1
Cheeters					
Low Carb All Flavors	1 pkg (1 oz)	104	8	4	1
Cheetos					
Cheddar	1 pkg	240	14	25	5
Dare					
Cabaret	3	70	4	9	1
Doritos					
Jalapeno Cheese	1 pkg	230	13	26	5
Nacho Cheesier	1 pkg	240	14	25	6

FOOD	PORTION	CALS	FAT	CARB	SUGAR
Dr. Kracker					
Flatbread Klassic 100% Whole Wheat 3 Seed	1	90	5	9	0
Flatbread Klassic Seed	1	100	4	11	tr
Flatbread Pumpkin Seed	1	100	4	10	0
Flatbread Seeded Spelt	1	110	5	10	0
Flatbread Seedlander	1	100	4	13	2
Flatbread Spelt Sunflower Cheese	1	100	5	11	0
Kribbons Krispy Graham	5	120	3	20	6
Kribbons Muesli	5	120	5	15	0
Foods Alive					
Golden Flax Maple & Cinnamon	5	150	8	12	4
Golden Flax Mexican Harvest	5	150	8	10	tr
Golden Flax Onion Garlic	5	140	7	11	1
Golden Flax Organic Hemp	5	130	6	12	tr
Golden Flax Regular	5	150	9	11	0
Gamesa					
Sabrisas	11	150	2	20	2
Heavenly					
All Flavors Cholesterol Free Sugar Free	1	16	4	3	0
Kashi					
TLC Country Cheddar	15 (1 oz)	130	3	21	1
TLC Honey Sesame	15 (1 oz)	130	3	22	5
TLC Natural Ranch	15 (1 oz)	130	3	22	3
TLC Original 7 Grain	15 (1 oz)	130	3	22	3
Keebler					
Sandwich Cracker Wheat & Cheddar	1 pkg	200	10	23	5

FOOD	PORTION	CALS	FAT	CARB	SUGAR
Kitchen Table Bakers					
Aged Parmesan	3	80	6	tr	0
Caraway Cheese	3	80	5	2	0
Sesame Cheese	3	80	5	2	0
Nature's Path					
Signature Tamari Flax	15	110	3	18	1
No-Carb Kitchen					
Cheese	1	25	3	0	0
Old London					
Mediterranean Toast	3	60	2	9	1
Pepperidge Farm					
Giant Goldfish Wheat	14	140	5	21	3
Goldfish Cheddar	55	140	5	20	tr
Goldfish Colors On The Go	1 pkg	170	7	24	1
Goldfish Original	55	140	6	20	tr
Goldfish Pretzel	43	130	3	24	tr
Goldfish w/ Whole Grain	55	140	5	19	tr
Peter Pan					
Peanut Butter Cheese	1 pkg	210	10	23	3
Peanut Butter Toast	1 pkg	210	11	23	3
Premium					
Saltine Fat Free	5	60	0	12	0
Saltine Unsalted Tops	5	60	2	11	0
Ritz					
Reduced Fat	5	70	2	11	1
Rykrisp					
Seasoned	2	60	2	10	0
SnackWell's					
Cracked Pepper	5	60	2	10	1
South Beach Diet					
Whole Wheat	1 pkg (0.8 oz)	100	4	16	2

FOOD	PORTION	CALS	FAT	CARB	SUGAR
Wasa					
Crispbread Fiber Rye	1 (0.4 oz)	30	1	7	0
Wheat Thins					
Harvest Crisps Five-Grain	13	140	4	23	4
Wheatsworth					
Crackers	5	80	4	10	1
Wisecrackers					
Low Fat Roasted Garlic	10	110	2	20	3
CRANBERRIES					
dried organic	⅓ cup	120	1	29	26
fresh chopped	1 cup	54	tr	14	–
Frieda's					
Dried	⅓ cup (1.4 oz)	110	1	28	26
Good Sense					
Cranberries 'N More	¼ cup	170	10	15	3
Dried Sweetened	½ cup	130	0	31	28
Jok'n'Al					
Cranberry Sauce	1 tbsp	8	0	2	1
Ocean Spray					
Craisins	⅓ cup	130	0	33	31
Cranberry Sauce Jellied	¼ cup	110	0	27	26
Cranorange	¼ cup	120	0	30	29
Whole Berry Sauce	¼ cup	110	0	28	27
Steel's					
Spiced Cranberry Sauce	⅓ cup	20	0	5	4
CRANBERRY JUICE					
Keto					
Kooler	½ tsp	0	0	0	0
Langers					
Cocktail	8 oz	140	0	35	32
Diet	8 oz	30	0	9	9
White	8 oz	120	0	28	28

FOOD	PORTION	CALS	FAT	CARB	SUGAR
Northland					
100% Juice	8 oz	130	0	33	29
Ocean Spray					
Cocktail	8 oz	140	0	34	34
Cocktail Reduced Calorie	8 oz	50	0	13	13
Cocktail Light Low Calorie	8 oz	40	0	10	10
Cranberry Drink	8 oz	130	0	32	32
Cranberry Spritzer	8 oz	160	0	41	40
Crantastic	8 oz	100	0	32	32
White Cranberry	8 oz	120	0	29	29
White Cranberry Peach	8 oz	120	0	30	30
White Cranberry Strawberry	8 oz	120	0	31	31
CRAYFISH					
cooked	3 oz	97	1	0	0
raw	8	24	tr	0	0
raw	3 oz	76	1	0	0
CREAM					
clotted cream	2 tbsp (1 oz)	164	18	1	—
creme fraiche	2 tbsp (1 oz)	100	11	1	—
half & half	1 tbsp (0.5 oz)	20	2	1	—
heavy whipping	1 tbsp (0.5 oz)	52	6	tr	—
heavy whipping whipped	1 cup (4.1 oz)	411	44	7	—
light coffee	1 tbsp (0.5 oz)	29	3	1	—
light whipping	1 tbsp (0.5 oz)	44	5	tr	—
Cabot					
Whipped	2 tbsp	30	2	2	1
Coffee-Mate					
Half & Half Fat Free	2 tbsp	20	0	3	2
Hood					
Half & Half	2 tbsp	40	4	1	1
Light	1 tbsp	30	3	tr	tr

FOOD	PORTION	CALS	FAT	CARB	SUGAR
Simply Smart Fat Free Half & Half	2 tbsp	15	0	2	2
Whipping Cream	1 tbsp	45	5	tr	1

CREAM CHEESE

cream cheese	1 oz	99	10	1	–
Philadelphia					
1/3 Less Fat	1 oz	70	6	tr	tr
Fat Free	1 oz	30	0	2	1

CREAM CHEESE SUBSTITUTE
WholeSoy & Co.

Soy Cream Cheese Organic Original & Flavored	2 tbsp	70	6	3	tr

CREAM OF TARTAR

cream of tartar	1 tsp	8	0	2	–

CREPES

basic crepe unfilled	1 (7 in)	112	6	11	2
Frieda's					
Ready-To-Use	1 (0.5 oz)	30	1	5	2

CROCODILE

cooked	3 oz	78	1	0	0

CROISSANT

plain	1 (2 oz)	232	12	26	–
plain	1 mini (1 oz)	115	6	13	–

CROUTONS
Cardini's

Italian	2 tbsp	30	2	4	0
Pepperidge Farm					
Whole Grain Caesar	6	35	1	5	1
Whole Grain Seasoned	6	30	1	5	tr

FOOD	PORTION	CALS	FAT	CARB	SUGAR
Rothbury Farms					
Seasoned	2 tbsp	30	1	5	0
CUCUMBER					
fresh raw sliced	½ cup (1.8 oz)	7	tr	1	
Frieda's					
Japanese	⅔ cup	10	0	2	1
Seedless Hothouse	⅔ cup	110	0	2	1
TAKE-OUT					
kimchee	½ cup (1.8 oz)	36	2	4	3
tzatziki	½ cup (3.4 oz)	72	6	4	3
CUMIN					
seed	1 tsp	8	tr	1	–
CURRANTS					
Sun-Maid					
Zante	¼ cup	130	0	31	29
CURRY					
curry powder	1 tsp	7	tr	1	tr
A Taste Of Thai					
Curry Paste Green	1 tsp	15	2	1	0
Curry Paste Panang	1 tsp	25	2	2	1
Curry Paste Red	1 tsp	20	2	1	0
Curry Paste Yellow	1 tsp	30	3	1	0
CUSK					
fillet baked	3 oz	106	1	0	0
CUSTARD					
READY-TO-EAT					
Kozy Shack					
Flan	1 pkg (4 oz)	145	4	25	23
TAKE-OUT					
baked	½ cup (5 oz)	148	7	15	–
flan	½ cup (5.4 oz)	220	6	35	–

FOOD	PORTION	CALS	FAT	CARB	SUGAR
flan de calabaza	1 piece (3.5 oz)	225	10	30	22
tocino del cielo heaven's delight	1 cup	856	21	156	154
zabaione	½ cup (57.2 g)	135	5	13	–

DANDELION GREENS

fresh cooked	½ cup	17	tr	3	–
Frieda's					
Dandelion Greens	2 cups	40	0	8	2

DANISH PASTRY
TAKE-OUT

cheese	1 (4¼ in) (2.5 oz)	266	16	26	–
cinnamon	1 (4¼ in) (2.3 oz)	262	15	29	–

DATES

jujube dried	1 oz	75	tr	19	–
jujube preserved in sugar	1 oz	91	tr	22	–
medjool	2-3 (1.4 oz)	120	0	31	25
Frieda's					
Medjool	2 to 3 (1.4 oz)	120	0	31	29
SunDate					
Fancy Medjool	3	120	0	31	25
Sunsweet					
California Pitted	5 to 6 (1.5 oz)	120	0	31	27

DELI MEATS/COLD CUTS

beerwurst beef	2 oz	155	13	2	0
berliner pork & beef	1 slice (0.8 oz)	53	4	1	1
blood sausage	1 slice (0.9 oz)	95	9	tr	tr
bologna beef	1 slice (1 oz)	88	8	1	0
bologna beef low fat	1 slice (1 oz)	57	4	1	0

FOOD	PORTION	CALS	FAT	CARB	SUGAR
bologna beef reduced sodium	1 slice (1 oz)	88	8	1	0
bologna beef & pork	1 slice (1 oz)	87	7	2	1
bologna beef & pork low fat	1 slice (1 oz)	64	5	1	0
braunschweiger pork	1 slice (1 oz)	92	8	1	0
dutch brand loaf pork & beef	1 slice (1.3 oz)	104	9	1	0
headcheese pork	1 slice (1.6 oz)	71	5	0	0
honey loaf pork & beef	1 slice (1 oz)	35	1	1	0
lebanon bologna beef	2 slices (1 oz)	105	6	tr	0
mortadella beef & pork	1 slice (0.5 oz)	47	4	tr	0
olive loaf pork	2 slice (2 oz)	134	9	5	0
pastrami beef	1 slice (1 oz)	41	2	tr	tr
peppered loaf pork & beef	1 slice (1 oz)	41	2	1	0
pepperoni pork & beef	15 slices (1 oz)	135	12	1	tr
salami cooked beef & pork	1 slice (0.8 oz)	58	5	1	0
salami hard pork	3 slices (0.9 oz)	14	8	1	0
salami hard pork & beef less sodium	1 slice (1 oz)	113	9	2	2
sandwich spread pork & beef	¼ cup	141	10	7	0
summer sausage thuringer cervilat	2 oz	203	17	2	tr
Hebrew National					
Bologna Beef	1 slice (1 oz)	80	8	0	0
Salami Beef	3 slices (2 oz)	150	13	0	0
DILL					
seed	1 tsp	6	tr	1	–
weed dry	1 tsp	3	tr	1	–

FOOD	PORTION	CALS	FAT	CARB	SUGAR
DINNER					
Banquet					
Turkey Meal	1 meal (9.25 oz)	290	13	28	6
Boston Market					
Glazed Rotisserie Chicken w/ Mashed Potatoes Gravy Vegetables	1 pkg (16 oz)	390	15	34	6
Meatloaf w/ Mashed Potatoes & Gravy	1 pkg (16 oz)	880	55	55	7
Golden Cuisine					
Beef Stew	1 pkg	350	10	32	7
Boneless Pork Patty	1 pkg	504	25	44	25
Breaded Baked Fish w/ Rice Pilaf	1 pkg	300	5	48	6
Chicken Cacciatore	1 pkg	417	10	56	4
Chicken & Noodles	1 pkg	331	8	39	10
Chicken Parmesan	1 pkg	430	19	47	7
Chicken w/ Marinara Sauce	1 pkg	329	8	37	13
Meatloaf Patty & Gravy	1 pkg	340	14	33	9
Mesquite Chicken	1 pkg	320	5	50	18
Pot Roast w/ Gravy	1 pkg	343	11	36	6
Salisbury Steak & Mushroom Sauce	1 pkg	350	10	47	5
Swedish Meatballs	1 pkg	440	26	32	5
Turkey Tetrazzini	1 pkg	304	6	29	5
Healthy Choice					
Beef Merlot	1 pkg	240	8	25	6
Beef Pot Roast	1 pkg	320	9	39	24
Beef Stroganoff	1 pkg	320	9	39	14
Beef Teriyaki	1 pkg	310	7	44	17
Beef Tips Portabello	1 pkg	280	8	28	16

FOOD	PORTION	CALS	FAT	CARB	SUGAR
Blackened Chicken	1 pkg	300	6	36	15
Boneless Beef Ribs w/ Classic BBQ Sauce	1 pkg	360	9	47	18
Charbroiled Beef Patty	1 pkg	310	9	37	9
Cheesy Rice & Chicken	1 pkg	250	5	27	7
Chicken Breast & Vegetables	1 pkg	260	7	30	4
Chicken Broccoli Alfredo	1 pkg	300	7	34	5
Chicken Carbonara	1 pkg	290	7	32	4
Chicken Margherita	1 pkg	340	8	42	11
Chicken Parmigiana	1 pkg	320	9	40	10
Chicken Piccata	1 pkg	260	5	36	5
Chicken Teriyaki	1 pkg	270	6	37	14
Chicken Tuscany	1 pkg	340	9	39	4
Country Breaded Chicken	1 pkg	370	9	55	23
Country Glazed Chicken	1 pkg	230	5	28	3
Country Herb Chicken	1 pkg	280	6	37	19
Creamy Herb Roasted Chicken	1 pkg	240	5	29	7
Grilled Basil Chicken	1 pkg	330	9	37	4
Grilled Chicken Breast & Pasta	1 pkg	250	7	25	6
Grilled Chicken Breast w/ Mashed Potatoes	1 pkg	190	5	19	0
Grilled Chicken Caesar	1 pkg	300	8	33	3
Grilled Chicken Marinara	1 pkg	270	5	35	8
Grilled Steak w/ Roasted Garlic Sauce	1 pkg	220	7	22	8
Grilled Turkey Breast	1 pkg	250	5	31	19
Grilled Whiskey Steak	1 pkg	280	6	38	18
Herb Baked Fish	1 pkg	360	9	51	12
Homestyle Chicken & Pasta	1 pkg	250	6	28	6

FOOD	PORTION	CALS	FAT	CARB	SUGAR
Honey Glazed Chicken	1 pkg	320	6	46	8
Lemon Pepper Fish	1 pkg	280	5	46	17
Mandarin Chicken	1 pkg	250	4	36	10
Mesquite Chicken BBQ	1 pkg	300	5	44	14
Mixed Grills Chicken Honey BBQ w/ Dipping Sauce	1 pkg	380	7	53	20
Mixed Grills Chicken Honey Mustard w/ Dipping Sauce	1 pkg	360	7	49	15
Mixed Grills Chicken Teriyaki w/ Dipping Sauce	1 pkg	340	7	48	21
Mixed Grills Chicken Tomato Garlic w/ Dipping Sauce	1 pkg	370	7	50	12
Mixed Grills Steak BBQ Sauce	1 pkg	420	8	59	24
Mixed Grills Steak Teriyaki w/ Dipping Sauce	1 pkg	350	9	39	23
Mixed Grills Steak w/ Zesty Steak Sauce	1 pkg	350	8	44	16
Oriental Style Beef	1 pkg	310	9	33	4
Oriental Style Chicken	1 pkg	240	5	28	5
Oven Roasted Beef	1 pkg	280	7	33	7
Princess Chicken	1 pkg	310	7	41	5
Roast Turkey Breast	1 pkg	220	6	23	1
Roasted Chicken Breast	1 pkg	280	8	32	8
Roasted Chicken Chardonnay	1 pkg	290	8	32	2
Salisbury Steak	1 pkg	360	9	45	19
Salisbury Steak w/ Red Skin Mashed Potatoes	1 pkg	200	6	20	5
Sesame Chicken	1 pkg	260	6	34	9

FOOD	PORTION	CALS	FAT	CARB	SUGAR
Slow Roasted Turkey Breast w/ Mashed Potatoes	1 pkg	210	7	17	1
Sweet & Sour Chicken	1 pkg	340	7	54	21
Traditional Meatloaf	1 pkg	300	9	36	17
Traditional Turkey Breast	1 pkg	330	5	50	26
Tuna Casserole	1 pkg	270	7	31	4
Kid Cuisine					
All American Fried Chicken	1 meal	500	21	48	14
All Star Chicken Breast Nuggets	1 meal	460	19	50	7
Bug Safari Chicken Breast Nuggets	1 meal	450	16	58	14
Carnival Corn Dog	1 meal	430	12	68	20
Deep Sea Adventure Fish Sticks	1 meal	400	12	56	16
Fiesta Beef Taco Dippers	1 meal	370	16	44	11
Pop Star Popcorn Chicken	1 meal	410	10	67	22
Laura's Lifestyle					
Carb Conscious Chicken Puttanesca	1 pkg (9 oz)	270	10	7	0
Carb Conscious Chicken Chow Mein	1 pkg (9 oz)	260	8	9	2
Carb Conscious Chicken Santa Fe	1 pkg (9 oz)	280	9	9	1
Carb Conscious Thai Chicken	1 pkg (9 oz)	280	8	11	2
Lean Cuisine					
Cafe Classics Baked Chicken Florentine	1 pkg (8 oz)	200	8	14	5
Cafe Classics Baked Lemon Pepper Fish	1 pkg (9 oz)	220	6	20	5

FOOD	PORTION	CALS	FAT	CARB	SUGAR
Cafe Classics Beef Peppercorn	1 pkg (8.75 oz)	220	7	25	8
Cafe Classics Beef Portabello	1 pkg (9 oz)	200	5	25	6
Cafe Classics Beef Pot Roast	1 pkg (9 oz)	190	6	23	4
Cafe Classics Bowl Creamy Basil Chicken	1 pkg (10.5 oz)	310	9	39	7
Cafe Classics Bowl Grilled Chicken Caesar	1 pkg (9 oz)	270	7	32	2
Cafe Classics Chicken & Vegetables	1 pkg (10.5 oz)	240	5	29	5
Cafe Classics Chicken Carbonara	1 pkg (9 oz)	280	7	33	5
Cafe Classics Chicken L'Orange	1 pkg (9 oz)	230	2	35	10
Cafe Classics Chicken Marsala	1 pkg (8.1 oz)	140	4	12	4
Cafe Classics Chicken Parmesan	1 pkg (10.9 oz)	280	5	36	9
Cafe Classics Chicken Tuscan	1 pkg (12 oz)	300	7	35	6
Cafe Classics Chicken w/ Almonds	1 pkg (8.5 oz)	260	4	38	12
Cafe Classics Chicken w/ Basil Cream Sauce	1 pkg (8.5 oz)	270	7	32	5
Cafe Classics Fiesta Grilled Chicken	1 pkg (9.5 oz)	250	6	31	6
Cafe Classics Garlic Beef & Broccoli	1 pkg (9 oz)	170	6	16	6
Cafe Classics Glazed Chicken	1 pkg (8.5 oz)	220	4	27	6

FOOD	PORTION	CALS	FAT	CARB	SUGAR
Cafe Classics Glazed Turkey Tenderloins	1 pkg (9 oz)	260	5	40	20
Cafe Classics Grilled Chicken	1 pkg (9.4 oz)	160	5	15	4
Cafe Classics Grilled Chicken w/ Teriyaki Glaze	1 pkg (10 oz)	270	3	42	11
Cafe Classics Herb Roasted Chicken	1 pkg (8 oz)	190	4	23	6
Cafe Classics Honey Dijon Grilled Chicken	1 pkg (8 oz)	220	4	22	10
Cafe Classics Honey Mustard Chicken	1 pkg (8 oz)	250	4	37	11
Cafe Classics Honey Roasted Pork	1 serv (9.5 oz)	230	9	18	8
Cafe Classics Lemon Garlic Shrimp	1 pkg (12 oz)	280	7	38	3
Cafe Classics Mandarin Chicken	1 pkg (9 oz)	270	4	46	11
Cafe Classics Meatloaf w/ Gravy & Whipped Potatoes	1 pkg (9.4 oz)	280	9	29	5
Cafe Classics Orange Peel Chicken	1 pkg (12 oz)	390	9	63	15
Cafe Classics Oven Roasted Beef	1 pkg (9.25 oz)	210	8	18	9
Cafe Classics Roasted Garlic Chicken	1 pkg (8.8 oz)	200	8	14	4
Cafe Classics Roasted Turkey & Vegetables	1 pkg (8 oz)	150	5	12	4
Cafe Classics Roasted Turkey Breast	1 pkg (12 oz)	280	6	39	9

FOOD	PORTION	CALS	FAT	CARB	SUGAR
Cafe Classics Roasted Turkey Breast w/ Dressing	1 pkg (9.75 oz)	270	2	51	30
Cafe Classics Salisbury Steak	1 pkg (12.5 oz)	310	8	34	9
Cafe Classics Salisbury Steak w/ Mac & Cheese	1 pkg (9.5 oz)	280	8	26	4
Cafe Classics Sesame Chicken	1 pkg (9 oz)	330	8	49	13
Cafe Classics Southern Beef Tips	1 pkg (8.75 oz)	250	5	36	11
Cafe Classics Steak Tips Portabello	1 pkg (7.5 oz)	180	7	13	4
Cafe Classics Steak Tips Dijon	1 pkg (12 oz)	320	8	44	12
Cafe Classics Stuffed Cabbage	1 pkg (9.5 oz)	200	6	26	5
Cafe Classics Swedish Meatballs	1 pkg (9.1 oz)	290	8	33	5
Cafe Classics Sweet & Sour Chicken	1 pkg (10 oz)	290	3	52	20
Cafe Classics Three Cheese Chicken	1 pkg (8 oz)	230	10	14	5
Comfort Classics Baked Chicken	1 pkg (8.6 oz)	230	5	32	5
Dinnertime Selects Balsamic Glazed Chicken	1 pkg (12 oz)	400	8	61	28
Dinnertime Selects Chicken Florentine	1 pkg (13.25 oz)	420	8	59	13
Dinnertime Selects Chicken Portabello	1 pkg (12 oz)	370	6	58	26
Skillets Beef Teriyaki & Rice	1 serv	190	3	32	10

FOOD	PORTION	CALS	FAT	CARB	SUGAR
Spa Cuisine Chicken Mediterranean	1 pkg (10.5 oz)	240	4	35	7
Spa Cuisine Chicken In Peanut Sauce	1 pkg (9 oz)	280	7	32	6
Spa Cuisine Chicken Pecan	1 pkg (9 oz)	260	6	34	5
Spa Cuisine Lemon Chicken	1 pkg (9 oz)	290	7	45	8
Spa Cuisine Lemongrass Chicken	1 pkg (9.4 oz)	240	6	29	4
Spa Cuisine Pork w/ Cherry Sauce	1 pkg (8.25 oz)	260	5	38	12
Spa Cuisine Rosemary Chicken	1 pkg (8.25 oz)	230	5	29	1
Spa Cuisine Salmon w/ Beef	1 pkg (9.5 oz)	360	8	31	4
Pacific Foods					
Beef Steak Stew	1 cup	250	7	29	5
Chicken Stew	1 cup	200	5	25	3
Quorn					
Meat Free Simply Saute Indian	½ pkg	240	4	47	3
Meat Free Simply Saute Mexican	½ pkg	340	7	61	5
Meat Free Simply Saute Thai	½ pkg	240	9	34	12
Savvy Faire					
Baja Jack Scramble	1 pkg (8.2 oz)	370	25	12	2
Braised Beef	1 pkg (9.4 oz)	320	18	15	4
Herb Crusted Chicken	1 pkg (9.7 oz)	430	21	34	4
South Beach Diet					
Beef & Broccoli & Asian Style Noodles	1 pkg	320	13	32	8

FOOD	PORTION	CALS	FAT	CARB	SUGAR
Caprese Style Chicken w/ Cauliflower & Broccoli	1 pkg	250	8	12	6
Cashew Chicken w/ Sugar Snap Peas	1 pkg	360	13	31	7
Garlic Herb Chicken w/ Green Beans	1 pkg	250	12	13	3
Mediterranean Style Chicken w/ Couscous	1 pkg	330	12	26	5
Savory Beef w/ Cheesy Broccoli	1 pkg	240	8	16	7
Savory Pork w/ Pecans & Green Beans	1 pkg	260	13	13	5
Swanson					
Turkey Breast & Stuffing Dinner	1 pkg (11.7 oz)	350	11	43	18
Tamarind Tree					
Alu Chole	1 pkg (9.25 oz)	320	7	57	6
Channa Dal Masala	1 pkg (9.25 oz)	290	3	55	6
Dal Makhani	1 pkg (9.25 oz)	350	6	63	6
Navratan Korma	1 pkg (9.25 oz)	370	15	55	10
Palak Paneer	1 pkg (9.25 oz)	350	17	43	6
Saag Chole	1 pkg (9.25 oz)	330	9	53	5
Vegetable Jalfrazi	1 pkg (9.25 oz)	280	7	50	6
DIP					
Cabot					
Bac'n Horseradish	2 tbsp	50	5	1	tr
Clam	2 tbsp	50	5	1	0
French Onion	2 tbsp	50	5	1	1
Ranch	1 tbsp	50	5	1	1
Salsa Grande	2 tbsp	50	5	1	1
Veggie	2 tbsp	50	5	2	1
Fritos					
Bean	2 tbsp	40	1	5	0

FOOD	PORTION	CALS	FAT	CARB	SUGAR
Chili Cheese	2 tbsp	45	3	3	1
Hot Bean	2 tbsp	40	1	56	0
Jalapeno Cheddar Cheese	2 tbsp	50	4	4	2
Mild Cheddar	2 tbsp	60	4	3	tr
Gringo Billy's					
Guacamole Mix	1 tsp	10	0	2	0
Guiltless Gourmet					
Black Bean Mild	2 tbsp	30	0	5	1
Black Bean Spicy	2 tbsp	30	0	5	0
Marzetti					
Veggie Fat Free Ranch	2 tbsp	35	7	6	2
Veggie Dip Light Veggie	1 pkg (3.25 oz)	170	17	3	2
Phillips Seafood					
Crab & Spinach	2 tbsp	50	5	1	0
Maryland Crab	2 tbsp	70	6	1	0
Racquet					
Hot Cheddar Jalapeno	2 tbsp	30	3	1	0
Ruffles					
French Onion	¼ cup	200	15	9	6
Ranch	2 tbsp	60	5	1	0
Walden Farms					
Low Carb Bruschetta	2 tbsp	35	3	0	1
Low Carb Pesto Bruschetta	1 tsp	10	1	9	9

DOUGHNUTS
Entenmann's

FOOD	PORTION	CALS	FAT	CARB	SUGAR
Crumb	1	260	12	36	21
Frosted Devil's Food	1	310	19	36	25
Frosted Mini	1 (1 oz)	150	11	12	7
Glazed	1	260	13	34	20
Plain Old Fashion	1	230	14	25	10
Rich Chocolate Frosted	1	280	18	29	16
Snack & Smile					
Mini Donuts Chocolate	6	370	19	45	23

FOOD	PORTION	CALS	FAT	CARB	SUGAR
Mini Donuts Glazed	6	340	16	46	28
Mini Donuts Powdered Sugar	6	320	13	46	22
Super Bakery					
Daily Donut	1 (2.2 oz)	250	14	26	11
Proballs Slam Powdered Baseballs	1 (1.3 oz)	130	6	17	6

DRINK MIXERS
Baja Bob's

FOOD	PORTION	CALS	FAT	CARB	SUGAR
Bloody Mary Mix Lean & Mean	4 oz	20	0	4	3
Pina Colada	4 oz	30	1	4	3
Sugar Free Margarita Mix	4 oz	10	0	tr	0
Sugar Free Margarita Mix Desert Lime	4 oz	10	0	tr	0
Sugar Free Margarita Mix Wild Strawberry	4 oz	10	0	tr	0
Sweet-n-Sour Mix	4 oz	10	0	tr	0

Ocean Spray

FOOD	PORTION	CALS	FAT	CARB	SUGAR
Bloody Mary Mix	4 oz	40	0	10	4
Margarita Mix	4 oz	160	0	40	28
Sour Mix	4 oz	140	0	34	34

DRUM

FOOD	PORTION	CALS	FAT	CARB	SUGAR
freshwater fillet baked	5.4 oz	236	10	0	0
freshwater baked	3 oz	130	5	0	0

DUCK

FOOD	PORTION	CALS	FAT	CARB	SUGAR
w/ skin roasted	1 cup (4.9 oz)	472	40	0	0
w/ skin w/ bone leg roasted	3 oz	184	10	0	0
w/ skin w/o bone breast roasted	3 oz	172	9	0	0
w/o skin roasted	1 cup (4.9 oz)	281	16	0	0

FOOD	PORTION	CALS	FAT	CARB	SUGAR
w/o skin w/ bone leg braised	1 cup (6.1 oz)	310	10	0	0
w/o skin w/o bone breast broiled	1 cup (6.1 oz)	244	4	0	0
wild w/ skin raw	½ duck (9.5 oz)	571	41	0	0
wild w/o skin breast raw	½ breast (2.9 oz)	102	4	0	0
Maple Leaf Farms					
Breast Filet	4 oz	360	33	0	0
Leg Quarters	4 oz	420	33	0	0
Orange Breast Filet	4 oz	320	28	1	1

DUMPLING
TAKE-OUT

FOOD	PORTION	CALS	FAT	CARB	SUGAR
bread dumpling	1 lg	330	10	28	–

EEL

FOOD	PORTION	CALS	FAT	CARB	SUGAR
fresh cooked	3 oz	200	13	0	0
smoked	3.5 oz	330	28	0	0

EGG
CHICKEN

FOOD	PORTION	CALS	FAT	CARB	SUGAR
hard or soft cooked	1	77	5	1	1
pickled	1	72	5	1	1
poached	1	73	5	tr	tr
scrambled plain	2	199	15	2	–
sunny side up	2	155	12	1	1
white cooked	1	17	tr	tr	tr
yolk cooked	1	55	4	1	tr
Egg-Land's Best					
Organic Brown	1	70	4	0	0
Sunny Fresh					
Eggs ASAP!	2	140	10	1	1
OTHER POULTRY					
duck 100 year old	1 (1 oz)	49	3	1	–

FOOD	PORTION	CALS	FAT	CARB	SUGAR
duck cooked	1 (2.5 oz)	129	10	1	1
duck preserved hard core	1 (1.8 oz)	80	6	1	0
duck preserved soft core	1 (1.8 oz)	80	6	1	0
duck salted	1 (1 oz)	54	4	2	–
goose cooked	1 (5 oz)	265	19	2	1
quail canned	1 (0.3 oz)	14	1	tr	tr
turkey raw	1 (2.8 oz)	135	9	1	–

EGG DISHES
TAKE-OUT

FOOD	PORTION	CALS	FAT	CARB	SUGAR
deviled	1 half	62	5	tr	tr
eggs benedict	2	825	64	26	3
omelet cheese	3 eggs	387	29	6	6
omelet mushroom	3 eggs	251	17	6	4
omelet mushroom & onion	3 eggs	294	20	7	5
omelet plain	3 eggs	338	25	4	4
omelet spanish	3 eggs	496	38	17	11
omelet spinach	3 eggs	279	19	6	4
omelet western	3 eggs	355	23	6	4
salad	½ cup	353	34	2	1
tortilla de amarillo omelet w/ plantain	3 eggs	536	35	43	21

EGG ROLLS
Frieda's

FOOD	PORTION	CALS	FAT	CARB	SUGAR
Egg Roll Wrappers	2 (1.6 oz)	130	1	28	1

Lean Cuisine

FOOD	PORTION	CALS	FAT	CARB	SUGAR
Cafe Classics Vegetable	1 pkg (9 oz)	310	5	60	17

Loompya

FOOD	PORTION	CALS	FAT	CARB	SUGAR
Lumpia Chicken & Vegetables	2	170	1	31	1

Nasoya

FOOD	PORTION	CALS	FAT	CARB	SUGAR
Egg Roll Wrapper	3	170	1	35	1

FOOD	PORTION	CALS	FAT	CARB	SUGAR
Pagoda					
Sweet & Sour Chicken	1 (2.7 oz)	170	6	25	5
Phillips					
Spring Rolls Crab & Shrimp w/ Sauce	3 (3.75 oz)	220	7	33	8
TAKE-OUT					
chicken	1 (3 oz)	140	4	20	5
lobster	1 (4.8 oz)	270	7	43	4
meat & shrimp	1 (4.8 oz)	320	12	41	3
pork & shrimp	1 (5 oz)	300	10	41	6
shrimp	1 (3 oz)	170	5	24	5
spicy pork	1 (3 oz)	200	9	23	3
vegetable	1 (3 oz)	170	4	28	4
EGG SUBSTITUTES					
Deb-El					
Just Whites	2 tsp	12	0	0	0
Egg Beaters					
Original	¼ cup	30	0	1	tr
Quick Eggs					
Fat Free Cholesterol Free	¼ cup	30	0	1	1
EGGNOG					
Hood					
Fat Free Sugar Free	1 cup	110	0	18	12
Golden	½ cup	180	9	22	20
Light	½ cup	140	4	22	21
TAKE-OUT					
eggnog	1 cup	306	22	16	—
EGGPLANT					
cubed cooked w/ oil	1 cup	133	8	17	6
pickled	½ cup	33	tr	7	3
slices grilled	1 (2 oz)	36	2	5	2

FOOD	PORTION	CALS	FAT	CARB	SUGAR
Frieda's					
Chinese	⅔ cup (3 oz)	20	0	5	3
Japanese Nasu	⅔ cup (3 oz)	20	0	3	2
TAKE-OUT					
baba ghannouj	¼ cup	55	4	5	–
caponata	2 tbsp (1 oz)	30	2	3	2
iman bayildi eggplant w/ onion & tomato	1 serv (15.6 oz)	345	28	25	6
indian eggplant runi	1 serv	180	14	13	1
papoutsakis little shoes	1 serv (15.5 oz)	245	16	15	1
ELDERBERRIES					
fresh	1 cup	105	1	27	–
ELK					
roasted	4 oz	215	4	0	0
ENERGY BARS					
All In One					
All Flavors	1 bar (1.8 oz)	180	5	20	1
Hooah!					
Chocolate Crisp	1 bar (2.29 oz)	280	9	40	18
LaraBar					
Apple Pie	1	190	9	23	16
Banana Cookie	1	210	10	24	19
Cashew Cookie	1	230	13	23	13
Cherry Pie	1	190	9	24	17
Chocolate Coconut Chew	1	220	12	24	18
Cocoa Mule	1	200	9	26	21
Ginger Snap	1	220	13	22	18
Luna					
Key Lime Pie	1 bar (1.7 oz)	180	4	29	15
Nature's Path					
Optimum Blueberry Flax & Soy	1 bar (2 oz)	200	3	37	20

FOOD	PORTION	CALS	FAT	CARB	SUGAR
Optimum Cranberry Ginger & Soy	1 bar (2 oz)	200	3	37	21
Optimum Peanut Butter	1 bar (2 oz)	230	8	33	14
Optimum ReBound	1 bar (2 oz)	190	4	33	20
Nutiva					
Organic Flax & Raisin	1	200	15	15	8
Original Organic Hempseed	1	210	14	11	5
PowerBar					
Harvest Apple Cinnamon Crisp	1 bar (2.3 oz)	240	4	45	18
Harvest Chunky Cherry Crunch	1 bar (2.3 oz)	240	4	45	18
Harvest Peanut Butter Chocolate Chip	1 bar (2.3 oz)	240	4	44	18
Harvest Strawberry Crunch	1 bar (2.3 oz)	230	4	45	18
Harvest Dipped Double Chocolate Crisp	1 bar (2.3 oz)	250	5	45	20
Harvest Dipped Oatmeal Raisin Cookie	1 bar (2.3 oz)	250	5	45	20
Harvest Dipped Toffee Chocolate Chip	1 bar (2.3 oz)	250	5	45	18
Performance Apple Cinnamon	1 bar (2.3 oz)	230	3	45	20
Performance Banana	1 bar (2.3 oz)	230	3	45	20
Performance Cappuccino	1 bar (2.3 oz)	230	2	45	18
Performance Chocolate	1 bar (2.3 oz)	230	2	45	18
Performance Chocolate Peanut Butter	1 bar (2.3 oz)	240	3	45	20
Performance Cookies & Cream	1 bar (2.3 oz)	240	4	45	20
Performance Malt Nut	1 bar (2.3 oz)	230	3	45	18

FOOD	PORTION	CALS	FAT	CARB	SUGAR
Performance Oatmeal Raisin	1 bar (2.3 oz)	230	3	45	20
Performance Peanut Butter	1 bar (2.3 oz)	230	4	45	16
Performance Strawberry Cream	1 bar (2.3 oz)	230	2	45	20
Performance Vanilla Crisp	1 bar (2.3 oz)	230	3	45	20
Performance Wild Berry	1 bar (2.3 oz)	230	3	45	18
Protein Plus Carb Select Chocolate	1 bar (2.5 oz)	260	7	30	1
Protein Plus Carb Select Chocolate Caramel Crunch	1 bar (2.6 oz)	270	11	32	1
Protein Plus Carb Select Chocolate Peanut Butter	1 bar (2.5 oz)	270	9	30	1
Protein Plus Carb Select Peanut Caramel	1 bar (2.6 oz)	270	11	32	1
Protein Plus Chocolate Fudge Brownie	1 bar (2.7 oz)	270	5	36	19
Protein Plus Chocolate Peanut Butter	1 bar (2.7 oz)	290	5	38	21
Protein Plus Cookies & Cream	1 bar (2.7 oz)	290	5	38	18
Protein Plus Vanilla Yogurt	1 bar (2.7 oz)	290	5	37	19
Triple Treat Caramel Peanut Crisp	1 bar (1.9 oz)	220	5	32	14
Triple Treat Caramel Peanut Fusion	1 bar (1.9 oz)	230	8	30	15
Triple Treat Chocolate Caramel Fusion	1 bar (1.9 oz)	230	8	30	15
Triple Treat Chocolate Peanut Butter Crisp	1 bar (1.9 oz)	220	5	32	14

FOOD	PORTION	CALS	FAT	CARB	SUGAR
Pria					
Carb Select Caramel Nut Brownie	1 bar (1.7 oz)	170	8	21	1
Carb Select Chocolate Mocha Crisp	1 bar (1.7 oz)	130	6	16	1
Carb Select Chocolate Peanut Butter Crisp	1 bar (1.7 oz)	130	6	16	1
Carb Select Cookies N' Caramel	1 bar (1.7 oz)	170	7	22	13
Carb Select Peanut Butter Caramel Nut	1 bar (1.7 oz)	170	8	21	1
Chocolate Peanut Crunch	1 bar (1 oz)	110	4	16	10
Complete Nutrition Chocolate Mint Crisp	1 bar (1.6 oz)	170	6	22	7
Complete Nutrition Chocolate Peanut Butter Crisp	1 bar (1.6 oz)	170	6	22	7
Complete Nutrition French Vanilla Crisp	1 bar (1.6 oz)	170	5	22	8
Creme Carmel Crisp	1 bar (1 oz)	110	3	17	10
Double Chocolate Cookie	1 bar (1 oz)	110	3	16	10
French Vanilla Crisp	1 bar (1 oz)	110	3	17	9
Mint Chocolate Cookie	1 bar (1 oz)	110	4	15	9
Strawberry Shortcake	1 bar (1 oz)	110	3	16	10
Slim-Fast					
Classic Meal Bar Chocolate Cookie Dough	1 bar	220	5	36	20
Classic Meal Bar Milk Chocolate Peanut	1 bar	220	5	37	24
High Protein Granola Bar Chocolate Chip	1 bar	190	6	20	9
High Protein Granola Bar Peanut	1 bar	200	7	21	8

FOOD	PORTION	CALS	FAT	CARB	SUGAR
Low Carb Breakfast Bar Apple Cobbler	1 bar	180	6	19	1
Low Carb Breakfast Bar Peanut Butter	1 bar	190	8	17	tr
Low Carb Snack Bar Caramel Nut	1 bar	120	5	19	1
Low Carb Snack Bar Coconut Almond	1 bar	120	5	15	tr
Low Carb Snack Bar Peanut Butter Crunch	1 bar	120	5	21	1
Optima Meal Bar Apple Crisp	1 bar	180	3	29	12
Optima Meal Bar Caramel Crispy Peanut	1 bar	220	6	33	15
Optima Meal Bar Chewy Granola Trail Mix	1 bar	210	5	34	16
Optima Snack Bar Banana Nut Muffin	1 bar	150	8	18	6
Optima Snack Bar Blueberry Muffin	1 bar	140	57	22	9
Optima Snack Bar Chocolate Peanut Nougat	1 bar	120	4	20	9
Optima Snack Bar Oatmeal Raisin Cookie	1 bar	120	4	19	8
Snickers Marathon					
Energy Chewy Chocolate Peanut	1 (1.9 oz)	220	7	26	18
Energy Multi Grain Crunch	1 (1.9 oz)	220	7	30	18
For Women Double Chocolate Nut	1 (2.8 oz)	150	4	23	10
For Women Honey Nut Oat	1 (2.8 oz)	150	4	24	12

FOOD	PORTION	CALS	FAT	CARB	SUGAR
Low Carb Chocolate Fudge Nut	1 (1.8 oz)	170	8	20	1
Low Carb Peanut Butter	1 (1.8 oz)	170	6	19	1
Protein Caramel Nut Surge	1 (2.8 oz)	290	8	41	23
Protein Chocolate Nut Burst	1 (2.8 oz)	290	7	36	15
Solo GI					
Berry Bliss	1 bar (1.6 oz)	190	5	23	16
Chocolate Charger	1 bar (1.6 oz)	190	6	24	16
Mint Mania	1 bar (1.6 oz)	190	6	24	16
Peanut Power	1 bar (1.6 oz)	200	7	22	14
South Beach Diet					
Chocolate Crisp	1 bar	210	6	26	0
Chocolate Peanut Butter	1 bar	210	8	26	tr
Cinnamon Creme	1 bar	220	7	26	tr
T.H.E. Bar					
Granola Raisin	1 (1.8 oz)	200	6	25	10

ENERGY DRINKS

Accelerade					
All Flavors	8 oz	80	0	16	16
Banzai					
Energy Drink	8 oz	120	0	30	27
Beaver Buzz					
Citrus	1 can	140	0	36	28
Bliss					
Energy Drink	1 can (8.4 oz)	110	0	27	26
Low Carb	1 can (8.4 oz)	26	0	5	4
Blu Fuel					
Energy Drink	1 can (10 oz)	133	0	33	33
BooKoo					
Energy Drink	8 oz	110	0	27	27
Shot All Flavors	1 can (5.57 oz)	80	0	19	19

FOOD	PORTION	CALS	FAT	CARB	SUGAR
Zero Carb	8 oz	0	0	0	0
Boost					
High Protein Vanilla	8 oz	240	6	33	16
Bossa Nova					
Acai Juice Mango	1 bottle (10 oz)	132	0	33	29
Acai Juice Original	1 bottle (10 oz)	138	1	34	29
Acai Juice Passion Fruit	1 bottle (10 oz)	132	1	33	29
Cascabel					
Energy Drink	1 can (8.4 oz)	110	0	28	27
Sugar Free	1 can (8.4 oz)	10	0	1	0
Cheetah					
Energy Drink	1 can (12 oz)	80	0	20	18
Cytomax					
Sport Drinks All Flavors	1 bottle (20 oz)	130	0	33	6
Defcon3					
Healthy Energy Soda	1 can (12 oz)	45	0	11	9
Defense					
Effervescent Supplement	1 can	150	0	39	36
Double Hit					
Maximum Energy Coffee Drink Sugar Free	1 can (12 oz)	0	0	0	0
Energy 69					
Energy Drink	1 can	110	0	28	28
Sugar Free	1 can	0	0	0	0
Everlast					
High Energy Citrus Blast	1 can (8.3 oz)	140	0	36	35
Full Throttle					
Energy Drink	8 oz	100	0	29	28
Fury	8 oz	110	0	29	29
Gatorade					
All Flavors	1 cup (8 oz)	50	0	14	14
Lemonade All Flavors	8 oz	50	0	14	14
Rain All Flavors	8 oz	50	0	14	14

FOOD	PORTION	CALS	FAT	CARB	SUGAR
Go Fast					
Energy Drink	1 can (8.4 oz)	90	0	23	21
Light	1 can (8.4 oz)	20	0	1	0
Sportsman's	1 can (8.4 oz)	90	0	23	21
Guaraviton					
Energy Drink	8 oz	98	0	20	19
Guru					
Energy Drink	1 can (8.3 oz)	100	0	25	22
Lite	1 can (8.3 oz)	5	0	1	1
Happy Bunny					
Spaz Juice	1 can (8.4 oz)	110	0	28	27
Her Energy					
Pink Lemonade	1 can (8.4 oz)	130	0	32	31
Pink Lemonade Sugar Free	1 can (8.4 oz)	0	0	0	0
Hiball					
All Flavors	1 bottle (10 oz)	10	0	0	0
Iron Energy					
All Flavors	8 oz	90	0	23	23
Jet Set					
Club Soda	1 can (12 oz)	0	0	0	0
Ginger Ale	1 can (12 oz)	150	0	37	36
Original	1 can (12 oz)	105	0	29	29
Tonic Water	1 can (12 oz)	150	0	37	36
Kabbalah					
Original	1 can (12 oz)	174	0	44	44
Sugar Free	1 can (12 oz)	<3	0	1	0
Krank'd					
All Flavors	1 bottle (16 oz)	80	0	18	13
Lost					
Big Gun	6 oz	100	–	26	26
Five-O	8 oz	70	–	16	16
Perfect 10	8 oz	10	–	3	3

FOOD	PORTION	CALS	FAT	CARB	SUGAR
Monster					
Energy Assault	8 oz	100	–	26	26
Energy Drink	8 oz	100	–	26	26
Khaos Energy Juice	8 oz	90	–	21	21
Lo Carb	8 oz	10	–	3	2
Nexcite					
Herbal Fizz	1 bottle	72	0	17	17
NOS					
High Performance	8 oz	110	0	28	27
Orange County Choppers					
High Octane Fuel	1 can (8.4 oz)	110	0	28	27
Pimp Juice					
Energy Drink	1 can (8 oz)	140	0	35	34
Tight	1 can (8 oz)	140	0	35	34
Powerade					
Arctic Shatter	8 oz	64	0	17	15
Flava 23	8 oz	63	0	17	15
Fruit Punch	8 oz	65	0	17	15
Green Squall	8 oz	64	0	17	15
Jagged Ice	8 oz	65	0	17	15
NASCAR Grape	8 oz	64	0	17	15
Olympic Citrus	8 oz	63	0	17	15
Option All Flavors	8 oz	10	0	2	2
PowerBar					
Endurance Sport Drink	1 pkg (0.6 oz)	70	0	17	9
Performance Recovery Drink	1 pkg (0.8 oz)	90	0	20	10
Rawlings EX2					
Sustained Energy	1 can (8.4 oz)	132	0	32	27
Red Eye					
Classic	1 bottle (12 oz)	208	0	50	49
Extreme	1 bottle (12 oz)	140	0	37	36
Gold	1 bottle (12 oz)	208	0	49	49

FOOD	PORTION	CALS	FAT	CARB	SUGAR
Passion	1 bottle (12 oz)	149	0	37	36
Platinum	1 bottle (12 oz)	149	0	37	36
Rip It					
Citrus X	8 oz	130	0	33	33
Citrus X Sugar Free	8 oz	0	0	0	0
Energy Fuel	8 oz	130	0	32	32
Energy Lite	8 oz	0	0	0	0
Rockstar					
Energy Cola	8 oz	120	0	30	29
Energy Drink	8 oz	110	0	29	27
Juiced	8 oz	90	0	22	21
Rox					
Energy Drink	1 can	110	0	28	27
Zero	1 can	10	0	1	0
Slim-Fast					
Classic Ready-To-Drink Creamy Milk Chocolate	1 can	220	3	40	34
Classic Ready-To-Drink French Vanilla	1 can	220	3	40	35
High Protein Ready-To-Drink All Flavors	1 can	190	5	23	13
Low Carb Diet Ready-To-Drink All Flavors	1 can	190	9	6	1
Snapple A Day					
Meal Replacement All Flavors	1 bottle (11.5 oz)	210	0	43	36
SoBe					
Lean Diet Citrus	8 oz	5	0	1	0
Source Burn					
2	8 oz	130	0	31	30
Energy Drink	8 oz	140	0	36	28
Sugar Free	8 oz	10	0	0	0

FOOD	PORTION	CALS	FAT	CARB	SUGAR
Speed Zone					
Energy Drink	1 can (8.4 oz)	110	0	28	28
Stewie's					
Domination Serum	1 can (8.45 oz)	110	0	28	27
Mind Erase Elixir	1 can (8.45 oz)	100	0	28	27
Stinger					
All Flavors	1 can (8.4 oz)	130	0	34	32
Sugar Free All Flavors	1 can (8.4 oz)	0	0	0	0
Swing Juice					
Energy Drink	8 oz	60	0	15	15
Tab					
Energy Drink	1 can (10.5 oz)	5	0	0	0
The Beast					
Energy Drink	1 can (8.3 oz)	120	0	28	28
Tornado					
Energy Drink	8 oz	110	0	30	27
Vault					
Enegry Drink	8 oz	120	0	32	32
Zero	8 oz	0	0	0	0
Wide Open Performance					
Energy Drink	1 can (8.3 oz)	120	0	27	27
Xcyto					
Sugar Free	1 can (12.5 oz)	10	0	2	0
Xtazy					
All Flavors	1 can	160	0	40	40
ENGLISH MUFFIN					
READY-TO-EAT					
Food For Life					
7 Sprouted Grains	1	160	2	32	0
Ezekiel 4:9 Cinnamon Raisin	1	160	0	36	10
Ezekiel 4:9 Sprouted Grain	1	160	1	30	0

FOOD	PORTION	CALS	FAT	CARB	SUGAR
Genesis 1:29 Original	1	180	4	30	0
Pepperidge Farm					
100% Whole Wheat	1	140	2	26	4
7 Grain	1	130	2	23	2
Sara Lee					
Heart Healthy Wheat w/ Honey	1	140	1	28	3
Original w/ Whole Grain	1	140	1	27	2
Thomas'					
Blueberry	1	140	1	29	5
Carb Consider	1	100	2	23	0
Hearty Grains 100% Whole Wheat	1	120	1	23	2
Hearty Grains Honey Wheat	1	130	1	27	3
Original	1	120	1	25	1
Raisin Bran	1	150	2	30	7
Raisin Cinnamon	1	140	1	30	8
Sourdough	1	120	1	25	2
Super Size	1	190	2	38	2
TAKE-OUT					
w/ butter	1 (2.2 oz)	189	6	30	—
FALAFEL					
Near East					
Falafel as prep	2½ patties	230	16	18	3
TAKE-OUT					
falafel	1 (1.2 oz)	57	3	5	—
FAT					
bacon grease	1 tbsp	116	13	0	0
beef shortening	1 tbsp	115	13	0	0
beef suet	1 oz	242	27	0	0
chicken	1 tbsp	115	13	0	0

FOOD	PORTION	CALS	FAT	CARB	SUGAR
duck	1 tbsp (13 g)	115	13	0	0
goose	1 tbsp	115	13	0	0
lard	1 tbsp (13 g)	115	13	0	0
meat pan drippings	½ tbsp	124	14	0	0
pork backfat	1 oz	230	25	0	0
salt pork	1 oz	212	23	0	0
shortening	1 tbsp	113	13	0	0
turkey	1 tbsp	115	13	0	0
Spectrum					
Organic Shortening	1 tbsp	110	13	0	0
FEIJOA					
fresh	1 (1.75 oz)	25	tr	5	—
FENNEL					
fresh bulb	1 (8.2 oz)	72	tr	17	—
fresh sliced	1 cup	27	tr	6	—
leaves	1 oz	7	tr	1	—
seed	1 tsp	7	tr	1	—
FENUGREEK					
seed	1 tsp	12	tr	2	—
FIBER					
apple fiber	0.5 oz	40	1	15	0
Choice					
Fiber Burst Lemon Lime	3 pieces	45	1	12	0
Fiber Burst Tropical Fruit	3 pieces	45	1	11	0
Metamucil					
Natural Fiber Regular Flavor	1 rounded tsp (7 g)	25	0	6	3
FIGS					
dried california	½ cup (3.5 oz)	200	1	58	—
fresh	1 med	50	tr	10	—

FOOD	PORTION	CALS	FAT	CARB	SUGAR
Jenny					
Sundried Kalamata	4	120	0	28	21
Trucco					
Kalamata	2	100	0	26	22
FIREWEED					
leaves chopped	1 cup (0.8 oz)	24	1	4	–
FISH					
CANNED					
Beach Cliff					
Fish Steaks In Louisiana Hot Sauce	1 can (3.7 oz)	160	7	2	0
Fish Steaks In Mustard Sauce	1 can (3.7 oz)	160	9	2	0
Fish Steaks In Soybean Oil	1 can (3.7 oz)	200	13	1	0
Fish Steaks w/ Hot Green Chilies	1 can (3.7 oz)	160	10	1	0
Fish Steaks w/ Jalapeno Peppers	1 can (3.7 oz)	130	14	1	0
Brunswick					
Fish Steaks In Louisiana Hot Sauce	1 can (3.7 oz)	160	7	2	0
Fish Steaks In Mustard Sauce	1 can (3.7 oz)	160	9	2	0
Fish Steaks In Soybean Oil	1 can (3.7 oz)	200	13	1	0
Fish Steaks In Spring Water	1 can (3.7 oz)	150	8	0	0
Fish Steaks w/ Hot Tabasco Peppers	1 can (3.7 oz)	220	14	1	0
Seafood Snacks Golden Smoked	1 can (3.2 oz)	170	11	0	0
Seafood Snacks In Lemon & Cracked Pepper	1 can (3.2 oz)	160	10	0	0

FOOD	PORTION	CALS	FAT	CARB	SUGAR
Seafood Snacks In Louisiana Hot Sauce	1 can (3.2 oz)	140	8	2	0
Seafood Snacks In Teriyaki Sauce	1 can (3.2 oz)	160	8	5	4
Seafood Snacks In Tomato & Basil Sauce	1 can (3.2 oz)	140	8	2	1
Seafood Snacks Kippered	1 can (3.2 oz)	160	9	0	0
Chicken Of The Sea					
Fish Steaks	½ can (2 oz)	70	3	1	1
FROZEN					
Gorton's					
Grilled Garlic Butter	1 piece (3.8 oz)	100	3	1	0
TAKE-OUT					
fish cake	1 (4.7 oz)	166	7	6	—
jamaican brown fish stew	1 serv	426	22	9	—
kedgeree	5.6 oz	242	11	15	—
mousse	1 serv (3.5 oz)	185	14	3	tr
stew	1 cup (7.9 oz)	157	4	10	—
taramasalata	2 tbsp	124	14	1	—
FISH OIL					
cod liver	1 tbsp	123	14	0	0
herring	1 tbsp	123	14	0	0
menhaden	1 tbsp	123	14	0	0
salmon	1 tbsp	123	14	0	0
sardine	1 tbsp	123	14	0	0
shark	1 oz	270	29	0	0
whale	1 oz	270	29	0	0
Cormega					
Omega-E Orange	1 pkg	20	2	0	0
Spectrum					
Cod Liver Oil w/ Lemon	1 tsp	40	5	0	0

FOOD	PORTION	CALS	FAT	CARB	SUGAR
FISH PASTE					
fish paste	2 tsp	15	1	tr	—
FLAXSEED					
Arrowhead					
Organic Flax Seeds	¼ cup	140	9	10	0
Bob's Red Mill					
Flax Seed Meal	2 tbsp	60	5	4	0
Cracker Flax					
Organic Apple Raisin	1 oz	130	5	16	4
Hodgson Mill					
Milled	2 tbsp	60	1	4	0
FLOUNDER					
FRESH					
cooked	3 oz	99	1	0	0
TAKE-OUT					
stuffed w/ crab	1 piece (7.6 oz)	332	11	14	2
FLOUR					
buckwheat whole groat	1 cup	402	4	85	3
potato	1 cup (6.3 oz)	628	1	143	—
white all-purpose	1 cup (4.4 oz)	455	1	95	—
white bread	1 cup (4.8 oz)	495	2	99	—
white cake unsifted	1 cup (4.8 oz)	496	1	107	—
white self-rising	1 cup (4.4 oz)	443	1	93	—
whole wheat	1 cup (4.2 oz)	407	2	87	—
Arrowhead					
Whole Grain Oat	⅓ cup	120	3	18	0
Bob's Red Mill					
Flour	⅓ cup	130	6	11	0
Heckers					
All Purpose Unbleached	¼ cup	100	0	22	tr
Whole Wheat	¼ cup	100	1	21	0

FOOD	PORTION	CALS	FAT	CARB	SUGAR
King Arthur					
All Purpose Unbleached	¼ cup	100	0	22	tr
FOOD COLORS					
blue	1 tsp	0	0	0	0
orange	1 tsp	0	0	0	0
red	1 tsp	tr	0	tr	0
yellow	1 tsp	tr	0	0	0
FRENCH TOAST					
TAKE-OUT					
plain	1 slice	151	7	16	–
w/ butter	2 slices	356	19	36	–
FROG LEGS					
TAKE-OUT					
as prep w/ seasoned flour & fried	1 (0.8)	70	5	15	–
FRUCTOSE					
Estee					
Fructose	1 tsp	15	0	4	4
Packet	1 pkg	10	0	3	3
FRUIT DRINKS					
READY-TO-DRINK					
Bolthouse Farms					
Berry Blast	8 oz	110	0	30	26
Green Goodness	8 oz	140	0	33	27
Passion Fruit Apple Carrot Juice	8 oz	120	0	29	28
Firefly					
Chill Out De-stress Drink	1 bottle (11.2 oz)	100	0	24	24
De-tox Morning After Drink	1 bottle (11.2 oz)	104	0	25	25

FOOD	PORTION	CALS	FAT	CARB	SUGAR
Five Alive					
Citrus	8 oz	120	0	30	28
Hawaiian Punch					
Bodacious Berry	8 oz	110	0	29	28
Fruit Juicy Red	8 oz	120	0	29	30
Green Berry Rush	8 oz	120	0	30	29
Mazin Melon Mix	8 oz	110	0	29	28
Tropical Vibe	8 oz	110	0	29	28
Wild Purple Smash	8 oz	110	0	29	28
Hi-C					
Blast Berry Blue	1 bottle	170	0	46	44
Blast Fruit Pow	1 bottle	180	0	46	45
Blast Wild Berry	1 pkg	100	0	26	25
Flashin' Fruit Punch	1 box	90	0	25	25
Shoutin' Orange Tangergreen	1 box	90	0	25	25
Strawberry Kiwi Kraze	1 box	100	0	27	26
Hog Wash					
All Flavors	1 bottle (10 oz)	37	0	10	8
Hood					
Fruit Punch	1 cup	120	0	30	28
Juici					
Sparkling All Flavors	1 bottle (12 oz)	105	0	28	28
Kool-Aid					
Jammers 10 All Flavors	1 pouch (6.75 oz)	10	0	2	2
Minute Maid					
Berry Kiwi	1 can (12 oz)	160	0	43	42
Cranberry Grape	8 oz	150	0	39	38
Light Guava Citrus	8 oz	5	0	2	tr
Light Mango Tropical	8 oz	5	0	2	tr
Light Orange Tangerine	8 oz	15	0	4	2
Orange Passion	8 oz	130	0	31	29

FOOD	PORTION	CALS	FAT	CARB	SUGAR
Orange Tangerine	8 oz	110	0	27	24
Tropical Punch Chilled	8 oz	110	0	30	29
Naked Juice					
Berry Blast	8 oz	120	0	30	26
Blue Machine	8 oz	170	1	41	30
Green Machine	8 oz	130	0	33	27
Mango Acai	8 oz	190	3	38	29
Power C	8 oz	120	1	29	23
Protein Zone	8 oz	210	4	27	25
Red Machine	8 oz	160	3	32	25
Strawberry Banana C	8 oz	120	0	28	23
Very Berry	8 oz	130	0	30	24
Very Pro Berry	8 oz	190	1	30	24
Well Being	8 oz	140	0	32	30
Northland					
Cranberry Blueberry	1 cup (8 oz)	140	0	34	30
Snapple					
Cranberry Raspberry	8 oz	120	0	29	27
Diet Carrot Apple	8 oz	10	0	3	1
Diet Plum-A-Granate	8 oz	0	0	0	0
Go Bananas	8 oz	120	0	30	26
Kiwi Strawberry	8 oz	110	0	28	26
Snapricot Orange	8 oz	120	0	30	28
TreeTop					
Apple Grape No Sugar Added	8 oz	130	0	32	26
Tropicana					
Just 10 Fruit Punch	1 pouch (6.75 oz)	10	0	3	2
Twister Orange Strawberry Banana Burst	8 oz	130	0	31	28
Wadda Juice					
All Flavors	8 oz	50	0	14	13

FOOD	PORTION	CALS	FAT	CARB	SUGAR
FRUIT MIXED					
CANNED					
Del Monte					
Carb Clever Fruit Cocktail	½ cup	40	0	11	10
Fruit Cocktail In 100% Juice	½ cup	60	0	15	14
Fruit Cocktail In Extra Light Syrup	½ cup	60	0	15	14
Fruit Cocktail In Heavy Syrup	½ cup	100	0	24	23
Fruit Naturals Tropical Medley	½ cup	70	0	18	16
Orchard Select Premium Mixed	½ cup	80	0	20	18
Snack Cups Strawberry Banana Peaches	1 pkg	70	0	17	16
SunFresh Citrus Salad	½ cup	80	0	20	17
Liberty Gold					
Fruit Cocktail In Heavy Syrup	½ cup	90	0	23	22
DRIED					
Goodniks					
Fruit Medley	¼ cup	110	2	24	20
FRUIT SNACKS					
fruit leather rolls	1 sm (0.5 oz)	49	tr	12	–
Betty Crocker					
Fruit By The Foot All Flavors	1 roll	80	2	17	10
Welch's					
White Grape Peach	20 pieces	110	0	24	21
GARLIC					
clove	1	4	tr	1	tr

FOOD	PORTION	CALS	FAT	CARB	SUGAR
fresh chopped	1 tbsp	18	tr	4	tr
powder	1 tsp	9	tr	2	1
Frieda's					
Elephant	1 tbsp	5	0	1	0
Vinegar Marinated	1 oz	30	0	7	0
McCormick					
Garlic Salt	¼ tsp	0	0	0	0

GEFILTE FISH

sweet	1 piece (1.5 oz)	35	1	3	–
Mrs. Adler's					
Pike'n Whitefish	1 piece (1.8 oz)	50	1	4	1

GELATIN
READY-TO-EAT
Del Monte

Mandarin Orange In Lite Orange Gel	1 pkg (4.5 oz)	60	0	14	12
Mixed Fruit In Cherry Gel	1 pkg (4.5 oz)	90	0	23	20
Peaches In Lite Strawberry Banana Gel	1 pkg (4.5 oz)	60	0	14	13
Peaches In Peach Gel	1 pkg (4.5 oz)	90	0	22	21
Peaches In Raspberry Gel	1 pkg (4.5 oz)	90	0	23	20
Hunt's					
Snack Pack Juicy Gels Raspberry Mixed Berry	1 serv (3.5 oz)	100	0	24	22
Snack Pack Juicy Gels Strawberry	1 serv (3.5 oz)	100	0	24	22
Snack Pack Juicy Gels Strawberry Orange	1 serv (3.5 oz)	100	0	24	22
Snack Pack Tropical Punch	1 serv (3.5 oz)	100	0	24	22
Jell-O					
Sugar Free Tropical Berry	1 serv (3.2 oz)	10	0	0	0

FOOD	PORTION	CALS	FAT	CARB	SUGAR
Kozy Shack					
Gel Treats Cherry	1 pkg (4 oz)	85	0	22	21
Gel Treats Lemon Lime	1 pkg (4 oz)	85	0	22	21
Gel Treats Orange	1 pkg (4 oz)	85	0	22	21
Gel Treats Strawberry	1 pkg (4 oz)	85	0	22	21
Gel Treats Sugar Free Orange	1 pkg (4 oz)	11	0	2	1
Gel Treats Sugar Free Strawberry	1 pkg (4 oz)	11	0	2	1
GIBLETS					
capon simmered	1 cup (5 oz)	238	8	0	0
chicken floured & fried	1 cup (5 oz)	402	19	6	—
chicken simmered	1 cup (5 oz)	228	7	1	—
turkey simmered	1 cup (5 oz)	243	7	3	—
GINGER					
ground	1 tsp	6	tr	1	tr
pickled	0.5 oz	5	0	1	—
root fresh	5 slices	9	tr	2	tr
root fresh sliced	¼ cup	19	tr	4	tr
Frieda's					
Crystallized	9 pieces (1.1 oz)	100	0	26	11
Galanga Thai Ginger	⅔ cup	60	1	13	0
GINSENG					
dried	1 oz	90	tr	20	—
fresh	1 oz	28	tr	6	—
GIZZARDS					
chicken simmered	1 cup (5 oz)	222	5	2	—
turkey simmered	1 cup (5 oz)	236	6	1	—
GNOCCHI					
Bellino					
W/ Potato	1 cup	240	1	55	2

FOOD	PORTION	CALS	FAT	CARB	SUGAR
GOAT					
roasted	3 oz	122	3	0	0
GOOSE					
w/ skin roasted	6.6 oz	574	41	0	0
w/ skin roasted	½ goose (1.7 lbs)	2362	170	0	0
w/o skin roasted	5 oz	340	18	0	0
w/o skin roasted	½ goose (1.3 lbs)	1406	75	0	0
GOOSEBERRIES					
fresh	1 cup	67	1	15	–
GRAPEFRUIT					
CANNED					
Del Monte					
Fruit Naturals Red	½ cup	60	0	16	13
SunFresh Red	½ cup	80	0	19	9
SunFresh White In Real Fruit Juice	½ cup	45	0	9	8
FRESH					
pink	½	37	tr	9	–
red	½	37	tr	9	–
white	½	39	tr	10	–
Sunkist					
Fresh	½ med	60	0	16	10
Oroblanco	½	100	1	22	17
GRAPEFRUIT JUICE					
Langers					
Diet Ruby Red	8 oz	40	0	9	9
Ruby Red	8 oz	130	0	33	30
Minute Maid					
Frozen + Calcium	8 oz	100	0	25	20
Ruby Red	8 oz	130	0	34	32

FOOD	PORTION	CALS	FAT	CARB	SUGAR
Ocean Spray					
100% Juice Pink	8 oz	110	0	28	28
100% White Juice	8 oz	100	0	24	24
Ruby Drink	8 oz	120	0	30	30
Ruby Red Drink	8 oz	130	0	33	33
Odwalla					
Juice	8 fl oz	90	0	20	16
Tao Tea					
Grapefruit Lemon Fusion	8 oz	72	0	18	14
GRAPE JUICE					
Ceres					
Hanepoot White Grape	8 oz	130	0	33	30
Hansen's					
White Grape 100% Juice	1 box (4.23 oz)	90	0	22	21
Keto					
Kooler	½ tsp	0	0	0	0
Langers					
Cocktail	8 oz	160	0	40	36
Nantucket Nectars					
Organic Concord Grape	8 oz	130	0	33	32
Welch's					
100% Juice	8 oz	170	0	42	40
100% White	8 oz	160	0	39	37
Light White Grape	8 oz	70	0	18	17
GRAPE LEAVES					
canned	1 (4 g)	3	tr	tr	—
TAKE-OUT					
dolmas	5 (4.2 oz)	200	11	23	3
GRAPES					
fresh	10	36	tr	9	—
Frieda's					
Champagne	½ cup (3 oz)	50	0	15	14

FOOD	PORTION	CALS	FAT	CARB	SUGAR
GRAVY					
CANNED					
Heinz					
Home Style Chicken	¼ cup	25	1	4	0
Pacific Foods					
Natural Beef	1 cup	20	0	4	0
Natural Turkey	¼ cup	25	1	4	0
MIX					
Bournvita					
Extract	2 heaping tsp	34	1	7	—
Bovril					
Extract	1 heaping tsp	9	0	tr	—
Marmite					
Extract	1 heaping tsp	9	0	tr	—
GREAT NORTHERN BEANS					
dried cooked	1 cup	209	1	37	—
GREEN BEANS					
CANNED					
Del Monte					
Cut	½ cup	20	0	4	2
Cut Italian	½ cup	30	0	6	2
Cut w/ Potatoes & Ham Flavor	½ cup	30	0	6	1
French Style	½ cup	20	0	4	2
Savory Sides Green Bean Casserole	½ cup	70	3	11	3
Whole	½ cup	20	0	4	2
FRESH					
raw	½ cup	17	tr	4	—
raw whole beans	10	17	tr	4	—
GreenLine					
Fresh Trimmed	3 oz	25	0	5	3

FOOD	PORTION	CALS	FAT	CARB	SUGAR
FROZEN					
Pictsweet					
Cut	⅔ cup	30	0	5	2
GREENS					
Ready Pac					
Microwave Leafy Greens as prep	½ cup	15	0	2	1
GROUPER					
cooked	1 fillet (7.1 oz)	238	3	0	0
GUAR GUM					
Bob's Red Mill					
Guar Gum	1 tbsp	20	0	6	0
GUAVA					
fresh	1	45	1	11	–
guava sauce	½ cup	43	tr	11	–
Frieda's					
Fresh	1 (3 oz)	45	1	10	5
GUAVA JUICE					
Ceres					
Guava	8 oz	120	0	29	29
GUINEA HEN					
w/ skin raw	½ hen (12.1 oz)	545	22	0	0
w/o skin raw	½ hen (9.3 oz)	292	7	0	0
HADDOCK					
fresh broiled	4 oz	127	1	0	0
smoked	1 oz	33	tr	0	0
TAKE-OUT					
breaded & fried	4 oz	229	10	10	1

FOOD	PORTION	CALS	FAT	CARB	SUGAR
HALIBUT					
atlantic & pacific cooked	3 oz	119	2	0	0
greenland baked	3 oz	203	15	0	0
HAM					
boneless extra lean roasted	3 oz	123	5	1	0
boneless roasted	3 oz	151	8	0	0
deviled	¼ cup	188	17	1	0
ham salad spread	2 tbsp	65	5	3	0
patty grilled	1 patty (2 oz)	205	19	1	0
prosciutto	4 slices (1.3 oz)	72	3	tr	0
sliced	3 slices (2.9 oz)	137	7	3	0
sliced extra lean	3 slices (2.2 oz)	69	2	2	0
westphalian smoked	1 oz	105	10	0	0
whole roasted	3 oz	207	14	0	0
Oscar Mayer					
Brown Sugar	3 slices (1.8 oz)	60	2	3	3
Lunchables Ham Bagels	1 pkg	410	10	64	27
Lunchables Ham Wraps	1 pkg	430	13	64	25
Smoked	3 slices (2.2 oz)	60	1	0	0
TAKE-OUT					
croquette	1 (2.2 oz)	149	9	8	2
thick slice fried	1 (2.2 oz)	140	9	tr	0
HAMBURGER					
Kid Cuisine					
Cheeseburger Builder	1 meal	390	11	58	11
Lean Pockets					
Cheeseburger	1 (4.5 oz)	280	7	42	11
TAKE-OUT					
cheeseburger + condiments	1 reg (4.5 oz)	347	17	28	5

FOOD	PORTION	CALS	FAT	CARB	SUGAR
double hamburger + condiments	1 reg (5.8 oz)	384	19	30	7
single patty + condiments	1 reg (4 oz)	299	11	35	8

HAMBURGER SUBSTITUTES
Boca Burgers
Flamed Grilled	1	90	4	5	0

Dr. Praeger's
California Burger	1 (2.7 oz)	100	3	10	0

Lightlife
Light Burgers	1 (3 oz)	120	2	11	0
Smart Menu Burger	1	80	1	14	1

Morningstar Farms
Garden Veggie Patties	1 patty (2.4 oz)	100	3	9	1
Harvest Burger	1	140	4	8	tr

HAZELNUTS
dry roasted	1 oz	188	19	5	–

Low Carb Creations
Soft Hazelnut Brittle	2 pieces (1 oz)	160	12	16	1

Torras
Hazelnut Chocolate Spread	1 tsp	27	2	3	0

Twist
Sugar Free Chocolate Hazelnut Spread	2 tbsp	180	14	2	0

HEART
beef simmered	3 oz	140	4	tr	0
chicken simmered	1 cup (5 oz)	268	11	tr	–
lamb braised	3 oz	158	7	2	–
pork braised	1 cup	215	7	1	–
pork braised	1	191	7	1	–
turkey simmered	1 cup (5 oz)	257	9	3	–
veal braised	3 oz	158	6	tr	–

FOOD	PORTION	CALS	FAT	CARB	SUGAR
HEARTS OF PALM					
Del Monte					
Hearts Of Palm	2–3 pieces	20	0	3	0
HEMP					
Nutiva					
Organic Protein Powder	2 scoops (1 oz)	120	3	14	0
Shelled Hempseed	2 tbsp	110	8	2	tr
HERBS/SPICES					
chinese five spice	1 tsp	7	tr	2	–
garam masala	1 tsp	8	tr	1	–
poultry seasoning	1 tsp	5	tr	1	–
pumpkin pie spice	1 tsp	6	tr	1	–
A Taste Of Thai					
Chicken & Rice Seasoning	¼ pkg (6 g)	15	0	3	3
Cut N Clean					
Greens Seasoning	1½ tsp	20	0	5	2
Gringo Billy's					
Meat Rubs Chipotle	¼ tsp	0	0	0	0
Meat Rubs Montreau	¼ tsp	0	0	0	0
Meat Rubs Ultimate	¼ tsp	0	0	0	0
Tuna Seasoning	1 tsp	5	1	1	0
McCormick					
Blends Bon Appetit	¼ tsp	0	0	0	0
Cajun Seasoning	¼ tsp	0	0	0	0
Greek Seasoning	¼ tsp	0	0	0	0
Jamaican Jerk Seasoning	¼ tsp	0	0	0	0
Seafood Seasoning	¼ tsp	0	0	0	0
Mrs. Dash					
Classic Italian	¼ tsp	0	0	0	0
Extra Spicy	¼ tsp	0	0	0	0
Garlic & Herb	¼ tsp	0	0	0	0
Grilling Blend Mesquite	¼ tsp	0	0	0	0

FOOD	PORTION	CALS	FAT	CARB	SUGAR
Grilling Blend Original Chicken	¼ tsp	0	0	0	0
Grilling Blend Original Steak	¼ tsp	0	0	0	0
Lemon Pepper	¼ tsp	0	0	0	0
Minched Onion Medley	¼ tsp	0	0	0	0
Original Blend	¼ tsp	0	0	0	0
Table Blend	¼ tsp	0	0	0	0
Tomato Basil Garlic	¼ tsp	0	0	0	0
Nueva Cocina					
Picadillo	2 tsp	15	0	3	2
Taco Fresco	2 tsp	15	0	3	1
HERRING					
atlantic baked	4 oz	230	13	0	0
dried salted	1 fillet (1.4 oz)	161	9	0	0
pickled	1 oz	74	5	3	–
pickled in cream sauce	1 oz	72	5	2	tr
roe	1 tbsp	39	2	tr	0
smoked kippered	1 oz	620	4	0	0
Beach Cliff					
Kippered Snacks	1 can (4 oz)	220	16	0	0
TAKE-OUT					
breaded fried	1 serv (4 oz)	225	14	9	1
HICKORY NUTS					
dried	1 oz	187	18	5	–
HOMINY					
CANNED					
white	1 cup (5.6 oz)	482	1	23	–
HONEY					
honey	1 cup (11.9 oz)	1031	0	279	270
honey	1 tbsp (0.7 oz)	64	0	17	17

FOOD	PORTION	CALS	FAT	CARB	SUGAR
orange blossom	1 tbsp	60	0	17	16
wild honey	1 tbsp	60	0	17	16
Frieda's					
Honeycomb	½ cup (3 oz)	260	0	70	70
Steel's					
Sugar Free	1 tbsp	24	0	6	0
SueBee					
Clover	1 tbsp	60	0	17	16
HONEYDEW					
FRESH					
cubed	1 cup	60	tr	16	–
HORSE					
roasted	3 oz	149	5	0	0
HORSERADISH					
wasabi root raw	1 (5.9 oz)	184	1	40	–
wasabi root raw sliced	1 cup (4.6 oz)	142	1	31	–
HOT CHOCOLATE					
Carnation					
Hot Cocoa Rich Chocolate as prep w/ 2% milk	1 pkg	200	8	27	12
Country Choice Naturals					
Irish Chocolate Mint Cocoa	1 pkg	100	0	23	20
Royal Chocolate Cocoa	1 pkg	100	0	23	20
Soy Cocoa Irish Chocolate Mint	1 pkg	100	1	23	17
Soy Cocoa Royal Chocolate	1 pkg	100	1	23	17
Keto					
Hot Cocoa	1 tsp	12	0	2	0

FOOD	PORTION	CALS	FAT	CARB	SUGAR
Low Carb Creations					
Cocoa as prep	1 cup	30	2	3	tr
White Hot Chocolate	1 cup	25	2	3	tr
Sipper Sweets					
Sugar Free Low Carb Mix	1 serv	50	3	3	0
Swiss Miss					
Caramel Cream	1 serv	110	3	21	18
Milk Chocolate	1 pkg	120	3	22	17
Milk Chocolate w/ Marshmallows	1 pkg	120	3	23	17
TAKE-OUT					
hot cocoa	1 cup	218	9	26	—
mexican hot chocolate	1 cup	173	6	20	—
HOT DOG					
beef	1 (1.5 oz)	149	13	2	2
beef & pork	1 (1.5 oz)	137	12	1	0
beef low fat	1 (2 oz)	133	11	1	0
chicken	1 (1.5 oz)	116	9	3	0
fat free	1 (2 oz)	62	1	6	0
low fat	1 (2 oz)	88	6	3	0
low sodium	1 (2 oz)	180	16	1	0
pork and beef cheese smokie	1 (1.5 oz)	141	12	1	1
turkey	1 (1.5 oz)	102	8	1	0
Boar's Head					
Beef Cocktail	5 (2 oz)	170	15	0	0
Healthy Choice					
Beef Low Fat	1 (1.8 oz)	70	3	7	2
Hebrew National					
97% Fat Free Beef	1 (1.7 oz)	45	2	3	0
Beef	1 (1.7 oz)	150	14	1	0
Cocktail Franks	5 (2 oz)	180	16	1	0
Dinner Frank	1 (4 oz)	350	32	1	0

FOOD	PORTION	CALS	FAT	CARB	SUGAR
Franks In A Blanket	5 (2.8 oz)	290	24	8	1
Reduced Fat Beef	1 (1.7 oz)	120	10	0	0
Oscar Mayer					
Corn Dogs	1 (3.2 oz)	260	15	25	9
State Fair					
Corn Dogs	1 (2.67 oz)	180	12	18	8
TAKE-OUT					
corndog	1	460	19	56	—
w/ bun chili	1	297	13	31	—
w/ bun plain	1	242	15	18	—

HOT DOG SUBSTITUTES
Lightlife

FOOD	PORTION	CALS	FAT	CARB	SUGAR
Smart Dogs	1	45	0	2	1
Smart Franks	1 (2 oz)	110	5	5	2
Tofu Pups	1 (1.5 oz)	60	3	2	0
Quorn					
Meat-Free Dogs	1 (1.5 oz)	70	4	3	0

HUMMUS
Athenos

FOOD	PORTION	CALS	FAT	CARB	SUGAR
Black Olive	2 tbsp	50	3	5	tr
Original	2 tbsp	50	3	5	tr
Travelers Hummus & Pita	1 pkg	325	13	48	5
Guiltless Gourmet					
Original	2 tbsp	35	2	4	0
Roasted Garlic	2 tbsp	35	2	4	0
TAKE-OUT					
hummus	⅓ cup	140	7	17	—

HYACINTH BEANS

FOOD	PORTION	CALS	FAT	CARB	SUGAR
dried cooked	1 cup	228	1	40	—

ICE CREAM AND FROZEN DESSERTS

FOOD	PORTION	CALS	FAT	CARB	SUGAR
chocolate	½ cup (4 fl oz)	143	7	19	13
dixie cup chocolate	1 (3.5 fl oz)	125	6	16	11

FOOD	PORTION	CALS	FAT	CARB	SUGAR
dixie cup strawberry	1 (3.5 fl oz)	112	5	16	9
dixie cup vanilla	1 (3.5 fl oz)	116	6	14	9
strawberry	½ cup (4 fl oz)	127	6	18	10
vanilla	½ cup (4 fl oz)	132	7	16	10
Breyers					
Bar Light Creamy Vanilla Chocolate Coated	1	160	8	21	15
Dove					
Beyond Vanilla	½ cup	260	16	25	21
Caramel Pecan Perfection	½ cup	310	18	32	27
Caramel Toffee Crunch	1 bar (2.8 oz)	270	16	29	26
Irresistibly Raspberry	½ cup	240	13	30	21
Milk Chocolate w/ Almonds	1 bar (2.7 oz)	270	18	23	20
Milk Chocolate w/ Vanilla Ice Cream	1 bar (2.7 oz)	260	17	25	22
Original Dove w/ Vanilla Ice Cream	1 bar (2.7 oz)	260	17	26	21
Original Dove Miniatures	5 pieces (3.1 oz)	300	20	32	25
Unconditional Chocolate	½ cup	300	18	31	28
Vanilla w/ A Chocolate Soul	½ cup	300	19	29	24
Edy's					
Carb Benefit Butter Pecan	½ cup	170	12	13	2
Carb Benefit Chocolate	½ cup	150	10	13	2
Carb Benefit Chocolate Chip	½ cup	160	11	14	2
Carb Benefit Mint Chocolate Chip	½ cup	160	11	14	2
Carb Benefit Vanilla Bean	½ cup	140	9	13	2
Dips Chocolate	26 pieces	420	32	28	25
Dips Vanilla	26 pieces	420	32	29	26
Grand Andes Cool Mint	½ cup	170	9	19	16

FOOD	PORTION	CALS	FAT	CARB	SUGAR
Grand Chocolate	½ cup	150	8	17	15
Grand Chocolate Chip	½ cup	160	8	19	16
Grand Chocolate Fudge Mousse	½ cup	160	8	20	15
Grand Coffee	½ cup	140	8	15	13
Grand Cookies 'N Cream	½ cup	160	8	19	14
Grand Dulce De Leche	½ cup	150	7	20	18
Grand French Vanilla	½ cup	160	9	16	11
Grand Ice Cream Sandwich	½ cup	150	7	19	13
Grand Peanut Butter Cup	½ cup	180	10	19	15
Grand Rocky Road	½ cup	170	10	19	14
Grand Toffee Bar Crunch	½ cup	170	9	19	18
Grand Turtle Sundae	½ cup	160	9	18	14
Grand Vanilla	½ cup	140	8	15	13
Slow Churned Light Butter Pecan	½ cup	120	5	16	12
Slow Churned Light Caramel Delight	½ cup	120	4	19	15
Slow Churned Light Chocolate	½ cup	110	4	16	11
Slow Churned Light Chocolate Chip	½ cup	120	5	17	13
Slow Churned Light Chocolate Fudge Chunk	½ cup	120	5	18	13
Slow Churned Light Coffee	½ cup	105	4	15	11
Slow Churned Light Cookie Dough	½ cup	130	5	20	14
Slow Churned Light Cookies 'N Cream	½ cup	120	4	18	13
Slow Churned Light French Silk	½ cup	130	5	20	15

FOOD	PORTION	CALS	FAT	CARB	SUGAR
Slow Churned Light French Vanilla	½ cup	100	4	15	11
Slow Churned Light Fudge Tracks	½ cup	120	5	18	13
Slow Churned Light Mint Chocolate Chips	½ cup	120	5	17	13
Slow Churned Light Mocha Almond Fudge	½ cup	120	5	16	12
Slow Churned Light Neapolitan	½ cup	100	3	15	11
Slow Churned Light Rocky Road	½ cup	120	4	17	12
Slow Churned Light Strawberry	½ cup	110	3	18	13
Slow Churned Light Vanilla	½ cup	100	4	15	11
Slow Churned No Sugar Added Butter Pecan	½ cup	120	5	15	3
Slow Churned No Sugar Added Chocolate	½ cup	95	3	14	4
Slow Churned No Sugar Added Cookie Dough	½ cup	110	4	16	3
Slow Churned No Sugar Added Fat Free Chocolate Fudge	½ cup	100	0	22	4
Slow Churned No Sugar Added Fat Free Raspberry Vanilla Swirl	½ cup	90	0	19	4
Slow Churned No Sugar Added Fat Free Vanilla	½ cup	90	0	20	4
Slow Churned No Sugar Added Fat Free Vanilla Chocolate Swirl	½ cup	100	0	20	4

FOOD	PORTION	CALS	FAT	CARB	SUGAR
Slow Churned No Sugar Added Fudge Tracks	½ cup	110	4	16	3
Slow Churned No Sugar Added Mint Chocolate Chips	½ cup	110	5	15	3
Slow Churned No Sugar Added Neapolitan	½ cup	95	3	14	4
Slow Churned No Sugar Added Triple Chocolate	½ cup	110	4	17	3
Slow Churned No Sugar Added Vanilla	½ cup	90	3	13	4
Healthy Choice					
Bar Sorbet & Cream	1	100	1	20	14
Brownie Bliss	½ cup	130	2	24	18
Butter Pecan Crunch	½ cup	100	2	18	4
Cappuccino Chocolate Chunk	½ cup	120	2	20	16
Caramel Fudge Brownie	½ cup	120	2	21	17
Cherry Chocolate Mambo	½ cup	130	2	23	19
Chocolate Chocolate Chunk	½ cup	120	2	21	17
Cookies 'N Cream	½ cup	120	2	21	16
Crazy Caramel	½ cup	120	2	23	17
Double Karma	½ cup	140	2	28	21
French Silk	½ cup	120	2	24	18
Happy Together	½ cup	150	2	29	21
Jumpin' Java	½ cup	130	2	25	20
Low Fat Bar Fudge	1	890	1	13	2
Low Fat Bar Mocha Fudge	1	90	2	17	14
Low Fat Bar Strawberry & Cream	1	90	2	17	15
Mint Chocolate Chip	½ cup	120	2	20	16

FOOD	PORTION	CALS	FAT	CARB	SUGAR
No Sugar Added Chocolate Fudge Brownie	½ cup	120	2	21	4
No Sugar Added Coffee Almond Fudge	½ cup	110	2	20	3
No Sugar Added Mint Chocolate Chip	½ cup	110	2	18	4
No Sugar Added Vanilla	½ cup	100	2	17	4
Peanut Butter Cup	½ cup	120	2	21	17
Praline & Caramel	½ cup	120	2	23	19
Rocky Road	½ cup	130	2	25	17
Sandwich Caramel	1	140	3	27	17
Sandwich Fudge Swirl	1	140	3	27	16
Sandwich Vanilla	1	130	3	24	14
Turtle Fudge Cake	½ cup	130	2	23	21
Vanilla	½ cup	110	2	19	15
Vanilla Bean	½ cup	120	2	21	16
Vanilla Caramel Fudge	½ cup	140	2	28	21
Hershey's					
French Vanilla	½ cup	170	10	17	16
Hood					
Butterscotch Blast	½ cup	160	7	20	15
Chocolate Eclair	1 bar (2.2 oz)	150	10	14	8
Creamy Coffee	½ cup	140	7	16	12
Fat Free Chocolate Passion	½ cup	100	0	22	14
Fat Free Very Vanilla	½ cup	100	0	23	14
Grasshopper Pie	½ cup	160	7	22	14
Light Butter Pecan	½ cup	140	6	18	11
Light Creamy Vanilla	½ cup	110	3	18	12
Low Fat No Sugar Added Vanilla Dream	½ cup	90	2	20	4
No Sugar Added Chocolate Chip	½ cup	100	3	21	4
Orange Cream	1 bar (2.2 oz)	90	2	19	13

FOOD	PORTION	CALS	FAT	CARB	SUGAR
Sandwich Vanilla Light	1 (2.2 oz)	160	3	29	14
Sandwich Vanilla Lowfat	1 (2.8 oz)	80	2	15	2
No Pudge!					
Giant Chocolate Eclair Low Fat	1 bar	110	2	23	14
Giant Cone Chocolate No Sugar Added	1	110	4	22	2
Giant Cone Cookies & Cream Low Fat	1	140	3	29	13
Giant Cone Fudgy Brownie Low Fat	1	140	3	32	15
Giant Cone Vanilla No Sugar Added	1	110	4	22	2
Giant Cookie & Cream Low Fat No Sugar Added	1 bar	100	3	21	2
Giant Fudgy Fat Free No Sugar Added	1 bar	60	0	17	3
Giant Sandwich Brownie Batter Low Fat	1	140	2	30	16
Giant Sandwich Brownie Chunk Low Fat	1	140	2	30	16
Giant Sandwich Vanilla & Chocolate No Sugar Added	1	130	5	22	2
Giant Strawberry Shortcake Low Fat	1 bar	110	2	23	14
Skinny Cow					
Sandwich Low Fat	1 (2.5 oz)	140	2	30	15
Tofutti					
Cuties Vanilla	1 (1.4 oz)	120	5	17	9
Turkey Hill					
Carb IQ Vanilla Bean	½ cup	110	8	15	3

FOOD	PORTION	CALS	FAT	CARB	SUGAR
Weight Watchers					
Smart Ones Giant Sundae	1 serv (8 oz)	150	1	39	24
TAKE-OUT					
gelato chocolate hazelnut	½ cup (5.3 oz)	370	29	26	21
gelato vanilla	½ cup (3 oz)	211	15	18	18

ICE CREAM CONES AND CUPS

FOOD	PORTION	CALS	FAT	CARB	SUGAR
wafer cone	1	17	tr	3	tr
waffle cone	1 lg	121	2	23	2

ICE CREAM TOPPINGS

FOOD	PORTION	CALS	FAT	CARB	SUGAR
nuts in syrup	2 tbsp	184	9	24	15
Colac					
Passion Fruit	1 tbsp	31	0	13	0
Strawberry	1 tbsp	31	0	13	0
Smucker's					
Butterscotch Caramel	2 tbsp	130	1	30	28
Dove Dark Chocolate	2 tbsp	140	5	22	15
Dove Milk Chocolate	2 tbsp	130	4	21	17
Dulce De Leche Milk Caramel Spread	2 tbsp	110	2	23	19
Hot Fudge	2 tbsp	140	4	22	16
Hot Fudge Sugar Free Fat Free	2 tbsp	90	0	23	0
Magic Shell Caramel	2 tbsp	220	18	14	13
Magic Shell Chocolate	2 tbsp	210	17	16	15
Magic Shell Chocolate Fudge	2 tbsp	120	14	19	11
Magic Shell Turtle Delight	2 tbsp	210	16	17	15
Magic Shell Twix	2 tbsp	210	15	18	15
Steel's					
Sugar Free Butterscotch	2 tbsp	60	0	21	0
Sugar Free Chocolate Fudge	2 tbsp	45	3	5	0

FOOD	PORTION	CALS	FAT	CARB	SUGAR
Sugar Free Hot Fudge	2 tbsp	65	3	18	0
Sugar Free Peanut Butter Fudge	2 tbsp	75	6	5	0

ICED TEA
MIX
Carb Options
| Lemon as prep | 1 serv | 0 | 0 | 0 | 0 |

READY-TO-DRINK
Arizona
| Green Tea w/ Ginseng & Honey | 8 oz | 70 | 0 | 18 | 17 |
| Lemon | 8 oz | 90 | 0 | 25 | 24 |

Bolthouse Farms
| Perfectly Protein Vanilla Chai Tea | 8 oz | 160 | 3 | 25 | 21 |

Brazil Gourmet
| Nectar Tea All Flavors | 8 oz | 90 | 0 | 23 | 21 |
| Nectar Tea Light Mango Passion | 8 oz | 60 | 0 | 17 | 16 |

Delta Blues
| Spearmint Tea Punch | 8 oz | 90 | 0 | 21 | 20 |

Fuze
LemonAID	8 oz	70	0	19	17
Slender Energy All Flavors	8 oz	20	0	5	5
Vitamin Tea Diet Peach	8 oz	5	0	1	0
Vitamin Tea Green Tea w/ Ginseng	8 oz	60	0	16	16
Vitamin Tea Lemon	8 oz	70	0	18	17
White Tea	8 oz	60	0	15	15
White Tea No Carb Diet Pomegranate	8 oz	0	0	0	0

Glaceau Vitamin Water
| Vital-T | 8 oz | 50 | 0 | 13 | 13 |

FOOD	PORTION	CALS	FAT	CARB	SUGAR
Hawaiian					
Iced Tea	1 can	120	0	35	35
Honest Tea					
Assam	8 oz	17	0	5	4
Black Forest Berry	8 oz	25	0	8	8
Gold Rush	8 oz	9	0	3	2
Green Dragon	8 oz	30	0	9	9
Kashmiri Chai	8 oz	17	0	6	5
Lori's Lemon	8 oz	30	0	9	9
Moroccan Mint	8 oz	17	0	5	5
Peach Oo-La-Long	8 oz	30	0	9	9
Hood					
Iced Tea	1 cup	100	0	25	24
Inko's					
White Tea All Flavors	1 bottle (16 oz)	56	0	14	14
White Tea Honeysuckle	1 bottle	0	0	0	0
Joe Tea					
All Flavors	8 oz	100	0	25	24
Kalahari					
Rooibos Red Tea All Flavors	8 oz	50	0	13	12
New Leaf					
All Flavors	8 oz	75	0	19	19
Republic Of Tea					
No Carb Unsweetened All Flavors	1 bottle (12 oz)	0	0	0	0
Snapple					
Diet Lemonade Ice Tea	8 oz	10	0	2	1
Diet Lime Green Tea	8 oz	0	0	1	0
Just Plain Tea	8 oz	0	0	0	0
Lemonade Ice Tea	8 oz	110	0	28	28
Lime Green Tea	8 oz	100	0	25	23
Mint	8 oz	110	0	27	25

FOOD	PORTION	CALS	FAT	CARB	SUGAR
Peach	8 oz	100	0	26	24
Very Cherry	8 oz	100	0	25	23
SoBe					
Lean Diet Green Tea	8 oz	0	0	1	0
Lean Diet Peach Tea	8 oz	5	0	1	0
Lemon	8 oz	90	0	25	24
Soy20					
Lemon Green Tea	1 bottle (12 oz)	90	0	22	22
Sri Lankan					
Apple	8 oz	70	0	17	17
Lemon	8 oz	60	0	15	15
Sweet Leaf Tea					
Diet Sweet	8 oz	0	0	0	0
Hibiscus Herbal	8 oz	25	0	8	8
Lemon & Lime	8 oz	0	0	0	0
Mint & Honey Green	8 oz	60	0	15	15
Peach	8 oz	75	0	19	19
Raspberry & Tangerine	8 oz	75	0	19	19
Sweet Tea	8 oz	75	0	19	19
T42					
A Classic Earl Grey	8 oz	60	0	14	14
Herbal All Flavors	8 oz	70	0	18	17
Jamaican Ginger Green Tea	8 oz	70	0	16	16
Lemon And Honey Green Tea	8 oz	60	0	12	12
Wake-Up Blend English Breakfast	8 oz	45	0	11	11
With Lemon	8 oz	60	0	14	14
Tao Tea					
Grapefruit Green Tea	8 oz	71	0	18	16
Lemon Green Tea	8 oz	67	0	17	16

FOOD	PORTION	CALS	FAT	CARB	SUGAR
Tradewinds					
Diet Green Tea	8 oz	0	0	0	0
Diet Raspberry	8 oz	0	0	0	0
Mango Green Tea	8 oz	80	0	20	20
XS Energy					
Energy Tea Berry Typhoon	1 can (8.4 oz)	12	0	1	0

ICES AND ICE POPS

FOOD	PORTION	CALS	FAT	CARB	SUGAR
Breyers					
Fruit Bars No Sugar Added	1 (1.75 oz)	25	0	5	2
Juice Bar Strawberry	1 (3.75 oz)	120	0	30	23
Soft Frozen Cup Lemonade	1 pkg (12 oz)	290	0	74	56
Soft Frozen Cup Strawberry	1 pkg (12 oz)	260	0	66	51
Edy's					
Sherbet Berry Rainbow	½ cup	130	2	29	23
Sherbet Key Lime	½ cup	130	2	28	23
Sherbet Orange Cream	½ cup	120	2	23	19
Sherbet Raspberry	½ cup	130	1	28	22
Sherbet Swiss Orange	½ cup	150	3	30	25
Sherbet Tropical Rainbow	½ cup	130	1	29	24
Whole Fruit Creamy Coconut	1 bar	120	3	21	16
Whole Fruit Lemonade	1 bar	80	0	20	19
Whole Fruit Lime	1 bar	80	0	20	19
Whole Fruit Orange & Cream	1 bar	80	2	16	15
Whole Fruit Peach	½ cup	90	0	23	21
Whole Fruit Strawberry	1 bar	80	0	21	20
Whole Fruit Tangerine	1 bar	80	0	20	19
Whole Fruit Tropical	1 bar	100	0	26	26
Whole Fruit Wild Berry	1 bar	80	0	21	20

FOOD	PORTION	CALS	FAT	CARB	SUGAR
Good Humor					
Great White	1 (3 oz)	70	0	18	14
Hyper Stripe	1 (2.7 oz)	80	0	19	15
Hawaiian Punch					
Arctic Surfers	1 pop	50	0	12	8
Hendrie's					
Citrus N' Berry Stix	1 (1.9 oz)	15	0	3	0
Fudge Stix Fat Free	1 bar (1.8 oz)	70	0	14	11
Hood					
Hoodsie Pop	1 (3.3 oz)	60	0	16	13
Minute Maid					
Fruit And Cream Swirl	1 tube (3 oz)	90	3	16	14
Fruit Bars	1 bar	60	0	15	14
Popsicle					
All Natural Ice Pops	1 (1.75 oz)	50	0	12	9
Bar Bart Simpson	1 (4 oz)	110	1	26	20
Bar Dora The Explorer	1 (4 oz)	100	0	25	20
Bar Fruti Holanda Lemon Lime	1 (3 oz)	90	0	23	18
Bar Fruti Holanda Strawberry	1 (3 oz)	90	0	23	19
Bar Incredible Hulk	1 (4 oz)	100	0	25	20
Bar Jimmy Neutron	1 (4 oz)	100	0	25	19
Bar Mega Warheads	1 (4 oz)	110	1	26	20
Bar Power Ranger	1 (4 oz)	100	0	23	18
Bar Spider Man	1 (4 oz)	100	0	25	20
Bar SpongeBob	1 (4 oz)	100	0	25	20
Big Stick Pops Big Reds	1 (3.5 oz)	70	0	17	12
Big Stick Pops Cherry Pineapple	1 (3.5 oz)	50	0	12	10
Bubble Play	1 (4 oz)	100	0	28	21
Creamsicle Bar	1 (2.5 oz)	100	3	18	14
Creamsicle Sugar Free	2 (3.3 oz)	40	2	10	0

FOOD	PORTION	CALS	FAT	CARB	SUGAR
Creamsicle Pop No Sugar Added	1 (1.75 oz)	25	0	6	1
Cup Cherry	1 (12 oz)	240	0	62	59
Cup Frostee Fudge	1 (10 oz)	280	11	41	33
Cup Lemon	1 (12 oz)	230	0	60	59
Cup Screwball	1 (3.75 oz)	110	0	27	22
Firecracker	1 (1.6 oz)	35	0	9	7
Fruita Holanda Coconut Bar	1 (3 oz)	120	3	25	21
Fudgsicle Bar	1 (2.5 oz)	90	2	16	13
Fudgsicle Bar Fat Free	1 (1.75 oz)	60	0	13	10
Fudgsicle Pop	1 (1.75 oz)	60	1	11	9
Fudgsicle Pops No Sugar Added	2 (1.75 oz)	90	1	19	3
Minis Fudge Bar	2 (2.4 oz)	80	2	16	13
Pop Great White	1 (1.75 oz)	45	0	11	9
Pop Lick-A-Color	1 (2 oz)	50	0	13	12
Pop Sherbet Cyclone	1 (1.8 oz)	50	1	11	10
Pop Towering Tornado	1 (3.5 oz)	90	0	21	10
Pop Ups Orange Burst	1 (2.75 oz)	80	1	19	15
Pop Ups Reckless Rainbow	1 (2.75 oz)	90	1	19	15
Pop Ups SpongeBob	1 (2.75 oz)	90	2	17	13
Pops Tropical Sugar Free	1 (1.75 oz)	15	0	3	0
Pops Wild Bunch	2 (2.2 oz)	60	0	14	11
Rainbow Floats	1 (1.75 oz)	60	2	11	8
Rainbow Pops	1 (1.75 oz)	45	0	11	11
Scribblers Juice Pops	2 (2.4 oz)	60	0	16	15
Shots	1 serv (1.7 oz)	40	1	9	9
Snow Cone	1 (7 oz)	30	0	7	5
Sugar Free Pops Orange Cherry Grape	1 (1.75 oz)	15	0	3	0
Super Mario Bros Bar	1 (4 oz)	100	0	25	20

FOOD	PORTION	CALS	FAT	CARB	SUGAR
Swirl Bar Cotton Candy	1 (2.6 oz)	60	0	13	10
Tingle Twister Ice Pops	1 (1.75 oz)	45	0	11	9
Torpedo Pop Cherry	1 (1.75 oz)	35	0	8	6
Tropicana					
Fruit Juice Bar Orange	1	45	0	11	9
Fruit Juice Bar Raspberry	1	45	0	11	8
Strawberry	1	45	0	11	8
Wawona					
Peach	1 pop	78	tr	19	16
Strawberry	1 pop	77	tr	18	16

JAM/JELLY/PRESERVES

FOOD	PORTION	CALS	FAT	CARB	SUGAR
all flavors jam	1 tbsp (0.7 oz)	48	0	13	10
all flavors jam	1 pkg (0.5 oz)	34	0	9	7
all flavors jelly	1 tbsp (0.7 oz)	52	0	14	12
all flavors jelly	1 pkg (0.5 oz)	38	0	10	9
all flavors preserve	1 tbsp (0.7 oz)	48	0	13	10
all flavors preserve	1 pkg (0.5 oz)	34	0	9	7
apple butter	1 tbsp (0.6 oz)	33	0	9	—
Colac					
Jelly All Flavors	1 tbsp	37	0	15	0
Jok'n'Al					
Low Carb Fruit Spreads All Flavors	1 tbsp	10	0	3	2
Matouk's					
Guava Jam	1 tbsp	50	0	13	12
Mango Jam	1 tbsp	50	0	12	12
Polaner					
All Fruit Grape	1 tbsp	40	0	10	10
Sarabeth's					
Spreadable Fruit Orange Apricot	1 tbsp	30	0	8	8
Spreadable Fruit Peach Apricot	1 tbsp	40	0	9	6

FOOD	PORTION	CALS	FAT	CARB	SUGAR
Smucker's					
Cider Apple Butter	1 tbsp	45	0	11	10
Jam Concord Grape	1 tbsp	50	0	13	12
Jam Red Plum	1 tbsp	50	0	13	12
Jam Seedless Red Raspberry	1 tbsp	50	0	13	12
Jam Seedless Strawberry	1 tbsp	50	0	13	12
Jelly Apple	2 tbsp	50	0	13	12
Jelly Concord Grape	1 tbsp	50	0	13	12
Jelly Currant	1 tbsp	50	0	13	12
Jelly Elderberry	1 tbsp	50	0	13	12
Jelly Guava	1 tbsp	50	0	13	12
Jelly Mixed Fruit	2 tbsp	50	0	13	12
Low Sugar All Flavors	1 tbsp	25	0	6	5
Preserves All Flavors	1 tbsp	50	0	13	12
Simply Fruit All Flavors	1 tbsp	40	0	10	8
Sugar Free All Flavors	1 tbsp	10	0	5	0
Welch's					
Grape Jam	1 tbsp	50	0	13	13
JAVA PLUM					
fresh	3	5	tr	1	—
JICAMA					
cooked	¾ cup	38	tr	9	—
Frieda's					
Jicama	¾ cup	35	0	7	0
JUTE					
cooked	1 cup	32	tr	6	1
KALE					
chopped cooked	½ cup	21	tr	4	—
KEFIR					
kefir	7 oz	132	8	10	—

FOOD	PORTION	CALS	FAT	CARB	SUGAR
KETCHUP					
banana	1 tsp	10	0	2	2
ketchup	1 tbsp	16	tr	4	–
Del Monte					
Ketchup	1 tbsp	15	0	4	4
Estee					
No Sugar Added	1 tbsp	15	0	5	1
Heinz					
Ketchup	1 tbsp	15	0	4	4
No Salt	1 tbsp	20	0	5	4
One Carb	1 tbsp	5	0	1	1
Organic	1 tbsp	20	0	5	4
Hunt's					
Ketchup	1 tbsp	15	0	4	4
No Salt Added	1 tbsp	20	0	4	4
Squeeze	1 tbsp	15	0	4	4
Keto					
Ketchup	1 tbsp	4	0	1	0
Steel's					
Sugar Free	1 tbsp	10	0	0	0
Stokelys					
Tomato	1 tbsp	15	0	4	4
Walden Farms					
Calorie Free	1 tbsp	0	0	0	0
KIDNEY					
beef simmered	3 oz	134	4	0	0
lamb braised	3 oz	116	3	1	–
pork cooked	3 oz	128	4	0	0
pork cooked	1 cup	211	7	0	0
veal braised	3 oz	139	5	0	0
KIDNEY BEANS					
canned	½ cup	105	1	19	2

FOOD	PORTION	CALS	FAT	CARB	SUGAR
dried cooked	½ cup	112	tr	20	tr
Bush's					
Light Red	½ cup	110	0	20	1
Goya					
Dark	½ cup	90	1	18	2
Progresso					
Red	½ cup	110	0	20	2
Rienzi					
Cannellini	½ cup	80	0	18	0
Red	½ cup	90	1	18	2
KIWIS					
fresh	1 med	46	tr	11	–
KNISH					
Gabila's					
Potato	1 (4.5 oz)	170	6	29	2
TAKE-OUT					
potato	1 med (3.5 oz)	166	6	25	2
potato	1 lg (7 oz)	332	12	49	5
KOHLRABI					
sliced cooked	½ cup	24	tr	5	–
Frieda's					
Kohlrabi	⅔ cup	25	0	5	2
KRILL					
fresh	1 oz	22	1	tr	–
KUMQUATS					
fresh	1	12	tr	3	–
LAMB					
cubed lean & fat braised	4 oz	253	10	0	0
cubed lean & fat broiled	4 oz	211	8	0	0
ground broiled	4 oz	321	22	0	0
leg roasted	4 oz	213	15	0	0

FOOD	PORTION	CALS	FAT	CARB	SUGAR
loin chop lean & fat broiled	1 chop (4 oz)	222	16	0	0
rib chop lean & fat broiled	1 chop (1.6 oz)	165	14	0	0
rib roast baked	4 oz	386	31	0	0
shank lean & fat braised	4 oz	360	20	0	0
shoulder chop lean & fat cooked	1 chop (5.5 oz)	274	20	0	0
shoulder w/ bone braised	4 oz	231	17	0	0

LAMB DISHES
TAKE-OUT

FOOD	PORTION	CALS	FAT	CARB	SUGAR
lamb curry	1 cup	257	14	4	1
moussaka	5.6 oz	312	21	16	–
stew	¾ cup	124	5	11	–

LAMBSQUARTERS

FOOD	PORTION	CALS	FAT	CARB	SUGAR
chopped cooked w/ salt	1 cup	58	1	9	–

LEEKS

FOOD	PORTION	CALS	FAT	CARB	SUGAR
chopped cooked	¼ cup	8	tr	2	–
raw chopped	¼ cup	16	tr	4	–
Frieda's					
Fresh	1 cup	50	0	12	3

LEMON

FOOD	PORTION	CALS	FAT	CARB	SUGAR
fresh	1 med	22	tr	12	–
lemon extract	½ tsp	12	tr	0	0
peel	1 tbsp	0	tr	1	–
wedge	1	5	tr	3	–
Sunkist					
Fresh	1 (2 oz)	15	0	5	1

LEMON EXTRACT
True Lemon

FOOD	PORTION	CALS	FAT	CARB	SUGAR
Crystallized Lemon	1 pkg (1 g)	0	0	tr	–

FOOD	PORTION	CALS	FAT	CARB	SUGAR
LEMON GRASS					
fresh	1 tbsp (5 g)	5	tr	1	—
LEMON JUICE					
bottled	1 tbsp	3	tr	1	—
fresh	1 tbsp	4	0	1	—
Adina					
Hibiscus Lemon Bissap	8 oz	80	0	28	19
LEMONADE					
MIX					
Keto					
Kooler Pink	½ tsp	0	0	0	0
Low Carb Creations					
Lemonade as prep	1 serv	10	0	2	tr
Raspberry as prep	1 serv	10	0	2	0
Sipper Sweets					
Sugar Free Low Carb	1 serv	8	0	1	0
READY-TO-DRINK					
Bolthouse Farms					
Mango Lemonade	8 oz	120	0	30	30
Hi-C					
Blast Pink	8 oz	120	0	31	31
Honest Ade					
Cranberry	8 oz	50	0	13	13
Hood					
Lemonade	1 cup	110	0	28	28
Langers					
Raspberry Lemonade	8 oz	120	0	29	26
White Cranberry Lemonade	8 oz	120	0	30	28
Minute Maid					
Chilled	8 oz	100	0	28	27
Coolers Pink	1 pouch (7 oz)	90	0	25	24

FOOD	PORTION	CALS	FAT	CARB	SUGAR
Light	8 oz	15	0	4	2
Naked Juice					
Just Made	8 oz	110	0	28	26
Ocean Spray					
Spritzer	8 oz	160	0	41	40
Santa Cruz					
Organic	1 can	160	0	40	39
Organic Raspberry	1 can	120	0	29	28
Snapple					
Lemonade	8 oz	110	0	28	27
Super Sour	8 oz	130	0	33	32
T42					
Lemonade	8 oz	90	0	25	25
Pink	8 oz	90	0	25	25
Three Drinks					
Sparkling	12 oz	12	0	3	2
Tropicana					
Sugar Free	1 can	10	0	tr	0
Zeigler's					
Old Fashioned	8 oz	120	0	30	27
LENTILS					
dried cooked	1 cup	231	1	40	–
Near East					
Lentil Pilaf as prep	1 cup	200	3	36	3
TAKE-OUT					
indian sambar	1 serv	236	5	37	–
yemiser selatta ethiopian lentil salad	1 serv (3 oz)	115	7	11	1
LETTUCE					
bibb	1 head (6 oz)	21	tr	4	–
boston	2 leaves	2	tr	tr	–
iceberg	1 leaf	3	tr	tr	–

FOOD	PORTION	CALS	FAT	CARB	SUGAR
iceberg	1 head (19 oz)	70	1	11	–
romaine shredded	½ cup	4	tr	1	–
Frieda's					
Limestone	⅔ cup	10	0	2	1
Green Giant					
Hearts Of Romaine	6 leaves (3 oz)	14	0	3	1
Mann's					
Romaine Jumbo Hearts	3 oz	15	0	3	2
Ocean Mist					
Romaine Hearts	6 leaves	20	1	3	2
Ready Pac					
Baby Arugula	4 cups	20	1	3	0
Bella Romaine	1½ cups	15	0	2	1
River Ranch					
Romaine Chopped	1½ cups	10	0	3	tr
Romaine Hearts	1½ cups	10	0	2	tr
LILY ROOT					
dried	1 oz	89	1	21	–
fresh	1 oz	32	tr	8	–
LIMA BEANS					
CANNED					
Del Monte					
Green	½ cup	80	0	15	0
DRIED					
cooked	½ cup	104	tr	20	–
LIME					
fresh	1	20	tr	7	–
Sunkist					
Fresh	1 (2 oz)	20	0	7	1
LIME JUICE					
bottled	1 tbsp	3	tr	1	–
fresh	1 tbsp	4	tr	1	–

FOOD	PORTION	CALS	FAT	CARB	SUGAR
Adina					
Lime Mint Mojita	8 oz	70	0	19	16
Honest Ade					
Limeade	8 oz	50	0	13	13
Minute Maid					
Light Limeade	8 oz	15	0	4	3
LING					
fresh baked	3 oz	95	1	0	0
LINGCOD					
baked	3 oz	93	1	0	0
LIQUOR/LIQUEUR					
7&7	1 serv	178	0	19	–
alabama slammer	1 serv	103	tr	7	–
amaretto sour	1 serv	295	tr	57	–
angel's kiss	1 serv	85	1	5	–
anisette	1 oz	111	0	11	–
apricot brandy	1 oz	96	0	9	–
apricot sour	1 serv	164	tr	8	–
aquavit	1 oz	65	0	0	0
b 52	1 serv	247	4	25	–
b&b	1 serv	75	0	0	0
bahama breeze	1 serv	70	tr	9	–
bahama mama	1 serv	153	tr	23	–
bailey's & amaretto	1 serv	184	5	16	–
bay breeze	1 serv	173	tr	18	–
bend me over	1 serv	242	tr	32	–
benedictine	1 oz	104	0	11	–
betsy ross	1 serv	206	0	5	–
black devil	1 serv	220	tr	1	–
black russian	1 serv	184	tr	12	–
bloody mary	1 serv	150	tr	5	–
bourbon & soda	1 serv (4 oz)	105	0	0	0

FOOD	PORTION	CALS	FAT	CARB	SUGAR
bourbon sour	1 serv	166	tr	8	—
brandy alexander	1 serv	266	6	12	—
brandy sour	1 serv	164	tr	8	—
bushwacker	1 serv	286	5	27	—
coffee liqueur	1 serv (1.5 oz)	175	tr	24	24
cognac	1 oz	67	0	tr	0
cosmopolitan martini	1 serv	126	tr	7	—
creme de menthe	1 serv (1.5 oz)	186	tr	21	21
daiquiri	1 serv (2 oz)	112	tr	4	3
dark & stormy	1 serv	64	0	0	0
doctor pepper	1 serv	95	0	12	—
fuzzy navel	1 serv	247	tr	10	—
gimlet vodka	1 serv	150	0	6	—
gin	1 serv (1.5 oz)	110	0	0	0
gin & tonic	1 serv (7.5 oz)	171	0	16	—
gin ricky	1 serv	114	tr	1	—
grasshopper	1 serv	275	5	26	—
harvey wallbanger	1 serv	198	tr	16	—
head banger	1 serv	165	0	4	—
hot buttered rum	1 serv	219	4	15	—
hot toddy	1 serv	188	1	13	—
hurricane	1 serv	205	tr	19	—
kamikaze	1 serv	136	0	2	—
long island iced tea	1 serv	292	tr	7	—
lynchburg lemonade	1 serv	465	tr	85	—
mai tai	1 serv	165	tr	17	—
manhattan	1 serv	171	tr	3	—
margarita	1 serv	173	0	11	—
martini	1 serv (3 oz)	206	0	2	tr
mellow yellow	1 serv	95	0	4	—
mint julep	1 serv	136	tr	17	—
mississippi mud	1 serv	496	12	46	—
mudslide	1 serv	566	10	46	—

FOOD	PORTION	CALS	FAT	CARB	SUGAR
narragansett	1 serv	168	0	2	—
nutcracker	1 serv	730	10	64	—
old fashioned	1 serv	223	tr	4	—
orange crush	1 serv	461	tr	65	—
pain killer	1 serv	277	tr	20	—
pina colada	1 serv (4.5 oz)	245	3	32	31
planter's cocktail	1 serv	105	0	3	—
planter's punch	1 serv	233	tr	34	—
presbyterian	1 serv	170	0	8	—
purple passion	1 serv	215	tr	22	—
rob roy	1 serv	171	0	3	—
rum	1 serv (1.5 oz)	97	0	0	0
rum cola	1 serv	209	tr	21	—
rum punch	1 serv	448	1	88	—
rusty nail	1 serv	159	0	6	—
sake	1 serv (1 oz)	39	0	1	0
salty dog	1 serv	210	tr	19	—
scotch & soda	1 serv	104	0	tr	—
screwdriver rum	1 serv	166	tr	16	—
sea breeze	1 serv	207	tr	19	—
sex on the beach	1 serv	190	tr	18	—
slippery nipple	1 serv	142	2	11	—
sloe gin fizz	1 serv (2.5 oz)	132	0	4	—
snake bite	1 serv	362	0	22	—
sour rum	1 serv	156	tr	8	—
swizzle rum	1 serv	187	0	15	—
tequila gimlet	1 serv	150	tr	6	—
tequila sour	1 serv	156	tr	8	—
tequila stinger	1 serv	221	tr	14	—
tequila sunrise	1 serv (6.8 oz)	232	tr	24	—
tom collins	1 serv (7.5 oz)	121	0	3	—
vodka	1 serv (1.5 oz)	97	0	0	0
vodka sour	1 serv	138	tr	3	—

FOOD	PORTION	CALS	FAT	CARB	SUGAR
vodka stinger	1 serv	378	tr	28	–
whiskey	1 serv (1.5 oz)	105	0	tr	–
whiskey sour	1 serv (3.5 oz)	162	tr	14	14
white russian	1 serv	290	8	17	–
zombie	1 serv	235	tr	10	–

LITCHI JUICE
Ceres
Litchi	8 oz	120	0	30	25

LIVER
beef pan-fried	3 oz	175	5	5	0
chicken stewed	1 cup (5 oz)	219	8	1	–
duck raw	1 (1.5 oz)	60	2	2	–
goose raw	1 (3.3 oz)	125	4	6	–
lamb braised	3 oz	199	13	0	0
lamb fried	3 oz	202	11	3	–
pork braised	3 oz	140	4	3	–
sheep raw	3.5 oz	131	4	0	–
turkey simmered	1 cup (5 oz)	237	8	5	–
veal braised	3 oz	154	5	3	0

LIVER SUBSTITUTES
Sabra
Vegetarian Liver	1 oz	70	7	1	1

LOBSTER
northern cooked	1 cup	142	1	2	–
spiny steamed	3 oz	122	2	3	–
spiny steamed	1 (5.7 oz)	233	3	5	–

FROZEN
Phillips Seafood
Lobster Cake	1 (3 oz)	230	15	7	1

TAKE-OUT
newburg	1 cup	485	27	13	–

FOOD	PORTION	CALS	FAT	CARB	SUGAR
LOGANBERRIES					
frzn	1 cup	80	tr	19	–
LONGANS					
fresh	1	2	0	tr	–
LOQUATS					
fresh	1	5	tr	1	–
LOTUS					
root raw sliced	10 slices	45	tr	14	–
root sliced cooked	10 slices	59	tr	14	–
seeds dried	1 oz	94	1	18	–
Frieda's					
Lotus Root Fresh	1 cup	50	0	15	0
LYCHEES					
Frieda's					
Fresh	6 to 8 (3.5 oz)	60	0	14	13
MACADAMIA NUTS					
dry roasted w/ salt	10 to 12 (1 oz)	200	22	4	2
Keto					
Chocolately Covered	1 oz	171	19	6	0
Maranatha					
Macadamia Butter	2 tbsp	230	24	5	1
Mauna Loa					
Chocolate Trio	9 pieces	200	15	19	17
Dry Roasted Salted	¼ cup	200	21	4	1
Dry Roasted Unsalted	¼ cup	200	21	4	1
Honey Roasted	¼ cup	210	21	6	4
Kona Coffee Glazed	¼ cup	190	15	10	6
Maui Onion & Garlic	¼ cup	200	16	18	14
Milk Chocolate Coated	3 pieces	230	16	18	16
Milk Chocolate Toffee	7 pieces	210	13	23	21

FOOD	PORTION	CALS	FAT	CARB	SUGAR
MACE					
ground	1 tsp	8	1	1	–
MACKEREL					
CANNED					
jack	1 cup	296	12	0	0
Brunswick					
Jack In Water	2 oz	100	5	5	0
Chicken Of The Sea					
Jack In Tomato Sauce	¼ cup	70	3	2	1
Jack In Water	⅓ cup	90	4	0	0
Orleans					
Jack	¼ cup	90	4	0	0
FRESH					
atlantic cooked	3 oz	223	15	0	0
atlantic raw	3 oz	174	12	0	0
jack baked	3 oz	171	9	0	0
king baked	3 oz	114	2	0	0
pacific baked	3 oz	171	9	0	0
spanish cooked	3 oz	134	5	0	0
SMOKED					
atlantic	3.5 oz	296	24	0	0
MAHI MAHI					
fresh baked	4 oz	192	13	1	tr
Phillips Seafood					
Coconut Mahi Mahi w/ Sauce	3 pieces	290	13	31	11
MALANGA					
dasheen mashed	1 cup	226	tr	53	1
dasheen pieces boiled	1 cup	212	tr	50	1
pieces fried	1 cup	304	11	52	1
Frieda's					
Malanga	⅔ cup	90	0	23	0

FOOD	PORTION	CALS	FAT	CARB	SUGAR
MALT					
malt liquor	1 bottle (12 oz)	148	0	13	tr
nonalcoholic	1 bottle (12 oz)	133	tr	29	29
MALTED MILK					
chocolate as prep w/ milk	1 cup	179	5	27	15
chocolate flavor powder	3 heaping tsp (0.7 oz)	79	1	18	5
natural flavor as prep w/ milk	1 cup	186	6	24	22
natural flavor powder	3 heaping tsp (0.7 oz)	87	2	1	12
MAMMY-APPLE					
fresh	1	431	4	106	–
MANGO					
Tomorrow's Tropicals					
Fresh	½ (3.6 oz)	70	1	17	15
MANGO JUICE					
Ceres					
Mango	8 oz	120	0	30	26
Langers					
Mongo Mango	8 oz	120	0	30	27
Naked Juice					
Mighty Mango	8 oz	120	0	30	18
MARGARINE					
squeeze	1 tsp	34	4	0	0
stick corn	1 tsp	34	4	0	0
tub corn	1 tsp	34	4	0	0
tub diet	1 tsp	17	2	0	0
Blue Bonnet					
Light Stick	1 tbsp	50	5	0	0
Soft Spread	1 tbsp	60	7	0	0

FOOD	PORTION	CALS	FAT	CARB	SUGAR
Soft Spread Light	1 tbsp	40	5	0	0
Stick	1 tbsp	80	9	0	0
Brummel & Brown					
Spread Made With Yogurt	1 tbsp	45	5	0	0
Fleischmann's					
Soft Spread Light	1 tbsp	40	5	0	0
Soft Spread Original	1 tbsp	70	8	0	0
Soft Spread Unsalted	1 tbsp	70	8	0	0
Soft Spread w/ Olive Oil	1 tbsp	70	8	0	0
I Can't Believe It's Not Butter					
Regular Stick	1 tbsp	90	10	0	0
Soft Fat Free	1 tbsp	5	0	0	0
Soft Light	1 tbsp	50	5	0	0
Soft Regular	1 tbsp	80	9	0	0
Soft w/ Calcium	1 tbsp	50	5	0	0
Spray	5 sprays	0	0	0	0
Squeeze	1 tbsp	60	7	0	0
Stick Light	1 tbsp	50	6	0	0
Parkay					
Light Spread	1 tbsp	50	5	0	0
Original Spread	1 tbsp	60	7	0	0
Original Stick	1 tbsp	90	10	0	0
Spray	5 sprays	0	0	0	0
Spread + Calcium	1 tbsp	45	5	0	0
Squeeze	1 tbsp	70	8	0	0
Stick Light	1 tbsp	50	5	0	0
Promise					
Buttery Spread	1 tbsp	80	8	0	0
Stick	1 tbsp	90	10	0	0
Smart Balance					
Buttery Spread No Trans Fat	1 tbsp	80	9	0	0

FOOD	PORTION	CALS	FAT	CARB	SUGAR
Spectrum					
Essential Omega	1 tbsp	80	10	0	0
Spread	1 tbsp	88	10	0	0
MARJORAM					
dried	1 tsp	2	tr	tr	–
MARLIN					
raw	3 oz	110	3	0	0
MARSHMALLOW					
marshmallow	1 reg (0.3 oz)	23	0	6	–
Gol D Lite					
Sugar Free	⅓ pkg (0.9 oz)	51	0	19	0
MATZO					
matzo ball	1 med	80	5	6	–
plain	1 (1 oz)	112	tr	24	–
whole wheat	1 (1 oz)	99	tr	22	–
Eddyleon					
Dark Chocolate Coated Egg Matzo	1 oz	97	3	17	16
Milk Chocolate Coated Egg Matzo	1 oz	97	4	16	15
Manischewitz					
Dark Chocolate Coated Egg	½ (1.5 oz)	90	5	31	6
Egg	1 (1.2 oz)	120	1	28	2
Streit's					
Egg	1 (1.1 oz)	120	1	25	1
Egg & Onion	1 (1 oz)	100	1	23	0
Passover	1 (1 oz)	110	1	25	0
MAYONNAISE					
Hellman's					
Mayonnaise	1 tbsp	90	10	0	0

FOOD	PORTION	CALS	FAT	CARB	SUGAR
Spectrum					
Canola Squeeze	1 tbsp	100	11	0	0
Canola Squeeze Light Eggless Vegan	1 tbsp	35	4	0	0
Organic Dijon	1 tbsp	90	10	1	0
Organic Olive Oil	1 tbsp	100	11	0	0
Organic Roasted Garlic	1 tbsp	100	11	0	0
Organic Squeeze	1 tbsp	100	11	0	0
Organic Wasabi	1 tbsp	100	11	0	0

MAYONNAISE TYPE SALAD DRESSING
Carb Options

FOOD	PORTION	CALS	FAT	CARB	SUGAR
Whipped Dressing	1 tbsp	50	5	0	0
Nasoya					
Fat Free Nayonaise	1 tbsp	10	0	2	1
Nayonaise	1 tbsp	35	4	1	0

MEAT STICKS

FOOD	PORTION	CALS	FAT	CARB	SUGAR
jerky beef	1 piece (0.7 oz)	82	5	2	2
Jack Link's					
Beef Jerky Teriyaki	1 oz	80	1	5	5
Pemmican					
Homestyle Tender All Flavors	1 oz	80	2	3	2
Kippered Beef Original	1 pkg (1 oz)	60	1	2	2
Kippered Beef Peppered	1 pkg (1 oz)	60	1	2	1
Kippered Beef Sweet & Hot	1 pkg (1 oz)	70	1	6	4
Kippered Beef Teriyaki	1 pkg (1 oz)	60	1	2	1
Long Lasting Hot & Spicy	1 oz	60	1	4	3
Long Lasting Original	1 oz	60	1	5	4
Long Lasting Peppered	1 oz	60	1	4	3
Long Lasting Teriyaki	1 oz	70	1	6	4
Premium Cut Beef Jerky	1 oz	80	1	4	2

FOOD	PORTION	CALS	FAT	CARB	SUGAR
Premium Cut Turkey Peppered	1 oz	70	1	5	4
Premium Cut Turkey Sweet Smoked	1 oz	70	1	5	4
Shredded Beef Jerky All Flavors	¼ cup	80	2	3	2
Steak Tips All Flavors	1 oz	70	2	5	4

MEAT SUBSTITUTES
Lightlife
Bologna	4 slices (2 oz)	60	0	0	0
Gimme Lean Ground Beef	1 serv (2 oz)	50	0	4	1
Smart BBQ	¼ cup	70	0	13	10
Smart Cutlet Salisbury Steak	1 (4.5 oz)	130	1	13	1
Smart Deli Country Ham	4 slices (2 oz)	90	0	5	0
Smart Deli Pastrami Style	4 slices (2 oz)	60	0	1	0
Smart Deli Pepperoni Style	13 slices (1 oz)	45	0	3	1
Smart Ground Original	⅓ cup (1.9 oz)	80	1	7	1
Smart Ground Taco Burrito	⅓ cup (2 oz)	70	0	5	1
Smart Menu Crumbles	⅓ cup	80	1	7	1
Smart Menu Meatless Meatballs	5	160	7	6	1
Smart Menu Steak Strips	1 serv (3 oz)	80	0	5	0
Smart Tex Mex	¼ cup	50	0	6	2

Quorn
Grounds	⅔ cup (3 oz)	80	3	5	1
Meatballs	4 (2.4 oz)	110	3	7	1

MELON
Frieda's
Camouflage	1 cup (5 oz)	50	0	13	7
SpriteMelon	1 (10.5 oz)	115	0	29	27

FOOD	PORTION	CALS	FAT	CARB	SUGAR
Temptation	1/10 melon (4.7 oz)	55	0	14	12

MILK
CANNED
Carnation
Evaporated	2 tbsp	40	2	3	3
Evaporated Fat Free	2 tbsp	25	0	4	4

Meyenberg
Evaporated Goat Milk	8 oz	145	8	10	10

DRIED
Carnation
Nonfat	1/3 cup	80	0	12	12

Meyenberg
Instant Goat Milk as prep	1 cup	142	7	11	11

REFRIGERATED
1%	1 cup	102	3	12	—
2%	1 cup	121	5	12	—
buttermilk	1 cup	99	2	12	—
goat	1 cup	168	10	11	—
human	1 cup	171	11	17	—
nonfat	1 cup	86	tr	12	—
whole	1 cup	150	8	11	—

Borden
Fat Free Skim	1 cup	80	0	12	11

Hood
1%	1 cup	110	3	13	12
2%	1 cup	130	5	13	12
Buttermilk Fat Free	1 cup	90	0	13	12
Carb Countdown 2%	8 oz	90	5	3	3
Carb Countdown Fat Free	8 oz	45	0	3	3
Fat Free	1 cup	80	0	13	12
Simply Smart 0% Fat	1 cup	90	0	13	12
Simply Smart 1% Fat	1 cup	120	3	13	12

FOOD	PORTION	CALS	FAT	CARB	SUGAR
Whole	1 cup	150	8	12	12
Lactaid					
1% Lowfat	1 cup	110	3	13	12
2% Reduced Fat	1 cup	130	5	12	12
Calcium Fortified	1 cup	80	0	13	12
Fat Free	1 cup	90	0	13	12
Whole	1 cup	150	8	12	12
Meyenberg					
Goat Milk	8 oz	142	7	11	11
Goat Milk Low Fat	8 oz	89	2	9	9
Skinny Cow					
Fat Free	8 oz	110	0	17	16
MILK DRINKS					
Cal-C					
Orange Tangerine	8 oz	70	0	19	14
Peach Mango	8 oz	70	0	19	14
Strawberry Citrus	8 oz	70	0	19	14
Cocio					
Chocolate Milk	1 bottle	225	7	32	28
Hershey's					
Chocolate Milk Fat Free	1 bottle	160	0	31	30
Chocolate Milk Reduced Fat	1 bottle	200	5	31	28
Hood					
Carb Countdown Chocolate 2%	8 oz	90	5	5	3
Chocolate Lowfat	1 cup	170	3	28	26
Chocolate Milk	1 cup	230	9	31	29
Coffee Lowfat Milk	1 cup	170	3	28	26
Keto					
Chocolate Milk Mix	1 scoop	36	1	3	0

FOOD	PORTION	CALS	FAT	CARB	SUGAR
Nesquik					
Chocolate as prep w/ lowfat milk	1 cup	210	5	30	18
Chocolate No Sugar as prep w/ lowfat milk	1 cup	130	1	18	3
Double Chocolate as prep w/ lowfat milk	1 cup	210	5	30	17
Ready-To-Drink Banana	1 cup	200	5	30	29
Ready-To-Drink Chocolate	1 cup	200	5	32	30
Ready-To-Drink Double Chocolate	1 cup	200	5	30	28
Ready-To-Drink Fat Free Chocolate	1 cup	160	0	32	30
Ready-To-Drink Strawberry	1 cup	200	5	33	31
Ready-To-Drink Very Vanilla	1 cup	200	5	30	29
Strawberry as prep w/ lowfat milk	1 cup	210	4	33	21
Vanilla as prep w/ lowfat milk	1 cup	210	4	33	13
Quaker					
Chocolate	8 oz	140	5	18	15
Strawberry	8 oz	130	5	18	16
Vanilla	8 oz	130	5	18	16
Rosa's Original					
Horchata All Flavors	8 oz	160	2	32	29
MILK SUBSTITUTES					
Almond Breeze					
Chocolate	8 oz	115	3	22	20
Original	8 oz	57	3	8	7
Original Unsweetened	8 oz	40	3	2	0
Vanilla	8 oz	91	3	16	15

FOOD	PORTION	CALS	FAT	CARB	SUGAR
Pacific Foods					
Almond Low Fat Original	1 cup	70	3	11	7
Almond Low Fat Vanilla	1 cup	100	3	15	11
Multi Grain Low Fat Original	1 cup	160	2	30	20
Oat Organic Low Fat Original	1 cup	130	3	24	19
Oat Organic Low Fat Vanilla	1 cup	130	3	24	19
Rice Low Fat Plain	1 cup	130	2	27	14
Rice Low Fat Vanilla	1 cup	130	2	27	14
Soy Organic Unsweetened Original	1 cup	90	5	4	2
Soy Select Low Fat Plain	1 cup	70	3	9	6
Soy Select Low Fat Vanilla	1 cup	80	3	11	9
Soy Ultra	1 cup	130	4	14	10
Soy Ultra Plain	1 cup	120	4	12	8
Vitasoy					
Classic Original	8 oz	120	5	11	5
Complete Original	8 oz	70	2	6	2
Complete Vanilla	8 oz	50	1	7	3
Creamy Original	8 oz	110	4	11	5
Green Tea Soymilk	8 oz	120	4	13	7
Light Original	8 oz	60	2	7	4
Light Chocolate	8 oz	100	2	17	14
Lite Vanilla	8 oz	70	2	10	7
Original Unsweetened	8 oz	80	4	5	tr
Rich Chocolate	8 oz	160	4	24	19
Smooth Vanilla	8 oz	120	4	13	8
Vanilla Delight	8 oz	120	4	13	8

MILKFISH (AWA)

FOOD	PORTION	CALS	FAT	CARB	SUGAR
baked	3 oz	162	7	0	0

FOOD	PORTION	CALS	FAT	CARB	SUGAR
MILKSHAKE					
chocolate	1 serv (10 oz)	393	14	60	52
malted milk shake	1 serv (10 oz)	402	14	62	58
vanilla	1 serv (10 oz)	379	13	60	59
Breyers					
Quick Vanilla	1 serv (10 oz)	320	17	37	36
Carb Options					
Chocolate Delite	1 can (11 oz)	190	9	6	1
Creamy Vanilla	1 can (11 oz)	190	9	6	1
Hershey's					
Chocolate	1 bottle	270	8	43	41
Cookies 'N' Cream	1 bottle	280	7	45	44
Strawberry	1 bottle	280	7	47	46
Vanilla Cream	1 bottle	320	7	55	44
Nesquik					
Ready-To-Drink Chocolate	1 cup	170	5	26	23
MILLET					
cooked	1 cup (6.1 oz)	207	2	41	–
MISO					
dried	1 oz	86	3	10	–
miso	½ cup	284	8	39	–
MOLASSES					
molasses	1 tbsp (0.7 oz)	53	0	14	12
Grandma's					
Robust	1 tbsp	60	0	15	14
MONKFISH					
baked	3 oz	82	2	0	0
MOOSE					
roasted	3 oz	114	1	0	0

FOOD	PORTION	CALS	FAT	CARB	SUGAR
MUFFIN					
MIX					
Carbsense					
Honey Bran not prep	1 serv (1.3 oz)	120	4	16	0
Jiffy					
Apple Cinnamon as prep	1	190	7	28	13
Banana Nut as prep	1	180	7	25	11
Blueberry as prep	1	190	7	28	13
Bran w/ Dates as prep	1	170	6	26	12
Corn as prep	1	180	6	30	8
Raspberry as prep	1	180	7	26	12
Ketogenics					
Apple Cinnamon Bran as prep	1	190	10	10	0
Chocolate Chip as prep	1	215	14	10	0
Wild Blueberry as prep	1	190	14	10	0
MiniCarb					
Apple Cinnamon as prep	1	225	16	7	2
Sweet Corn as prep	1	225	16	80	1
Miracle Maize					
Country Style as prep	1	155	6	22	2
Sweet as prep	1	180	6	29	10
READY-TO-EAT					
Fred's Incredible Muffins					
All Flavors	1 (2.5 oz)	100	3	26	8
Natural Ovens					
Blueberry	1 (2.5 oz)	180	5	29	10
Carrot Nut	1 (2.5 oz)	170	6	35	15
Raisin Bran	1 (2.5 oz)	170	3	36	15
Otis Spunkmeyer					
Apple Cinnamon	1 (4 oz)	420	22	54	32
Cheese Streusel	½ muffin (2 oz)	220	10	30	18

FOOD	PORTION	CALS	FAT	CARB	SUGAR
TAKE-OUT					
corn	1 lg (2.5 oz)	214	7	32	5
raisin bran lowfat	1 (4 oz)	270	1	61	35
MULBERRIES					
fresh	1 cup	61	1	14	–
MULLET					
striped cooked	3 oz	127	4	0	0
MUNG BEANS					
dried cooked	1 cup	213	1	39	–
MUNGO BEANS					
dried cooked	1 cup	190	1	33	–
MUSHROOMS					
CANNED					
pieces	½ cup	19	tr	4	–
Green Giant					
Pieces & Stems	½ cup	30	0	4	1
Sunny Dell					
Portabella Sliced	½ cup	20	0	4	0
DRIED					
chanterelle	1 oz	25	tr	tr	–
cloud ear	1 (5 g)	13	tr	3	–
shiitake	4 (½ oz)	44	tr	11	–
straw	1 piece (6 g)	2	tr	tr	–
tree ear	½ cup (0.4 oz)	36	tr	10	–
wood ear mok yee	½ cup (0.4 oz)	25	tr	8	–
Frieda's					
Chanterelle	2 pieces (4 g)	15	0	2	0
Wood Ear	3 pieces (4 g)	15	0	2	0
FRESH					
chanterelle	3.5 oz	11	tr	tr	–
enoki raw	1 (4 in)	2	tr	tr	–

FOOD	PORTION	CALS	FAT	CARB	SUGAR
oyster raw	1 sm (0.5 oz)	6	tr	1	–
raw sliced	½ cup	9	tr	2	–
sliced cooked	½ cup	21	tr	4	–
Frieda's					
Enoki	¼ pkg (1 oz)	10	0	2	1

MUSKRAT

roasted	3 oz	199	10	0	0

MUSSELS

blue raw	1 cup	129	3	6	–
fresh blue cooked	3 oz	147	4	6	–

MUSTARD

dry mustard	1 tsp	15	1	1	–
organic yellow	1 tsp	5	0	0	0
Country Cupboard					
Smokey Garlic or Horseradish	1 tsp	10	0	2	1
French's					
Classic Yellow	1 tsp	0	0	0	0
Gulden's					
Spicy Brown	1 tsp	5	0	0	0
Hebrew National					
Deli	1 tsp	4	0	0	0

MUSTARD GREENS

fresh chopped cooked	½ cup	11	tr	1	–

NATTO

natto	½ cup	187	10	13	–

NAVY BEANS

DRIED

cooked	1 cup	259	1	48	–

FOOD	PORTION	CALS	FAT	CARB	SUGAR
NECTARINE					
fresh	1	67	1	16	—
NEUFCHATEL					
neufchatel	1 oz	74	7	1	—
Back To Nature					
Organic	⅛ pkg (1 oz)	70	6	tr	tr
NOODLES					
egg cooked	1 cup (5.6 oz)	213	2	40	—
japanese soba cooked	1 cup (4 oz)	113	tr	24	—
japanese somen cooked	1 cup (6.2 oz)	231	tr	48	—
rice cooked	1 cup (6.2 oz)	192	tr	44	—
A Taste Of Thai					
Rice Wide	2 oz	200	0	46	0
Azumaya					
Asian Style Thin Cut	1 cup	210	1	43	1
Manischewitz					
Fine Yolk Free	1½ cups	210	1	40	2
Wide Yolk Free	1¾ cups	210	1	40	2
Nasoya					
Chinese	1 cup	210	1	43	1
Japanese	1 cup	210	1	43	1
Spinach	1 cup	210	1	42	1
Pennsylvania Dutch					
Yolk Free Ribbons as prep	1½ cups	210	1	41	2
NOPALES					
cooked	1 cup (5.2 oz)	23	tr	5	—
NUTMEG					
ground	1 tsp	12	1	1	—
NUTRITION SUPPLEMENTS					
Boost					
Breeze	8 oz	160	0	31	31

FOOD	PORTION	CALS	FAT	CARB	SUGAR
Diabetic	8 oz	250	12	20	–
DiabetiTrim					
Shake French Vanilla	1 pkg	90	1	10	5
Ensure					
Creamy Milk Chocolate Shake	1 can (8 oz)	350	11	50	18
Plus Vanilla Shake	1 bottle (8 oz)	350	11	50	16
PowerBar					
Powergel All Flavors	1 pkg (1.4 oz)	120	2	26	7
Pria					
Complete Shake Creamy Milk Chocolate	1 pkg (11.6 oz)	170	5	21	13
Complete Shake French Vanilla	1 pkg (11.6 oz)	170	5	22	14
Resource					
Beneprotein Protein Powder	1 scoop	25	0	0	0
Optisource High Protein Drink	1 box (4 oz)	100	3	6	0
Slim-Fast					
Optima Ready-To-Drink All Flavors	1 can	180	5	24	17
Optima Shake Mix Chocolate Royale as prep w/ fat free milk	1 serv	190	5	29	21
Optima Shake Mix French Vanilla as prep w/ fat free milk	1 serv	200	4	30	22
Vitasoy					
Weight Management Meal All Flavors	1 bottle (10 oz)	200	1	39	31

FOOD	PORTION	CALS	FAT	CARB	SUGAR
NUTS MIXED					
oil roasted w/o peanuts salted	¼ cup	221	20	8	2
Estee					
Chocolate Covered Fruit & Nut Mix Fructose Sweetened	¼ cup	210	12	19	10
Good Sense					
Deluxe Mix	¼ cup	180	13	8	2
Here's Howe					
Royal Mixed Nuts	1 oz	180	17	7	2
Judy's					
Sugar Free Mixed Nut Brittle	¼ piece (1 oz)	120	7	3	0
Kind					
Nut Delight	1 bar (1.4 oz)	203	15	12	8
Mauna Loa					
Macadamia Mixed	¼ cup	190	15	8	1
Macadamias & Cashews	¼ cup	180	15	8	1
Organic Trails					
Tamari Roasted Nuts & Seeds	¼ cup	190	15	10	1
Planters					
NUT-rition Heart Healthy Mix	1 pkg (1.5 oz)	260	23	8	2
OCA					
Frieda's					
Oca	½ cup	70	0	15	0
OCTOPUS					
fresh steamed	3 oz	140	2	4	–
OHELOBERRIES					
fresh	1 cup	39	tr	10	–

FOOD	PORTION	CALS	FAT	CARB	SUGAR
OIL					
almond	1 tbsp	120	14	0	0
apricot kernel	1 tbsp	120	14	0	0
avocado	1 tbsp	124	14	0	0
butter oil	1 tbsp	112	13	0	0
canola	1 tbsp	124	14	0	0
coconut	1 tbsp	117	14	0	0
corn	1 tbsp	120	14	0	0
cottonseed	1 tbsp	120	14	0	0
garlic oil	1 tbsp	150	17	0	0
grapeseed	1 tbsp	120	14	0	0
hazelnut	1 tbsp	120	14	0	0
mustard	1 tbsp	124	14	0	0
olive	1 tbsp	119	14	0	0
peanut	1 tbsp	119	14	0	0
peppermint	1 tsp	42	4	0	0
rice bran	1 tbsp	120	14	0	0
safflower	1 tbsp	120	14	0	0
sesame	1 tbsp	120	14	0	0
soybean	1 tbsp	120	14	0	0
sunflower	1 tbsp	120	14	0	0
teaseed	1 tbsp	120	14	0	0
walnut	1 tbsp	120	14	0	0
wheat germ	1 tbsp	120	14	0	0
Alpha					
Hazelnut	1 oz	257	29	0	0
Consorzio					
Dipping Oil	1 tbsp	120	14	0	0
Olive Basil	1 tbsp	120	14	0	0
Olive Roasted Pepper	1 tbsp	120	14	0	0
Organic Extra Virgin Olive Meyer Lemon	1 tbsp	120	14	0	0

FOOD	PORTION	CALS	FAT	CARB	SUGAR
Enova					
Oil	1 tbsp	120	14	0	0
Hollywood					
Safflower	1 tbsp	120	14	0	0
Mazola					
Corn	1 tbsp	120	14	0	0
No Stick Spray	⅓ sec spray	0	0	0	0
Pure Cooking Spray Canola All Flavors	¼ sec spray	0	0	0	0
Right Blend	1 tbsp	120	14	0	0
Vegetable	1 tbsp	120	14	0	0
Nutiva					
Coconut Organic Extra Virgin	1 tbsp	120	14	0	0
Hemp Organic Cold Pressed	1 tbsp	120	14	0	0
Orville Redenbacher's					
Popping & Topping	1 tbsp	120	14	0	0
Pam					
Cooking Spray All Types	⅓ sec spray	0	0	0	0
Spectrum					
Almond	1 tbsp	120	14	0	0
Apricot Kernel	1 tbsp	120	14	0	0
Avocado	1 tbsp	120	14	0	0
Canola Organic	1 tbsp	120	14	0	0
Coconut Organic	1 tbsp	120	14	0	0
Corn	1 tbsp	120	14	0	0
Grapeseed	1 tbsp	120	14	0	0
Grapeseed Oil Spray	⅓ sec spray	0	0	0	0
Hazelnut Toasted Organic	1 tbsp	120	14	0	0
Mediterranean Olive Organic	1 tbsp	120	14	0	0

FOOD	PORTION	CALS	FAT	CARB	SUGAR
Organic Extra Virgin Oil Spray	⅓ sec spray	0	0	0	0
Peanut	1 tbsp	120	14	0	0
Pumpkin Seed Organic	1 tbsp	120	14	0	0
Sesame Organic	1 tbsp	120	14	0	0
Sesame Toasted Organic	1 tbsp	120	14	0	0
Soy Organic	1 tbsp	120	14	0	0
Sunflower Organic	1 tbsp	120	14	0	0
Walnut	1 tbsp	120	14	0	0
Walnut Organic	1 tbsp	120	14	0	0
Wesson					
Canola	1 tbsp	120	14	0	0
OKRA					
CANNED					
pickled	6 pods (2.3 oz)	18	tr	4	1
Glory					
Cut	½ cup	25	0	6	2
FRESH					
cooked w/ salt	8 pods	19	tr	4	2
luffa chinese okra cooked	1 cup	39	tr	8	4
sliced cooked w/ salt	½ cup	18	tr	4	2
TAKE-OUT					
batter dipped fried	10 pieces (2.6 oz)	142	10	12	3
OLIVES					
green	4 med	15	2	tr	—
green olive tapenade	1 tbsp	25	3	1	1
ripe	1 sm	4	tr	tr	—
spanish stuffed	5 (0.5 oz)	15	1	1	0
ONION					
DRIED					
flakes	1 tbsp	16	tr	4	—

FOOD	PORTION	CALS	FAT	CARB	SUGAR
powder	1 tsp	7	tr	2	–
shallots	1 tbsp	3	0	1	–
FRESH					
chopped cooked	½ cup	47	tr	11	–
raw chopped	1 tbsp	4	tr	1	–
scallions raw chopped	1 tbsp	2	tr	tr	–
shallots raw chopped	1 tbsp	7	tr	2	–
Antioch Farms					
Vidalia	1 med	60	0	14	–
Frieda's					
Cipolline	3 (3 oz)	30	0	7	5
Maui	⅓ cup (1.1 oz)	10	0	3	2
Pearl	⅔ cup (3 oz)	30	0	7	5
Nature's Harvest					
Onion	1 med (5.2 oz)	60	0	14	9
TAKE-OUT					
fried	½ cup (7.5 oz)	176	11	17	–
rings breaded & fried	8 to 9	275	16	31	–

OPOSSUM

roasted	3 oz	188	9	0	0

ORANGE
CANNED
Del Monte

SunFresh Mandarin	½ cup	80	0	19	17

Dole

Fruit Bowls Mandarin Oranges	1 pkg	70	0	18	17

FRESH

california navel	1	65	tr	16	–
california valencia	1	59	tr	14	–
florida	1	69	tr	17	–
peel	1 tbsp	6	tr	2	–

FOOD	PORTION	CALS	FAT	CARB	SUGAR
sections	1 cup	85	tr	21	—
Frieda's					
Cara Cara	1 med (5 oz)	70	0	16	12
Mandarin Delite	1 cup (5 oz)	60	0	16	12
Mandarin Page	1 cup (5 oz)	60	0	12	12
Mandarin Pixie	1 cup (5 oz)	60	0	16	12
Mandarin Satsuma	1 (5 oz)	60	0	16	12
Melogold	½ (6 oz)	50	0	13	10
Seville	1 (3 oz)	40	0	10	8
Sunkist					
Cara Cara Navel	1 med	80	0	21	14
Minneola Tangelo	1 (3.8 oz)	70	0	13	11
Moro	1 (5.4 oz)	70	0	16	13
Orange	1 med	80	0	21	14
Satsuma Mandarin	1 (3.8 oz)	50	0	11	9

ORANGE JUICE
Bright & Early

FOOD	PORTION	CALS	FAT	CARB	SUGAR
Orange Drink	8 oz	110	0	30	28
Dole					
100% Juice	8 oz	110	0	27	23
Hi-C					
Blast Orange Drink	8 oz	120	0	33	30
Orange Lavaburst	1 box	90	0	25	25
Hood					
100% Juice	1 cup	120	0	30	30
Italian Volcano					
Blood Orange Organic	1 serv (6.75 oz)	84	0	21	19
Minute Maid					
Country Style	8 oz	110	0	27	24
Heart Wise	8 oz	110	0	27	24
Kids+	8 oz	110	0	27	24
Light	8 oz	50	0	13	10
Original	8 oz	110	0	27	24

FOOD	PORTION	CALS	FAT	CARB	SUGAR
Plus Calcium	8 oz	110	0	27	24
W/ Extra Vitamin C & E Plus Zinc	8 oz	110	0	27	24
Naked Juice					
Just OJ	8 oz	110	0	25	25
Ocean Spray					
100% Juice	8 oz	120	0	31	31
Simply Orange					
Pulp Free w/ Calcium	8 oz	110	0	26	22
Snapple					
Orangeade	8 oz	120	0	29	29
Tropicana					
Grovestand	8 oz	110	0	26	22
Healthy Heart	8 oz	110	0	26	22
Healthy Kids	8 oz	110	0	26	22
HomeStyle	8 oz	110	0	26	22
Immunity Defense	8 oz	110	0	26	22
Light'N Healthy	8 oz	50	0	13	10
Low Acid	8 oz	110	0	26	22
With Calcium + Vitamin D	8 oz	110	0	26	22
TAKE-OUT					
orange julius	1 serv (24 oz)	443	tr	118	–
OREGANO					
ground	1 tsp	5	tr	1	–
OYSTERS					
canned eastern	1 cup	112	4	6	0
eastern baked	6 med	47	1	4	–
eastern raw	6 med	50	1	5	–
eastern sauteed	6 med	76	5	3	0
smoked	6	33	1	2	0

FOOD	PORTION	CALS	FAT	CARB	SUGAR
Brunswick					
Smoked	1 can (3 oz)	140	8	7	0
Bumble Bee					
Smoked	¼ cup	120	7	6	0
Whole	¼ cup	70	3	3	0
Chicken Of The Sea					
Smoked In Oil	1 can (3.75 oz)	140	8	8	0
Smoked In Water	1 can (3.75 oz)	120	3	10	0
Smoked Teriyaki	1 can (3.75 oz)	120	3	12	6
Whole	½ can (2 oz)	80	3	6	0
TAKE-OUT					
breaded & fried	6	368	18	40	–
fritter	1 (1.4 oz)	121	6	12	tr
oysters rockefeller	1 cup	302	17	22	2
PANCAKE/WAFFLE SYRUP					
lite	¼ cup	98	0	27	20
pancake syrup	1 pkg (2 oz)	156	tr	41	38
pancake syrup	¼ cup	209	tr	55	50
Aunt Jemima					
Original	¼ cup	210	0	52	32
Country Cupboard					
Boysenberry	¼ cup	0	0	0	0
Maple Butter	¼ cup	0	0	2	0
Strawberry	¼ cup	0	0	1	0
Estee					
Maple	¼ cup	30	0	7	0
Karo					
Pancake Syrup	¼ cup	240	0	63	25
Keto					
Maple Butter	¼ cup	0	0	1	1
Ketogenics					
Zero Carb	¼ cup	0	0	0	0

FOOD	PORTION	CALS	FAT	CARB	SUGAR
Log Cabin					
Lite	¼ cup	100	0	25	24
Mrs. Butter-worth's					
Lite	¼ cup	100	0	25	24
Original	¼ cup (2 oz)	230	0	56	35
Smucker's					
Breakfast Syrup Sugar Free	¼ cup	30	0	8	0
Stonewall Kitchen					
Maine Maple	¼ cup	210	0	54	51
PANCAKES					
FROZEN					
Golden					
Potato	1 (1.3 oz)	70	3	10	2
Inland Valley					
Potato	1 (2 oz)	120	8	12	tr
MIX					
Aunt Jemima					
Buttermilk Pancake & Waffle Mix not prep	⅓ cup	160	3	31	6
Pancake & Waffle Mix Whole Wheat as prep	3 pancakes	200	7	30	4
Aunt Paula's					
Pancake & Waffle Mix as prep	2	132	8	6	0
Big Train					
Low Carb Pancake & Waffle Mix as prep	3	190	10	12	0
Carbolite					
Low Carb Mix not prep	⅓ cup	100	tr	10	0
Carbsense					
Buckwheat not prep	½ cup	140	3	10	0
Buttermilk not prep	½ cup	140	3	10	0

FOOD	PORTION	CALS	FAT	CARB	SUGAR
Hungry Jack					
Buttermilk Pancake & Waffle as prep	3 (4-inch) pancakes	150	2	31	7
Keto					
Banana not prep	⅓ cup	114	2	6	0
Original not prep	⅓ cup	114	2	5	0
Ketogenics					
Low Carb not prep	⅔ cup	185	4	15	1
TAKE-OUT					
buckwheat	1 (7 in)	142	5	19	4
plain	1 (7 in)	183	3	35	10
potato	1 (1.3 oz)	70	4	8	tr
w/ butter & syrup	2 (8.1 oz)	520	14	91	—
whole wheat	1 (7 in)	183	8	23	5
PAPAYA					
fresh	1	117	tr	30	—
fresh cubed	1 cup	54	tr	14	—
Del Monte					
In Extra Light Syrup w/ Passion Fruit Puree	½ cup	70	0	17	16
Frieda's					
Mexican	1 cup (5 oz)	50	0	14	8
PAPAYA JUICE					
nectar	1 cup	142	tr	36	—
Ceres					
Papaya	8 oz	120	0	30	27
PAPRIKA					
paprika	1 tsp	6	tr	1	—
PARSLEY					
dry	1 tsp	1	tr	tr	—
fresh chopped	½ cup	11	tr	2	—

FOOD	PORTION	CALS	FAT	CARB	SUGAR
Frieda's					
Parsley Root	⅔ cup	10	1	2	0
PARSNIPS					
fresh cooked	1 (5.6 oz)	130	tr	31	–
fresh sliced cooked	½ cup	63	tr	15	–
Frieda's					
Sliced	1 cup	100	0	24	6
PASSION FRUIT JUICE					
Ceres					
Passion Fruit	8 oz	120	0	31	28
PASTA					
DRY					
Barilla					
Pastina	2 oz	210	2	40	tr
Penne	1 cup (2 oz)	200	1	42	1
Plus Penne	2 oz	200	1	38	1
Tortelloni Ricotta & Spinach	¾ cup	240	8	31	3
Catelli					
Bistro Cracked Black Pepper Fettucine	¼ pkg	320	1	65	7
Bistro Italian Herb Fettuccine	¼ pkg	310	2	64	5
Bistro Lemon Pepper Linguine	¼ pkg	320	2	64	9
Bistro Rainbows	3 oz	320	1	66	6
Bistro Spinach Lasagne	3 oz	320	2	64	4
Bistro Sun Dried Tomato & Basil Spaghettini	¼ pkg	320	2	65	7
Bistro Vegetable Fusilli	3 oz	320	1	65	4
Healthy Harvest Flax Omega-3	3 oz	290	3	60	17

FOOD	PORTION	CALS	FAT	CARB	SUGAR
Healthy Harvest Multigrain	3 oz	310	2	60	3
Healthy Harvest Organic Whole Wheat	3 oz	320	2	64	3
Healthy Harvest Whole Wheat All Shapes	3 oz	310	2	62	4
Darielle					
All Shapes not prep	2 oz	160	1	18	3
DaVinci					
Spaghetti	2 oz	210	1	43	3
Dreamfields					
All Shapes not prep	2 oz	190	1	42	1
Food For Life					
Ezekiel 4:9 Sprouted Grain	2 oz	210	2	39	0
Keto					
Elbows not prep	1.6 oz	108	0	5	0
Spaghetti not prep	1.3 oz	130	1	7	0
LifeStream					
Organic All Shapes	2 oz	208	4	36	3
Notta Pasta					
Rice Pasta All Shapes	2 oz	200	0	48	0
Pastalia					
Heart Health Low Carb not prep	2 oz	176	2	10	tr
Ronzoni					
Healthy Harvest Whole Wheat Blend Thin Spaghetti	½ pkg (2 oz)	180	1	42	1
Lasagne	2½ pieces (2 oz)	210	1	42	2
Tradizione D'Italia All Shapes	2 oz	210	1	42	2
San Giorgio					
Elbows not prep	½ cup	210	1	42	2

FOOD	PORTION	CALS	FAT	CARB	SUGAR
Whey Cool					
High Protein Xtreme Rotini	1 serv (2 oz)	210	2	8	4
REFRIGERATED					
Buitoni					
Angel Hair	1¼ cups	230	3	43	1
Fettuccine	1¼ cups	240	3	45	1
Fettuccine Spinach	1¼ cups	260	3	45	1
Linguine	1¼ cups	240	3	45	1
Ravioletti Three Cheese	1 cup	270	6	43	3
Ravioli Doublestuffed Mozzarella & Herb	1½ cups	340	12	43	3
Ravioli Four Cheese	1¼ cups	330	14	40	3
Ravioli Chicken & Roasted Garlic	1¼ cups	340	11	47	3
Ravioli Chicken Parmesan	1¼ cups	310	8	45	3
Ravioli Classic Beef	1¼ cups	340	10	48	4
Ravioli Garden Vegetable	1 cup	250	5	39	4
Ravioli Light Four Cheese	1¼ cups	230	4	37	3
Tortellini Herb Chicken	1 cup	340	9	52	3
Tortellini Mixed Cheese	1 cup	320	7	50	3
Tortellini Spinach Cheese	1 cup	330	8	49	3
Tortellini Three Cheese	1 cup	320	7	50	4
Tortelloni Cheese & Roasted Garlic	1 cup	270	8	37	2
Tortelloni Chicken & Prosciutto	1 cup	330	9	47	2
Tortelloni Mozzarella & Herb	1 cup	330	9	47	3
Tortelloni Mozzarella & Pepperoni	1 cup	330	10	45	3
Tortelloni Portabello Mushroom & Cheese	1 cup	270	6	46	2

FOOD	PORTION	CALS	FAT	CARB	SUGAR
Tortelloni Sun Dried Tomato	1 cup	310	9	46	4
Tortelloni Sweet Italian Sausage	1 cup	330	9	48	5

PASTA DINNERS
CANNED
Annie's Homegrown

Organic All Stars	1 cup	150	1	31	11
Organic BernieOs	1 cup	150	1	31	11
Organic Cheesy Ravioli	1 cup	180	4	31	9
Organic P'sghetti Loops	1 cup	190	4	29	9

Chef Boyardee

Beefaroni	1 cup	260	9	35	6

FROZEN
Golden Cuisine

Cheese Manicotti	1 pkg	360	12	43	11
Spaghetti & Meatballs	1 pkg	490	22	51	16
Tuna Casserole	1 pkg	386	8	53	7

Healthy Choice

Breaded Chicken Breast w/ Mac & Cheese	1 pkg	290	5	35	5
Fettuccine Alfredo	1 pkg	280	7	40	5
Fettuccine Alfredo Chicken	1 pkg	290	7	32	3
Lasagna Bake	1 pkg (9 oz)	270	7	38	13
Macaroni & Cheese	1 pkg	290	7	44	5
Manicotti	1 pkg	280	5	44	16
Rigatoni w/ Broccoli & Chicken	1 pkg	270	7	29	4
Spaghetti w/ Meat Sauce	1 pkg	310	6	48	8
Stuffed Pasta Shells	1 pkg	290	6	40	10

FOOD	PORTION	CALS	FAT	CARB	SUGAR
Kid Cuisine					
Cheese Blaster Mac & Cheese	1 meal	380	11	58	11
Twist & Twirl Spaghetti w/ Mini Meatballs	1 meal	460	14	66	23
Lean Cuisine					
Cafe Classics Bow Tie Pasta & Chicken	1 pkg (9.5 oz)	240	5	33	7
Cafe Classics Bowl Three Cheese Stuffed Ragatoni	1 pkg (10 oz)	260	7	38	8
Cafe Classics Cheese Lasagna w/ Chicken Breast Scallopini	1 pkg (10 oz)	290	8	36	7
Cafe Classics Four Cheese Cannelloni	1 pkg (9.1 oz)	260	7	30	9
Cafe Classics Grilled Chicken & Penne Pasta	1 pkg (12 oz)	320	5	52	25
Cafe Classics Jumbo Rigatoni w/ Meatballs	1 pkg (15.4 oz)	400	8	58	12
Cafe Classics Lasagna w/ Meat Sauce	1 pkg (10.5 oz)	310	7	43	9
Cafe Classics Macaroni & Beef	1 pkg (9.5 oz)	270	5	39	10
Cafe Classics Macaroni & Cheese	1 pkg (10 oz)	300	7	43	8
Cafe Classics Penne Pasta w/ Tomato Basil Sauce	1 pkg (10 oz)	270	3	51	13
Cafe Classics Roasted Chicken w/ Lemon Pepper Fettuccini	1 pkg (8.1 oz)	250	6	32	3
Cafe Classics Shrimp & Angel Hair Pasta	1 pkg (10 oz)	240	5	35	8

FOOD	PORTION	CALS	FAT	CARB	SUGAR
Cafe Classics Spaghetti w/ Meat Sauce	1 pkg (11.5 oz)	280	4	48	9
Cafe Classics Spaghetti w/ Meatballs	1 pkg (9.5 oz)	270	5	38	7
Dinnertime Selects Chicken Fettuccini	1 pkg (12 oz)	360	7	54	26
One Dish Favorites Alfredo Pasta w/ Chicken & Broccoli	1 pkg (10 oz)	270	6	38	6
One Dish Favorites Angel Hair Pasta Marinara	1 pkg (10 oz)	260	4	48	10
One Dish Favorites Cheese Ravioli	1 pkg (8.5 oz)	250	6	38	10
One Dish Favorites Chicken Fettuccini	1 pkg (9.25 oz)	280	7	33	6
One Dish Favorites Lasagna Cheese Florentine Bake	1 pkg (10 oz)	270	6	35	8
One Dish Favorites Lasagna Chicken Florentine	1 pkg (10 oz)	270	6	35	8
One Dish Favorites Lasagna Classic Five Cheese	1 pkg (11.5 oz)	330	7	48	11
Skillet Chicken Alfredo	1 serv	180	4	25	5
Michelina's					
Lasagna w/ Meat Sauce	1 pkg (9 oz)	280	8	40	7
Savvy Faire					
Lasagna Florentine	1 pkg (9.2 oz)	300	19	14	4
Slim-Fast					
Fettuccine Alfredo	1 pkg	240	6	41	4

FOOD	PORTION	CALS	FAT	CARB	SUGAR
Rotini w/ Tomato & Italian Herb	1 pkg	240	2	45	7
Shells & Creamy Cheese Sauce	1 pkg	240	6	40	5
South Beach Diet					
Penne & Chicken In Roasted Red Pepper Sauce	1 pkg	290	13	26	5
Stouffer's					
Lasagna w/ Meat Sauce	1 cup	250	8	27	5
MIX					
A Taste Of Thai					
Coconut Ginger	1 cup	280	7	5	2
Pad Thai For Two	½ pkg	345	1	89	8
Peanut Noodles as prep	1 cup	330	10	53	11
Red Curry Noodles as prep	1 cup	280	8	51	6
Annie's Homegrown					
Gluten Free Rice Pasta & Cheddar as prep	1 cup	330	5	60	4
Organic Shells & Real Aged Wisconsin Cheddar as prep	1 cup	370	15	48	2
Organic Skillet Meals Beef Stroganoff as prep	1 cup	320	13	16	4
Organic Skillet Meals Cheddar & Herb Chicken as prep	1 cup	310	7	30	35
Organic Skillet Meals Cheeseburger Macaroni as prep	1 cup	350	13	27	4
Organic Skillet Meals Cheese Lasagna as prep	1 cup	280	9	25	75

FOOD	PORTION	CALS	FAT	CARB	SUGAR
Organic Skillet Meals Chicken Fettucine as prep	1 cup	330	8	27	3
Organic Skillet Meals Creamy Tuna Spirals as prep	1 cup	260	7	30	3
Organic Whole Wheat Shells & Cheddar as prep	1 cup	360	15	48	2
Shells & Real Aged Wisconsin Cheddar as prep	1 cup	290	5	51	5
Shells & White Cheddar as prep	1 cup	290	5	51	5
Aramana					
Cheddar Cheeseburger as prep	1 cup	260	17	11	2
Creamy Chicken Alfredo as prep	1 cup	260	16	12	2
Mild Mexican as prep	1 cup	260	16	12	2
Back To Nature					
Alfredo & Gemelli as prep	1 cup	340	11	48	6
Macaroni & Cheese as prep	1 cup	320	10	48	7
White Cheddar & Spirals as prep	1 cup	330	12	48	8
Keto					
Macaroni & Cheese not prep	1 serv	112	10	5	0
Near East					
Angel Hair w/ Spicy Tomato as prep	1 cup	240	6	39	3
Radiatore Basil & Herb as prep	1 cup	240	6	39	2

FOOD	PORTION	CALS	FAT	CARB	SUGAR
Vermicelli Garlic & Oil as prep	1 cup	310	9	48	3
Whey Cool					
High Protein Macaroni & Cheese as prep	1 serv	260	5	12	7
REFRIGERATED					
Country Crock					
Elbow Macaroni & Cheese	1 cup	380	17	40	5
TAKE-OUT					
bami goreng indonesian noodle dish	1 cup	170	3	25	4
lasagna	1 piece (2.5 in x 2.5 in)	374	21	25	—
macaroni & cheese	1 cup	230	10	26	—
manicotti	¾ cup (6.4 oz)	273	12	28	—
rigatoni w/ sausage sauce	¾ cup	260	12	28	—
spaghetti w/ meatballs & cheese	1 cup	407	19	38	—

PASTA SALAD
TAKE-OUT

FOOD	PORTION	CALS	FAT	CARB	SUGAR
pasta salad w/ crab vegetables mayonnaise	1 cup	317	16	33	2

PATE

FOOD	PORTION	CALS	FAT	CARB	SUGAR
chicken liver canned	1 tbsp (13 g)	109	2	1	—
duck pate	1 oz	96	8	1	tr
mushroom anchovy pate	1 can (2.25 oz)	130	11	7	1
pate foie gras	1 oz	127	13	1	—
pork pate	1 oz	107	10	1	1
pork pate en croute	1 oz	91	7	3	tr
shrimp	1 can (2.25 oz)	140	10	7	1

FOOD	PORTION	CALS	FAT	CARB	SUGAR

PEACH
CANNED

FOOD	PORTION	CALS	FAT	CARB	SUGAR
peachsauce	½ cup	120	0	32	31
Del Monte					
Freestone Lite Slices	½ cup	60	0	14	13
Freestone Sliced	½ cup	100	0	24	23
Fruit Naturals Chunks	½ cup	70	0	17	16
Halves In Heavy Syrup	½ cup	100	0	24	23
Orchard Select Sliced Cling	½ cup	80	0	22	19
Sliced In 100% Juice	½ cup	60	0	15	14
Dole					
All Natural Yellow Cling Sliced	½ cup	80	0	17	16
Liberty Gold					
Sliced Cling In Heavy Syrup	½ cup	100	0	24	23
S&W					
Slices Lightly Sweetened Juice	½ cup	80	0	19	18

DRIED

FOOD	PORTION	CALS	FAT	CARB	SUGAR
halves	10	311	1	80	–
Crispy Green					
Crispy Peaches	1 pkg (0.36 oz)	38	0	9	7

FRESH

FOOD	PORTION	CALS	FAT	CARB	SUGAR
peach	1	37	tr	10	–

PEACH JUICE

FOOD	PORTION	CALS	FAT	CARB	SUGAR
nectar	1 cup	134	tr	35	–
Ceres					
Peach	8 oz	120	0	30	26

PEANUT BUTTER
Carb Options

FOOD	PORTION	CALS	FAT	CARB	SUGAR
Creamy	2 tbsp	190	17	5	tr

FOOD	PORTION	CALS	FAT	CARB	SUGAR
Estee					
Creamy Low Sodium	2 tbsp	180	16	6	1
Jif					
Creamy	2 tbsp	190	16	7	3
Reduced Fat Creamy	2 tbsp (1.3 oz)	190	12	15	4
Maranatha					
Crunchy	2 tbsp	190	16	7	2
Salted	2 tbsp	190	16	7	2
Peanut Butter & Co.					
Cinnamon Raisin Swirl	2 tbsp	143	7	10	4
Crunch Time	2 tbsp	200	16	7	2
Dark Chocolate Dreams	2 tbsp	175	12	8	3
Smooth Operator	2 tbsp	200	16	7	2
The Heat Is On	2 tbsp	164	10	9	4
White Chocolate Wonderful	1 tbsp	165	12	8	3
Skippy					
Creamy	2 tbsp	190	17	7	3
Reduced Fat Creamy	2 tbsp	190	12	15	5
Roasted Honey Nut	2 tbsp	190	17	7	3
Roasted Honey Nut Super Chunk	2 tbsp	190	17	7	3
Squeeze Stix	1 pkg	140	12	5	3
Squeeze Stix Chocolate	1 pkg	140	10	9	7
Squeez'It	2 tbsp	190	17	7	3
Super Chunk	2 tbsp	190	17	7	3
Super Chunk Reduced Fat	2 tbsp	190	12	14	4
Smucker's					
Goober All Flavors	3 tbsp	240	13	24	21
Natural Chunky	2 tbsp	210	16	6	1
Natural Creamy	2 tbsp	210	16	6	1
Natural Honey	2 tbsp	200	16	9	4

FOOD	PORTION	CALS	FAT	CARB	SUGAR
Natural No Salt Added Creamy	2 tbsp	210	16	7	6
Natural Reduced Fat Creamy	2 tbsp	200	12	12	2
PEANUTS					
chocolate coated	10 (1.4 oz)	208	13	20	–
cooked	½ cup	102	7	7	–
dry roasted w/ salt	30 nuts (1 oz)	170	14	6	2
A Taste Of Thai					
Spicy Peanut Bake	¼ pkg	45	2	7	5
At Last!					
Chocolate Covered	1 pkg (0.9 oz)	150	11	18	0
Brach's					
Double Dippers Chocolate Covered	15 pieces	210	12	23	19
Estee					
Chocolate Coated Fructose Sweetened	¼ cup	170	9	23	6
Frito Lay					
Salted	1 oz	160	14	6	1
Salted w/ Shells	½ cup	160	14	6	1
Judy's					
Sugar Free Coconut Peanut Brittle	¼ piece (1 oz)	90	5	2	0
Low Carb Creations					
Soft Peanut Brittle	2 pieces (1 oz)	140	10	8	<2
Planters					
Honey Roasted	1 oz	160	13	8	4
Sweet Delight					
Peanut Roasters	⅓ pkg (1 oz)	160	12	7	tr

FOOD	PORTION	CALS	FAT	CARB	SUGAR
PEAR					
CANNED					
Del Monte					
Carb Clever Sliced	½ cup	40	0	10	9
Halves In 100% Juice	½ cup	60	0	15	14
Halves In Light Syrup	½ cup	60	0	15	14
Orchard Select Sliced Bartlett	½ cup	80	0	20	19
S&W					
Halves In Lightly Sweetened Juice	½ cup	80	0	21	17
DRIED					
halves	10	459	1	122	—
FRESH					
asian	1 (4.3 oz)	51	tr	13	—
pear	1	98	1	25	—
sliced w/ skin	1 cup	97	1	25	—
PEAR JUICE					
nectar	1 cup	149	tr	39	—
Ceres					
Pear	8 oz	120	0	30	29
PEAS					
CANNED					
Del Monte					
Sweet	½ cup	60	0	13	6
Sweet Very Young Small	½ cup	60	0	10	5
Green Giant					
Sweet	½ cup	60	0	12	5
Libby's					
No Salt No Sugar Added	½ cup	70	1	10	5
DRIED					
split cooked	1 cup	231	1	41	-

FOOD	PORTION	CALS	FAT	CARB	SUGAR
FRESH					
green cooked	½ cup	67	tr	13	—
green raw	½ cup	58	tr	11	—
snap peas cooked	½ cup	34	tr	6	—
snap peas raw	½ cup	30	tr	5	—
Frieda's					
Snow Peas	1 cup	35	0	6	3
Sugar Snap	⅔ cup (3 oz)	35	0	6	3
River Ranch					
Sugar Snap	1½ cups	35	0	6	4
FROZEN					
Green Giant					
Sweet	⅔ cup	70	1	12	6
Pictsweet					
Green Peas	⅔ cup	70	0	12	4
TAKE-OUT					
pea & potato curry	1 serv (7 oz)	284	22	19	—
pea curry	1 serv (4.4 oz)	438	42	11	—
PECANS					
candied	1 oz	190	17	10	4
halves dry roasted w/ salt	20 (1 oz)	200	21	4	1
Keto					
Chocolately Covered	1 oz	207	19	6	0
Sweet Delights					
Pecan Roasters	⅓ pkg (1 oz)	210	21	4	1
PEPEAO					
dried	½ cup	36	tr	10	—
PEPPER					
black	1 tsp	5	tr	1	—
cayenne	1 tsp	6	tr	1	—
red	1 tsp	6	tr	1	—
white	1 tsp	7	tr	2	—

FOOD	PORTION	CALS	FAT	CARB	SUGAR
McCormick					
Lemon & Pepper Seasoning Salt	¼ tsp	0	0	0	0
PEPPERS					
FRESH					
banana	1 (4 in) (1.2 oz)	9	tr	2	–
chili green hot	1	18	tr	4	–
chili red hot	1 (1.6 oz)	18	tr	4	–
green	1 (2.6 oz)	20	tr	5	–
green chopped cooked	½ cup	19	tr	5	–
habanero chile	1 tsp	9	tr	2	–
jalapeno	1 (0.5 oz)	4	tr	1	–
red	1 (2.6 oz)	20	tr	5	–
red chopped cooked	½ cup	19	tr	5	–
serrano	1 (6 g)	2	tr	tr	–
yellow	1 (6.5 oz)	50	tr	12	–
PERCH					
FRESH					
cooked	3 oz	99	1	0	0
ocean perch atlantic cooked	3 oz	103	2	0	0
PERSIMMONS					
dried japanese	1	93	tr	25	–
fresh	1	32	tr	8	–
fresh japanese	1	118	tr	31	–
Frieda's					
Dried Fuyu	⅓ cup (1.4 oz)	140	0	35	27
PHEASANT					
breast w/o skin raw	½ breast (6.4 oz)	243	6	0	0
leg w/o skin raw	1 (3.6 oz)	143	5	0	0
roasted	3.5 oz	215	9	0	0

FOOD	PORTION	CALS	FAT	CARB	SUGAR
w/ skin raw	½ pheasant (14 oz)	723	37	0	0
w/o skin raw	½ pheasant (12.4 oz)	470	13	0	0

PHYLLO
Ekizian
Sheets	¼ lb	433	9	76	2

PICKLES
bread & butter	6 slices	39	tr	9	4
dill	1 lg (4.7 oz)	24	tr	6	5
dill sliced	6 slices	7	tr	2	1
sweet gherkin	1 (1.2 oz)	41	tr	11	5
tsukemono japanese pickles sliced	¼ cup	10	tr	2	1

Claussen
Kosher Dills Whole	½ (1 oz)	5	0	1	0

Del Monte
Dill Halves	1 piece (1 oz)	5	0	1	0
Hamburger Dill Chips	1 serv (1 oz)	0	0	0	0
Sweet	1 serv (1 oz)	40	0	10	10
Sweet Gerkins	1 serv (1 oz)	40	0	10	10
Tiny Kosher Dill	1 serv (1 oz)	5	0	1	0

Hebrew National
Dill	1	23	0	4	2

Mt Olive
Bread & Butter No Sugar Added	1 oz	0	0	tr	0

PIE
FROZEN
Edwards
Pie Slices Oreo Cream	1 slice (2.6 oz)	290	17	32	22

FOOD	PORTION	CALS	FAT	CARB	SUGAR
Mrs. Smith's					
Dutch Apple	1 slice (3.3 oz)	260	10	40	19
TAKE-OUT					
apple	⅛ of 9 in pie (5.4 oz)	411	19	58	–
banana cream	⅛ of 9 in pie (5.2 oz)	398	20	49	–
blueberry	⅛ of 9 in pie (5.2 oz)	360	18	49	–
butterscotch	⅛ of 9 in pie (4.5 oz)	355	18	42	–
cherry	⅛ of 9 in pie (6.3 oz)	486	22	69	–
chocolate creme	1 slice (4 oz)	344	22	38	–
coconut creme	⅛ of 9 in pie (4.7 oz)	396	21	46	–
coconut custard	⅙ of 8 in pie (3.6 oz)	271	14	32	–
custard	⅛ of 9 in pie (4.5 oz)	262	11	34	–
key lime	1 slice (5 oz)	420	14	71	28
lemon meringue	1 slice (4.5 oz)	303	10	53	–
mince	⅛ of 9 in pie (5.8 oz)	477	18	79	–
pecan	1 slice (4 oz)	452	21	65	–
pumpkin	1 slice (3.8 oz)	229	10	30	–
vanilla cream	⅛ of 9 in pie (4.4 oz)	350	18	41	–
PIE CRUST					
FROZEN					
baked	9 in crust	884	56	85	17
baked	⅛ of 9 in pie	113	7	11	2
puff pastry shell	1 (1.4 oz)	223	15	18	tr

FOOD	PORTION	CALS	FAT	CARB	SUGAR
tart shell	1 (1 oz)	149	10	14	3
MIX					
Jiffy					
Pie Crust Mix	½ crust	180	10	19	0
MiniCarb					
Pie Crust Mix	1 slice	105	7	1	0
READY-TO-EAT					
chocolate crumb	⅛ of 9 in pie	132	8	14	6
chocolate crumb	1 (9 in crust)	1063	65	114	46
graham cracker	1 (9 in crust)	1037	52	137	81
graham cracker	⅛ of 9 in pie	109	5	14	8
graham cracker dessert shell	1 (1.1 oz)	148	7	20	12
PIE FILLING					
apple	⅛ can (2.6 oz)	74	tr	19	18
Colac					
All Flavors	1 tbsp	19	0	7	0
Comstock					
Light Cherry	⅓ cup	60	0	15	14
PIEROGI					
Mrs. T's					
Potato & Cheddar	3 (4.2 oz)	180	3	34	3
PIG'S EARS AND FEET					
ear simmered	1	184	12	tr	—
feet pickled	1 oz	58	5	tr	—
feet pickled	1 lb	921	73	tr	—
feet simmered	3 oz	165	11	0	0
PIKE					
northern cooked	3 oz	96	1	0	0
walleye baked	3 oz	101	1	0	0

FOOD	PORTION	CALS	FAT	CARB	SUGAR
PIMIENTOS					
canned	1 tbsp	3	tr	1	—
PINE NUTS					
pignolia dried	1 tbsp	51	5	1	—
Frieda's					
Pine Nuts	¼ cup	150	15	4	0
Good Sense					
Pignolias	¼ cup	190	15	9	0
PINEAPPLE					
CANNED					
Del Monte					
Chunks In Heavy Syrup	½ cup	90	0	24	22
Chunks In Its Own Juice	½ cup	70	0	17	15
Crushed In Heavy Syrup	½ cup	90	0	24	22
Crushed In Its Own Juice	½ cup	70	0	17	15
Fruit Naturals Chunks	½ cup	70	0	18	15
Dole					
All Natural Chunks	½ cup	60	0	16	13
Chunks Juice Pack	½ cup	60	0	15	13
Liberty Gold					
Slices Natural Juice	½ cup	80	0	21	19
FRESH					
slice	1 slice	42	tr	10	—
Cala Fruit					
Golden Sliced	1 serv (3.5 oz)	50	0	12	11
Frieda's					
Zululand Queen	1 cup (5 oz)	70	1	17	16
Frosty Fresh					
Peeled & Cored	½ cup	60	0	14	13
PINEAPPLE JUICE					
Adina					
Pineapple Ginger Gin-Jah	8 oz	80	0	19	18

FOOD	PORTION	CALS	FAT	CARB	SUGAR
Ceres					
Pineapple	8 oz	120	0	29	25
PINK BEANS					
dried cooked	1 cup	252	1	47	–
PINTO BEANS					
DRIED					
cooked	1 cup	235	1	44	–
PISTACHIOS					
dry roasted w/ salt	47 nuts (1 oz)	160	13	8	2
dry roasted w/ shells unsalted	½ cup	180	14	9	3
American Almond					
Pistachio Paste	2 tbsp	160	11	14	10
Sweet Delights					
Pistachio Roasters	⅓ pkg (1 oz)	190	14	9	3
PITANGA					
fresh	1	2	tr	1	–
PIZZA					
Celeste					
Cheese	1 (5.5 oz)	360	14	42	5
Freschetta					
Pepperoni	½ pie (5.8 oz)	470	21	51	5
Healthy Choice					
French Bread Cheese	1 pie	340	5	51	8
French Bread Pepperoni	1 pie	340	5	52	8
French Bread Supreme	1 pie	340	5	52	8
French Bread Vegetable	1 pie	320	5	51	8
Jeno's					
Crisp 'N Tasty Cheese	1 pie (6.8 oz)	460	19	52	6
Jiffy					
Crust Mix as prep	⅕ crust	180	4	33	2

FOOD	PORTION	CALS	FAT	CARB	SUGAR
Kid Cuisine					
Cheese Pizza Painter	1 meal	320	6	53	25
Dip & Dunk Cheese Pizza Strips	1 meal	510	14	74	27
Primo Pepperoni Pizza	1 meal	400	7	71	30
Lean Cuisine					
Causal Eating Deluxe	1 pkg (6 oz)	370	9	55	7
Causal Eating Four Cheese	1 pkg (6 oz)	400	9	59	7
Casual Eating French Bread Cheese	1 serv (6 oz)	320	7	47	7
Casual Eating French Bread Deluxe	1 pkg (6.1 oz)	310	9	44	7
Casual Eating French Bread Pepperoni	1 pkg (5.25 oz)	300	7	44	5
Casual Eating Margherita	1 pkg (6 oz)	320	9	48	5
Casual Eating Pepperoni	1 pkg (6 oz)	380	9	55	7
Casual Eating Roasted Vegetable	1 pkg (6 oz)	330	5	58	7
Casual Eating Spinach & Mushroom	1 pkg (6.1 oz)	310	7	46	4
Casual Eating Three Meat	1 pkg (6.4 oz)	350	9	48	6
Lean Pockets					
Pepperoni	1 (4.5 oz)	280	7	42	7
Sausage & Pepperoni	1 (4.5 oz)	280	7	41	9
Red Baron					
Deep Dish Single Pepperoni	1 pizza	460	22	41	3
French Bread Supreme	1 pie (5.8 oz)	370	15	43	3
South Beach Diet					
Deluxe	1 pie (6.8 oz)	280	8	34	6
Four Cheese	1 pie (6.3 oz)	290	9	33	6
Grilled Chicken & Vegetable	1 pie (6.8 oz)	280	8	34	6

FOOD	PORTION	CALS	FAT	CARB	SUGAR
Pepperoni	1 pie (6.3 oz)	290	10	33	6
Totino's					
Crisp Crust Cheese	½ pie	320	14	34	4
TAKE-OUT					
cheese	12 in pie	1121	26	164	–
cheese	⅛ of 12 in pie	140	3	21	–
cheese deep dish individual	1 (5.5 oz)	460	24	47	4
cheese meat & vegetables	12 in pie	1472	43	170	–
cheese meat & vegetables	⅛ of 12 in pie	184	5	21	–
pepperoni	⅛ of 12 in pie	181	7	20	–
pepperoni	12 in pie	1445	56	157	–

PIZZA CRUST

FOOD	PORTION	CALS	FAT	CARB	SUGAR
crust	1 slice (1.7 oz)	130	2	25	1
whole wheat	⅛ crust	140	1	27	0
Alvarado Street Bakery					
Sprouted Wheat California Style	⅛ pie	190	3	35	1
Carbsense					
Garlic & Herb as prep	1 slice	100	1	7	0
Keto					
Dough Mix as prep	1 slice	79	1	5	tr
MiniCarb					
Parmesan Herb Mix as prep	1 slice	130	5	6	0

PIZZA SAUCE

FOOD	PORTION	CALS	FAT	CARB	SUGAR
Hunt's					
Family Favorites	¼ cup	25	0	5	3

PLANTAINS

FOOD	PORTION	CALS	FAT	CARB	SUGAR
cooked mashed	1 cup	232	tr	62	28
sliced cooked	1 cup	179	tr	48	22

FOOD	PORTION	CALS	FAT	CARB	SUGAR
Chester's					
Chips	1 oz	150	9	17	0
TAKE-OUT					
mofongo	1 serv	320	3	71	31
ripe fried	2.8 oz	214	7	38	–
sweet baked w/ ice cream	1 serv	285	8	57	35
PLUMS					
canned in heavy syrup	1 cup	163	tr	42	39
canned purple juice pack	1 cup	146	tr	38	35
canned purple water pack	1 cup	102	tr	27	25
dried japanese	1	9	tr	2	1
fresh	1	30	tr	8	7
pickled	1	34	tr	9	9
POI					
poi	½ cup	134	tr	33	–
POKEBERRY SHOOTS					
cooked	½ cup	16	tr	3	–
POLENTA					
Frieda's					
Organic	2 slices (3.5 oz)	70	0	15	1
POLLACK					
atlantic baked	3 oz	100	1	0	0
POMEGRANATE					
fresh	1	104	tr	26	–
POMEGRANATE JUICE					
Naked Juice					
Pomegranate Passion	8 oz	150	0	38	37
Odwalla					
PomaGrand Berry	8 oz	140	0	35	27
PomaGrand Mango	8 oz	160	0	39	29

FOOD	PORTION	CALS	FAT	CARB	SUGAR
POM					
100% Juice	8 oz	140	0	35	34
Pomegranate Blueberry	8 oz	140	0	34	24
Pomegranate Cherry	8 oz	140	0	33	28
Pomegranate Mango	8 oz	140	0	34	28
Pomegranate Tangerine	8 oz	150	0	37	31
POMPANO					
broiled	4 oz	192	13	1	tr
smoked	2 oz	109	6	0	0
steamed	4 oz	232	13	0	0
TAKE-OUT					
battered & fried	4 oz	304	21	8	tr
breaded & fried	4 oz	361	22	14	1
POPCORN					
air-popped	1 cup (0.3 oz)	31	tr	6	–
caramel coated	1 cup (1.2 oz)	152	5	28	14
caramel coated w/ peanuts	⅔ cup (1 oz)	114	2	23	11
oil popped	1 cup (0.4 oz)	55	3	6	tr
Cape Cod					
White Cheddar	2⅓ cups	170	12	13	2
Chester's					
Microwave Butter	3 cups	170	12	16	tr
Microwave Cheddar Cheese	3 cups	200	13	17	2
Cracker Jack					
Butter Toffee	¾ cup	140	4	22	12
Original	½ cup	120	2	23	15
Dale & Thomas					
Caramel	½ cup	75	4	17	15
Hall Of Fame Kettlecorn	½ cup	34	1	6	6

FOOD	PORTION	CALS	FAT	CARB	SUGAR
North Country Cheddar	½ cup	73	5	7	1
Peanut Butter & White Chocolate Drizzlecorn	½ cup	115	6	15	12
Purepopped Natural	½ cup	26	2	3	0
Sweet Georgia Pecan	½ cup	96	3	18	10
Toffee Crunch Drizzlecorn	½ cup	107	5	15	11
Jolly Time					
American's Best White	5 cups	100	1	24	0
American's Best Yellow	5 cups	100	1	24	tr
America's Best 94% Fat Free	5 cups	100	2	20	tr
Blast O Butter Light	4 cups	120	6	16	tr
Butter Licious Light	5 cups	125	5	20	0
Crispy & White Light	5 cups	125	5	20	0
Healthy Pop 94% Fat Free	5 cups	100	2	20	tr
Healthy Pop Caramel Apple	5 cups	100	2	20	tr
Healthy Pop Kettle	4 cups	100	2	24	tr
White	5 cups	100	1	24	0
Yellow	5 cups	100	1	24	tr
Judy's					
Sugar Free Popcorn Nut Brittle	¼ piece (1 oz)	100	5	3	0
Mauna Loa					
Macadamia Nut Butter Corn Crunch	1 oz	150	8	18	11
Orville Redenbacher's					
Hot Air	1 cup	15	0	3	0
Kernel Original	1 cup	15	0	3	0
Microwave Butter Light	1 cup	20	1	3	0
Microwave Kettle Korn Sweet	1 cup	35	3	3	0

FOOD	PORTION	CALS	FAT	CARB	SUGAR
Microwave Movie Theater Butter Light	1 cup	20	1	3	0
Microwave Movie Theater Extra Butter	1 cup	35	3	3	0
Microwave Natural Light	1 cup	20	1	3	0
Microwave Pour Over Butter	1 cup	40	3	3	0
Microwave Pour Over Cheddar	1 cup	50	3	6	0
Microwave Regular Butter	1 cup	35	2	3	0
Microwave Regular Corn On the Cob	1 cup	35	3	3	0
Microwave Regular Natural	1 cup	15	2	3	0
Microwave Regular Old Fashioned Butter	1 cup	35	2	3	0
Microwave Regular Tender White	1 cup	40	3	3	0
Microwave Smart Pop Butter	1 cup	15	0	3	0
Microwave Smart Pop Kettle Korn	1 cup	20	0	3	0
Microwave Smart Pop Movie Theater Butter	1 cup	20	0	3	0
Microwave Sweet Cinnabon	1 cup	50	3	6	1
Microwave Sweet Honey Butter	1 cup	35	3	3	0
Microwave Sweet 'N Buttery	1 cup	40	3	3	0
Microwave Ultimate Butter	1 cup	30	3	3	0

FOOD	PORTION	CALS	FAT	CARB	SUGAR
Microwave Sweet Caramel	1 cup	90	5	15	4
White	1 cup	15	0	3	0
Poppycock					
The Original	½ cup	160	8	20	13
Smart Balance					
No Trans Fat Low Sodium Low Fat	1 cup	20	0	6	0
Smartfood					
Reduced Fat White Cheddar	3 cups	140	6	19	1
White Cheddar	1 pkg	160	10	14	2

POPCORN CAKES
Orville Redenbacher's

FOOD	PORTION	CALS	FAT	CARB	SUGAR
Butter	2	60	1	14	0
Caramel	1	40	0	10	3
Chocolate	1	45	0	10	4
Mini Butter	8	60	1	12	0
Mini Caramel	7	50	0	13	4
Mini Peanut Caramel Crunch	6	60	1	12	4
Mini Peanut Crunch	6	60	1	12	4
Mini Sour Cream & Onion	8	60	1	12	0
White Cheddar	2	60	1	13	0

POPPY SEEDS

FOOD	PORTION	CALS	FAT	CARB	SUGAR
poppy seeds	1 tsp	15	1	1	–
American Almond					
Baker's Style Poppy Seed Filling	2 tbsp	120	5	18	16

PORGY

FOOD	PORTION	CALS	FAT	CARB	SUGAR
fresh	3 oz	77	tr	0	0

FOOD	PORTION	CALS	FAT	CARB	SUGAR

PORK

FRESH

FOOD	PORTION	CALS	FAT	CARB	SUGAR
boston blade roast lean & fat cooked	3 oz	229	16	0	0
boston blade steak lean & fat cooked	3 oz	220	14	0	0
center loin roast lean bone in cooked	3 oz	169	8	0	0
center loin chop lean bone in cooked	3 oz	172	7	0	0
center rib chop lean & fat bone in cooked	3 oz	213	13	0	0
center rib roast lean & fat bone in cooked	3 oz	217	13	0	0
fresh ham rump lean roasted	3 oz	175	7	0	0
fresh ham rump lean & fat roasted	3 oz	214	12	0	0
fresh ham shank lean roasted	3 oz	183	9	0	0
fresh ham shank lean & fat roasted	3 oz	246	17	0	0
fresh ham whole lean roasted	3 oz	179	8	0	0
fresh ham whole lean roasted diced	1 cup	285	13	0	0
fresh ham whole lean & fat roasted	3 oz	232	15	0	0
fresh ham whole lean & fat roasted diced	1 cup	369	24	0	0
ground 97% fat free	4 oz	130	3	0	0
ground cooked	3 oz	252	18	0	0

FOOD	PORTION	CALS	FAT	CARB	SUGAR
loin chop lean bone in braised	3 oz	191	11	0	0
loin chop lean bone in broiled	3 oz	199	12	0	0
loin roast lean bone in roasted	3 oz	210	13	0	0
loin whole lean & fat braised	3 oz	203	12	0	0
loin whole lean & fat broiled	3 oz	206	12	0	0
loin whole lean & fat roasted	3 oz	211	12	0	0
lungs braised	3 oz	84	3	0	0
pancreas cooked	3 oz	186	9	0	0
ribs country style lean & fat braised	3 oz	252	18	0	0
shoulder arm picnic lean & fat roasted	3 oz	269	20	0	0
shoulder whole lean & fat roasted	3 oz	248	18	0	0
shoulder whole lean & fat roasted diced	1 cup	394	29	0	0
shoulder whole lean roasted	3 oz	196	12	0	0
shoulder whole lean roasted diced	1 cup	311	18	0	0
sirloin chop lean & fat bone in braised	3 oz	208	13	0	0
sirloin roast lean & fat bone in cooked	3 oz	222	14	0	0
spareribs braised	3 oz	338	26	0	0
spleen braised	3 oz	127	3	0	0
tail simmered	3 oz	336	30	0	0

FOOD	PORTION	CALS	FAT	CARB	SUGAR
tenderloin lean roasted	3 oz	139	4	0	0
top loin chop boneless lean & fat cooked	3 oz	198	11	0	0
top loin roast boneless lean & fat cooked	3 oz	192	10	0	0
TAKE-OUT					
chicharrones pork cracklings fried	1 cup	844	72	22	–

PORK DISHES
Hormel

Center Cut Loin Lemon Garlic	1 serv (4 oz)	130	5	1	0
Extra Lean Apple Burbon	1 serv (4 oz)	140	5	5	5
Pork Roast Au Jus	1 serv (5 oz)	180	7	0	0

Morton's Of Omaha

Tender Pork Roast w/ Gravy & Vegetables	1 serv (5 oz)	210	10	10	2

Smithfield

Tenderloin Garlic & Herb	3 oz	100	3	2	0
Tenderloin Hickory Sweet	4 oz	110	3	6	4
TAKE-OUT					
pork vandaloo curry	1 serv	620	47	3	–
tourtiere	1 piece (4.9 oz)	451	34	21	–

POT PIE
TAKE-OUT

beef	1 serv (6.9 oz)	449	24	44	–
chicken	⅓ of 9 in pie (8.1 oz)	545	31	42	–
ham	1 serv (11 oz)	752	45	58	3
oyster	1 serv (11.5 oz)	817	53	67	6

FOOD	PORTION	CALS	FAT	CARB	SUGAR
POTATO					
CANNED					
Del Monte					
New Whole	2 med (5.5 oz)	60	0	13	0
Savory Sides Au Gratin	½ cup	80	3	13	1
FRESH					
baked w/ skin	1 (6.5 oz)	220	tr	51	—
boiled	½ cup	68	tr	16	—
Arrowfarms					
Yukon Gold	1 med (5 oz)	100	0	26	3
Dole					
Idaho	1 (5.3 oz)	100	0	26	3
Frieda's					
Fingerling	4 (5 oz)	100	0	25	3
Green Giant					
Red Potatoes	1 med (5 oz)	100	0	26	3
Lucinda's					
Red "C"	1 med (5.2 oz)	100	0	26	3
SunLite					
SunLite	1 (5 oz)	87	0	18	0
FROZEN					
Healthy Choice					
Cheddar Broccoli Potatoes	1 pkg	270	7	41	7
Inland Valley					
Crinkle Cuts	15 pieces (3 oz)	150	5	25	tr
Crisscut Fries	13 pieces (3 oz)	160	7	22	tr
Curly QQQ's	1⅓ cups (3 oz)	180	8	25	tr
Fajita Fries	17 pieces (3 oz)	170	8	22	1
French Fries	15 pieces (3 oz)	130	4	21	tr
Hash Browns	⅔ cup	70	0	16	tr
Home Browns	1 patty (2.2 oz)	130	7	15	tr
Mashed Homestyle	⅔ cup	160	6	22	2
Simply Shreds	1 cup	70	0	15	tr

FOOD	PORTION	CALS	FAT	CARB	SUGAR
Stix	5 pieces (3 oz)	170	10	19	tr
Stuffed Spudz w/ Cheese	5 pieces	210	11	20	tr
Tater Babies	8 pieces (3 oz)	130	5	19	tr
Tater Puffs	10 pieces	160	7	20	tr
Twice Baked	1 (5.2 oz)	230	12	23	3
Twice Baked Sour Cream Bacon & Chives	1 (5.2 oz)	240	8	36	2
Twice Baked Triple Cheese	1 (5.2 oz)	250	10	33	3
Lean Cuisine					
One Dish Favorites Deluxe Cheddar	1 pkg (10.4 oz)	260	7	36	8
MIX					
Betty Crocker					
Mashed Butter & Herb	½ cup	160	7	21	1
Hungry Jack					
Mashed Potato Flakes as prep	½ cup	160	7	21	0
Idahoan					
AuGratin as prep	½ cup	150	6	20	2
Hash Browns as prep	½ cup	160	8	18	0
Hash Browns Cheesy not prep	½ cup	120	2	23	1
Mashed Baked as prep	½ cup	110	3	19	2
Mashed Butter & Herb as prep	½ cup	110	3	20	2
Mashed Buttery Homestyle as prep	½ cup	110	3	20	2
Mashed Four Cheese as prep	½ cup	100	3	19	2
Mashed Southwest as prep	½ cup	110	3	20	2
Roasted Garlic as prep	½ cup	600	3	20	3
Scalloped as prep	½ cup	150	7	21	2

FOOD	PORTION	CALS	FAT	CARB	SUGAR
REFRIGERATED					
Country Crock					
Garlic Mashed	⅔ cup	170	7	23	1
Homestyle Mashed	⅔ cup	190	9	23	1
TAKE-OUT					
au gratin w/ cheese	½ cup	178	10	17	—
baked topped w/ cheese sauce	1	475	29	47	—
baked topped w/ sour cream & chives	1	394	22	50	—
curry	1 serv (6 oz)	292	16	36	—
french fries	1 reg	235	12	29	—
hash brown	½ cup (2.5 oz)	151	9	16	—
indian yogurt potatoes	1 serv	315	9	52	—
mashed	½ cup	111	4	18	—
o'brien	1 cup	157	3	30	—
potato dumpling	3.5 oz	334	1	74	—
potato pancakes	1 (1.3 oz)	101	7	11	—
potato salad	½ cup	179	10	14	—
red new boiled	5 sm (5 oz)	120	0	27	3
scalloped	½ cup	127	5	18	—
twice baked w/ cheese	1 half (10 oz)	392	18	48	—
POTATO STARCH					
potato starch	1 oz	96	tr	24	—
POUT					
ocean baked	3 oz	86	1	0	0
PRETZELS					
milk chocolate covered twists	4 (1 oz)	140	7	19	11
Aramana					
Soy Pretzels	15 (1 oz)	100	3	12	0

FOOD	PORTION	CALS	FAT	CARB	SUGAR
Cape Cod					
Pretzels	25	130	1	27	tr
Goodniks					
Yogurt Pretzels	15	180	7	28	15
Rold Gold					
Braided Twists	8	110	1	22	tr
Braided Twists Honey Wheat	8	110	1	22	tr
Checkers	20	110	2	22	tr
Rods	3	110	1	22	1
Sourdough Hard	1	100	1	21	tr
Sourdough Specials	5	110	1	23	1
Sticks	48	100	0	23	1
Thins	9 pieces	110	1	23	tr
Tiny Twists	18 pieces	110	0	23	tr
Tiny Twists Cheddar	20	110	1	22	tr
Tiny Twists Honey Mustard	13	110	1	23	1
Snyder's Of Hanover					
Snaps	24 (1 oz)	110	1	24	0

PRUNE JUICE

jarred	1 cup	182	tr	45	42
Ocean Spray					
100% Juice	8 oz	180	0	44	42

PRUNES

cooked w/o sugar	½ cup	133	tr	35	31
dried	1	20	tr	5	3
American Almond					
Baker's Style Ledvar	2 tbsp	90	0	21	17
St Dalfour					
French Prunes	3	100	0	22	9
Sunsweet					
Dried Plums	5	100	0	24	12

FOOD	PORTION	CALS	FAT	CARB	SUGAR
PUDDING					
MIX					
Keto					
Banana not prep	½ scoop	62	3	3	0
Chocolate not prep	½ scoop	66	3	4	0
French Vanilla not prep	½ scoop	62	3	3	0
READY-TO-EAT					
Hunt's					
Dessert Favorites Banana Cream Pie	1 serv (3.5 oz)	140	6	20	13
Dessert Favorites Chocolate Brownie	1 serv (3.5 oz)	190	7	28	22
Dessert Favorites Chocolate Mud Pie	1 serv (3.5 oz)	170	7	25	20
Dessert Favorites Chocolate Peanut Butter Pie	1 serv (3.5 oz)	190	8	27	21
Dessert Favorites Dulce De Leche Caramel Cream	1 serv (3.5 oz)	140	5	23	17
Dessert Favorites Lemon Meringue Pie	1 serv (3.5 oz)	130	3	26	21
Snack Pack Butterscotch	1 serv (3.5 oz)	130	5	20	15
Snack Pack Chocolate	1 serv (3.5 oz)	104	5	22	17
Snack Pack Chocolate Fudge	1 serv (3.5 oz)	150	5	23	16
Snack Pack Chocolate Marshmallow	1 serv (3.5 oz)	130	5	21	16
Snack Pack Fat Free Chocolate	1 serv (3.5 oz)	90	0	20	15
Snack Pack Fat Free Tapioca	1 serv (3.5 oz)	80	0	18	13
Snack Pack Fat Free Vanilla	1 serv (3.5 oz)	80	0	19	13

FOOD	PORTION	CALS	FAT	CARB	SUGAR
Snack Pack Lemon	1 serv (3.5 oz)	120	3	23	20
Snack Pack Swirl Chocolate Caramel	1 serv (3.5 oz)	140	5	22	17
Snack Pack Swirl S'mores	1 serv (3.5 oz)	140	5	21	17
Snack Pack Tapioca	1 serv (3.5 oz)	130	5	20	14
Snack Pack Vanilla	1 serv (3.5 oz)	130	5	21	18
Jell-O					
Fat Free Chocolate Vanilla Swirl	1 serv (4 oz)	100	0	23	17
Fat Free Tapioca	1 serv (4 oz)	100	0	23	17
Fat Free Vanilla Caramel	1 serv (4 oz)	100	0	23	16
Tapioca	1 serv (4 oz)	110	2	25	19
Kozy Shack					
Banana	1 pkg (4 oz)	132	3	22	18
Chocolate	1 pkg (4 oz)	139	4	24	19
Chocolate No Sugar Added	1 pkg (4 oz)	93	3	14	5
Rice	1 pkg (4 oz)	135	3	23	14
Tapioca	1 pkg (4 oz)	134	3	23	17
Tapioca No Sugar Added	1 pkg	90	3	11	5
Vanilla	1 pkg (4 oz)	130	3	22	17
Vanilla No Sugar Added	1 pkg (4 oz)	90	2	14	5
Swiss Miss					
Low Fat Tapioca	1 pkg (4 oz)	130	3	24	19
Low Fat Vanilla	1 serv (4 oz)	120	2	24	18
TAKE-OUT					
bread w/ raisins	1 cup	306	9	47	29
coconut	1 cup	291	9	45	38
corn	1 cup	328	13	43	17
indian pudding	½ cup	156	4	25	16
noodle pudding kugel	1 cup	297	10	44	15
plum pudding	1 slice (1.5 oz)	125	5	20	12
rice pudding	1 cup	302	4	60	37

FOOD	PORTION	CALS	FAT	CARB	SUGAR
tapioca	1 cup	236	7	35	31
yorkshire	1 serv (3 oz)	177	8	22	–

PUMMELO
fresh	1	228	tr	59	–
sections	1 cup	71	tr	18	–
Sunkist					
Fresh	¼	90	1	20	14

PUMPKIN
butter	1 tbsp	32	0	8	8
cooked mashed	½ cup	24	tr	6	–
flowers cooked	½ cup	10	tr	2	–
Libby's					
Puree	½ cup	40	1	9	4

PUMPKIN SEEDS
roasted	¼ cup	296	24	8	–
whole roasted	¼ cup	71	3	9	–
David					
All Natural	¼ cup	160	13	3	0
Good Sense					
Roasted & Salted	½ cup	160	13	3	0

PURSLANE
cooked	1 cup	21	tr	4	–

QUAIL
w/ skin raw	1 quail (3.8 oz)	210	13	0	0

QUICHE
TAKE-OUT
cheese	⅛ of 9 in pie	566	44	27	1
lorraine	⅛ of 9 in pie	568	44	27	1
spinach	⅛ of 9 in pie	342	26	17	1

FOOD	PORTION	CALS	FAT	CARB	SUGAR
QUINCE					
fresh	1	53	tr	14	–
QUINOA					
quinoa not prep	1 cup (6 oz)	636	10	117	–
RABBIT					
domestic w/o bone roasted	3 oz	167	7	0	0
wild w/o bone stewed	3 oz	147	3	0	–
RACCOON					
roasted	3 oz	217	12	0	0
RADICCHIO					
raw shredded	½ cup	5	tr	1	–
RADISHES					
chinese dried	½ cup	157	tr	37	–
chinese raw sliced	½ cup	8	tr	2	–
chinese sliced cooked	½ cup	13	tr	3	–
daikon dried	½ cup	157	tr	37	–
daikon raw sliced	½ cup	8	tr	2	–
daikon sliced cooked	½ cup	13	tr	3	–
red raw	10	7	tr	2	–
white icicle raw sliced	½ cup	7	tr	1	–
Frieda's					
Black	¾ cup	15	0	3	2
Chinese Lo Bok	⅔ cup	25	0	5	3
Daikon	½ cup	15	1	1	0
Korean Moo	⅔ cup	15	0	3	2
TAKE-OUT					
korean kimchee	½ cup	31	1	6	–
moo namul saengche korean salad	1 serv (3.7 oz)	34	tr	8	6

FOOD	PORTION	CALS	FAT	CARB	SUGAR
RAISINS					
chocolate coated	10 (0.4 oz)	39	2	7	—
jumbo golden	¼ cup	130	0	31	29
seedless	1 tbsp	27	tr	7	—
Brach's					
California Chocolate Covered	35 pieces	170	6	28	26
Estee					
Chocolate Covered Fructose Sweetened	¼ cup	180	6	27	16
Goodniks					
Yogurt Raisins	3 tbsp	145	5	23	17
Sun-Maid					
California Golden	¼ cup	130	0	31	29
California Seedless	¼ cup	130	0	31	29
RASPBERRIES					
fresh	1 cup	61	1	14	—
frzn unsweetened	¾ cup	130	0	29	6
Frieda's					
Dried	⅓ cup (1.4 oz)	145	1	36	25
RASPBERRY JUICE					
Naked Juice					
Raspberry Ade	8 oz	90	0	22	19
Nantucket Nectars					
Organic Very Raspberry	8 oz	120	0	30	29
RELISH					
Del Monte					
Hamburger	1 tbsp	20	0	5	5
Hot Dog	1 tbsp	15	0	4	3
Sweet Pickle	1 tbsp	20	0	5	5
Frieda's					
Kim Chee	¼ cup	15	0	2	0

FOOD	PORTION	CALS	FAT	CARB	SUGAR
Matouk's					
Hot Chow	2 tbsp	20	0	5	2
Kuchela	1 tsp	9	1	tr	0
RENNIN					
tablet	1 (0.9 g)	1	0	tr	—
RHUBARB					
fresh	½ cup	13	tr	3	—
frzn as prep w/ sugar	½ cup	139	tr	37	—
RICE					
glutinous cooked	1 cup (6.1 oz)	169	tr	37	—
starch	1 oz	98	0	24	—
A Taste Of Thai					
Coconut Garlic Basil as prep	¾ cup	160	0	35	2
Coconut Ginger as prep	¾ cup	190	0	42	2
Jasmine not prep	¼ cup	160	0	36	0
Yellow Curry as prep	¾ cup	180	2	38	2
Buitoni					
Risotto Garden Vegetable	1 serv	210	1	47	1
Risotto Portobello Mushrooms	1 serv	210	0	48	0
Risotto Rosemary & Potatoes	1 serv	210	1	47	0
Risotto Tomato Basil	1 serv	210	1	46	1
Carolina					
Black Beans & Rice Mix as prep	1 serv	200	2	39	0
Gold as prep	1 cup	160	0	37	0
Spanish Rice Mix as prep	1 serv	180	1	42	1
Country Crock					
Chicken Rice w/ Herbs	1 cup	210	4	42	1

FOOD	PORTION	CALS	FAT	CARB	SUGAR
Gourmet House					
Brown & White not prep	¼ cup	160	10	34	1
Mahatma					
Jambalaya as prep	1 cup	190	1	42	1
Nacho Cheese Mix as prep	1 serv	250	3	49	5
Thai Jasmine as prep	¾ cup	160	0	36	0
Near East					
Creative Grains Chicken & Herb as prep	1 cup	270	6	51	2
Creative Grains Creamy Parmesan as prep	1 cup	280	8	48	2
Creative Grains Roasted Garlic as prep	1 cup	220	5	41	1
Creative Grains Roasted Pecan as prep	1 cup	240	8	37	1
Long Grain & Wild Rice Roasted Vegetable & Chicken as prep	1 cup	220	5	43	1
Long Grain & Wild Rice Garlic & Herb as prep	1 cup	220	5	43	1
Pilaf Brown Rice as prep	1 cup	210	5	41	1
Pilaf Chicken as prep	1 cup	220	5	43	1
Pilaf Mix Curry as prep	1 cup	220	5	44	0
Pilaf Mix Garlic & Herb as prep	1 cup	220	3	44	0
Pilaf Mix Long Grain & Wild as prep	1 cup	220	5	43	0
Pilaf Mix Rice as prep	1 cup	220	5	44	0
Pilaf Mix Roasted Chicken & Garlic as prep	1 cup	220	4	44	1
Pilaf Mix Spanish Rice as prep	1 cup	310	8	54	2

FOOD	PORTION	CALS	FAT	CARB	SUGAR
Pilaf Mix Toasted Almond as prep	1 cup	230	6	40	1
Pilaf Mix Wild Mushroom & Herb as prep	1 cup	220	5	44	1
Nueva Cocina					
Arroz A La Mexicana	1 cup	190	1	41	2
Arroz Con Pollo	1 cup	150	0	35	1
Gallo Pinto	⅓ pkg	220	0	47	1
Moros Y Cristianos	⅓ pkg	220	0	47	tr
Paella	⅕ pkg	160	0	35	1
Pacific Foods					
Ready-To-Serve Lemon & Herb	½ pkg	240	3	48	2
Ready-To-Serve Roasted Chicken	½ pkg	240	6	45	1
Ready-To-Serve Spanish Style	½ pkg	230	3	45	1
Ready-To-Serve Wild Rice & Mushroom	½ pkg	230	3	46	1
Rice Expressions					
Indian Basmati	1 cup	180	tr	40	0
Organic Brown	1 cup	160	1	34	0
Organic Long Grain	1 cup	180	tr	40	0
Organic Rice Pilaf	1 cup	170	3	32	1
Organic Tex Mex	1 cup	190	2	40	0
River Rice					
Brown Long Grain not prep	¼ cup	150	1	32	0
S&W					
Arborio as prep	¾ cup	150	0	35	0
Basmati Mix as prep	¾ cup	160	0	36	0
Brown Long Grain not prep	¼ cup	150	1	32	0

FOOD	PORTION	CALS	FAT	CARB	SUGAR
Long Grain Organic not prep	¼ cup	150	0	35	0
Success					
Beef Mix as prep	1 cup	240	7	42	2
Grilled Chicken & Broccoli Mix as prep	1 cup	240	6	42	1
Red Beans & Rice Mix as prep	1 cup	300	7	51	1
White as prep	1 cup	190	0	44	0
Yellow Mix as prep	1 cup	170	3	33	0
Uncle Ben's					
White Converted as prep	1 cup	170	0	38	0
Water Maid					
White Medium Grain not prep	¼ cup	160	0	37	0
TAKE-OUT					
coconut rice	1 serv	500	42	30	–
congee	½ cup (4.1 oz)	44	–	10	–
nasi goreng (fried rice)	1 serv	206	4	35	–
nasi goreng indonesian rice & vegetables	1 cup (4.9 oz)	130	0	28	1
paella	1 serv (7 oz)	308	16	17	–
pilaf	½ cup	84	3	11	–
risotto	1 serv (6.6 oz)	426	18	65	–
spanish	¾ cup	363	27	19	–
RICE CAKES					
Mr. Krispers					
Baked Rice Krisps Barbecue	37	110	3	21	3
Baked Rice Krisps Nacho	37	120	3	21	3
Baked Rice Krisps Sea Salt & Pepper	37	110	4	20	2

FOOD	PORTION	CALS	FAT	CARB	SUGAR
Baked Rice Krisps Sour Cream & Onion	37	110	4	19	2
Tastemorr					
Rice Crisps Caramel	7	55	0	12	3
ROCKFISH					
pacific cooked	3 oz	103	2	0	0
ROE					
fresh baked	1 oz	58	2	1	–
ROLL					
FROZEN					
Pepperidge Farm					
Hearth Fired Hearty Wheat Dinner Roll	1	120	1	25	3
READY-TO-EAT					
brioche sweet roll	1 (3.5 oz)	410	23	41	5
dinner	1 (1 oz)	85	2	14	–
hotdog whole wheat	1 (1.5 oz)	110	2	19	2
Alvarado Street Bakery					
Sprouted Wheat Burger Bun	1 (2.2 oz)	140	2	27	4
Country Kitchen					
Wheat Light	1	80	2	17	1
Natural Ovens					
Best Burger Bun	1	178	4	29	3
Better Wheat Buns	1	140	2	30	4
Gourmet Dinner	1	70	1	15	3
Pepperidge Farm					
Kaiser Soft 100% Whole Wheat	1	200	3	35	5
Super Bakery					
Daily Donut Reduced Fat	1 (2.2 oz)	200	6	35	11
Organic Sandwich Bun	1 (3.6 oz)	250	3	42	1

FOOD	PORTION	CALS	FAT	CARB	SUGAR
Sub Roll	1 (3.6 oz)	250	3	42	1
REFRIGERATED					
Pillsbury					
Crescent	1 (1.7 oz)	170	10	20	4
ROSE HIP					
fresh	1 oz	26	0	5	—
ROSEMARY					
dried	1 tsp	4	tr	1	—
ROUGHY					
orange baked	3 oz	75	1	0	0
RUTABAGA					
cooked mashed	½ cup	41	tr	9	—
SABLEFISH					
baked	3 oz	213	17	0	0
smoked	1 oz	72	6	0	0
SAFFRON					
saffron	1 tsp	2	tr	tr	—
SAGE					
ground	1 tsp	2	tr	tr	—
SALAD					
MIX					
Fresh Express					
Baby Spinach Trio	4 cups (3 oz)	20	0	4	1
Krakus					
Bordeaux	1 pkg (5 oz)	35	0	5	1
Ready Pac					
All American	2.5 cups	15	0	3	1
Bowl Salad Chef	1 pkg	350	25	9	5
Bowl Salad Chicken Caesar	1 pkg	380	27	8	3

FOOD	PORTION	CALS	FAT	CARB	SUGAR
Bowl Salad Greek	1 pkg	400	35	5	2
Bowl Salad Spinach Bacon	1 pkg	300	17	22	13
Bowl Salad Spring Mix Veggie	1 pkg	330	23	18	6
Caesar Romaine	1½ cups	15	0	2	1
Classic Crisp Salad	2¼ cups	10	0	2	tr
Continental	3 cups	20	0	4	2
Costa Brava	3 cups	15	0	3	2
Hearty Green Salad	2½ cups	10	0	2	tr
Lafayette	3 cups	10	0	3	1
Milano	3 cups	15	0	3	0
Organic Caesar Romaine	2¼ cups	15	0	2	tr
Organic Mesclun Blend	1 pkg (4.5 oz)	35	0	7	0
Organic Monterey	3 cups	15	0	3	1
Parisian	2 cups	20	0	4	1
Portofino	1 pkg (5 oz)	25	0	4	0
Santa Barbara	3½ cups	15	0	3	1
Spring Mix	1 pkg (5 oz)	35	0	7	0
River Ranch					
American Blend	1½ cups	15	0	3	1
Caesar Kit	1½ cups	110	12	7	1
European Blend	1¾ cups	10	0	2	tr
Garden	1½ cups	15	0	3	1
Garden Supreme	1½ cups	15	0	3	1
Italian Blend	1¾ cups	15	0	2	tr
Raspberry Vinaigrette Kit	1¾ cups	130	8	13	7
Riviera Blend	1½ cups	10	0	2	1
TAKE-OUT					
caesar	2 cups	337	28	13	3
chef w/o dressing	1½ cups	386	28	9	–
cobb w/ dressing	4 cups	635	49	23	9
greek w/ dressing	2 cups	210	15	6	4
tossed 7-layer	2 cups	557	51	15	8

FOOD	PORTION	CALS	FAT	CARB	SUGAR
tossed w/o dressing	1½ cups	32	tr	7	—
waldorf	1 cup	242	21	15	10

SALAD DRESSING
MIX
A Taste Of Thai
Peanut Dressing as prep	2 tbsp	40	2	7	5

Good Seasons
Italian as prep	2 tbsp	130	14	3	1
Italian not prep	⅛ pkg (3 g)	5	0	1	tr

READY-TO-EAT
Carb Options
Italian	2 tbsp	70	8	0	0
Ranch	2 tbsp	150	17	0	0

Consorzio
Balsamic Vinaigrette	2 tbsp	60	1	2	2
Honey Mustard	2 tbsp	100	8	6	5
Italian	2 tbsp	60	7	1	1
Mango	1 tbsp	15	0	4	3
Raspberry & Balsamic	1 tbsp	15	0	4	3
Strawberry Balsamic	1 tbsp	10	0	2	2

Drew's
Low Carb Garlic Italian	1 tbsp	80	9	0	0
Low Carb Lemon Tahini Goddess	1 tbsp	80	9	1	0
Low Carb Sesame Orange	1 tbsp	80	9	2	0

Kraft
Free Thousand Island	2 tbsp	45	0	10	5

Nasoya
Creamy Dill	1 tbsp	30	3	1	0
Creamy Italian	2 tbsp	70	7	1	1
Garden Herb	2 tbsp	60	7	1	1
Sesame Garlic	2 tbsp	60	7	1	1

FOOD	PORTION	CALS	FAT	CARB	SUGAR
Spectrum					
Honey Dijon	2 tbsp	35	2	4	4
Organic Creamy Dill	2 tbsp	25	0	4	2
Organic Creamy Garlic	2 tbsp	20	0	4	3
Organic Greek Goddess	2 tbsp	110	11	2	0
Organic Omega 3 Balsamic Vinaigrette	2 tbsp	80	8	3	1
Organic Omega 3 Ginger Garlic Vinaigrette	2 tbsp	80	8	2	0
Organic Omega 3 Raspberry Vinaigrette	2 tbsp	80	8	3	2
Organic Porcini Mushroom Vinaigrette	2 tbsp	70	6	2	0
Organic Rocky Mountain Ranch	2 tbsp	130	14	1	0
Organic Sweet Onion & Garlic	2 tbsp	15	0	3	2
Organic Toasted Sesame	2 tbsp	15	0	3	2
Provencal Garlic Lover's	2 tbsp	50	5	2	0
Zesty Italian	2 tbsp	30	2	1	0
Steel's					
Honey Mustard	1 tbsp	90	7	0	0
Sweet Ginger Lime	1 tbsp	68	7	1	0
Wishbone					
Italian	2 tbsp	80	8	3	2
Just 2 Good! Creamy Caesar	2 tbsp	45	2	7	2
Thousand Island	2 tbsp	130	12	6	6

SALAD TOPPINGS

FOOD	PORTION	CALS	FAT	CARB	SUGAR
Salad Pizazz!					
Asian Medley	1 tbsp	40	3	2	2
Cherry Cranberry Pecano	1 tbsp	35	2	4	3
Honey Toasted Delites	1 tbsp	40	3	2	2

FOOD	PORTION	CALS	FAT	CARB	SUGAR
Orange Cranberry Almondine	1 tbsp	35	2	4	3
Raspberry Cranberry Walnut Frisco	1 tbsp	30	2	4	3
Tomato 'N Bacon Parmesano	1 tbsp	30	1	3	1
Tomato Pinenut Tuscano	1 tbsp	130	2	2	1
SALMON					
CANNED					
w/ bone	½ cup	106	5	0	0
Bumble Bee					
Blueback	¼ cup	110	7	0	0
Keta	¼ cup	90	4	0	0
Pink	¼ cup	90	5	0	0
Red	¼ cup	110	7	0	0
Skinless & Boneless	¼ cup	50	1	0	0
Smoked Fillets In Oil	⅓ cup	150	9	0	0
Chicken Of The Sea					
Pink	1 pkg (3 oz)	90	3	0	0
Pink Skinless Boneless	¼ cup	60	2	0	0
Red	¼ cup	110	7	0	0
Smoked Pacific	1 pkg (3 oz)	120	4	1	1
Libby's					
Alaskan Sockeye Red	¼ cup	110	7	0	0
Pink Skinless Boneless	¼ cup	50	1	0	0
Red	¼ cup	110	7	0	0
FRESH					
atlantic farmed baked	4 oz	233	14	0	0
coho wild poached	4 oz	209	9	0	0
pink baked	4 oz	169	5	0	0
roe raw	1 oz	59	3	tr	–
sockeye baked	4 oz	245	12	0	0

FOOD	PORTION	CALS	FAT	CARB	SUGAR
FROZEN					
Phillips Seafood					
Salmon Cakes	1 (3 oz)	180	13	3	1
SMOKED					
lox	1 oz	33	1	0	0
TAKE-OUT					
guisado stew salmon	1 serv (7.4 oz)	320	16	18	3
roulette w/ spinach stuffing	1 serv (4 oz)	160	6	10	0
salmon cake	1 (4.2 oz)	264	16	14	1
salmon loaf	1 slice (3.7 oz)	206	11	9	2
SALSA					
black bean & corn	2 tbsp	15	0	3	1
citrus	2 tbsp (1 oz)	10	0	2	2
peach	2 tbsp	15	0	4	4
tomato-less corn & chile	2 tbsp	45	0	10	6
Cape Cod					
Medium & Mild	2 tbsp	15	0	3	1
Del Salsa					
Fire Roasted All Flavors	2 tbsp	8	0	2	0
Gringo Billy's					
Salsa Mix	1 tsp	5	1	1	0
Guiltless Gourmet					
Roasted Red Pepper	2 tbsp	10	0	2	1
Southwestern Grill	2 tbsp	15	0	2	0
Tostitos					
All Natural	2 tbsp	15	0	3	2
Con Queso	2 tbsp	40	3	5	tr
Monterey Jack Queso	2 tbsp	40	3	4	0
Restaurant Style	2 tbsp	15	0	3	1

FOOD	PORTION	CALS	FAT	CARB	SUGAR
SALSIFY					
Frieda's					
Salsify	¾ cup	70	0	16	2
SALT/SEASONED SALT					
salt	1 tbsp (18 g)	0	0	0	0
salt	1 tsp (6 g)	0	0	0	0
McCormick					
Celery Salt	¼ tsp	0	0	0	0
SALT SUBSTITUTES					
Molly McButter					
Lite Sodium	1 tsp	5	0	2	—
SANDWICHES					
Lean Pockets					
Bacon Egg & Cheese	1 (4.5 oz)	150	5	21	2
Barbecue Sauce w/ Beef	1 (4.5 oz)	290	7	47	11
Chicken Cheddar & Broccoli	1 (4.5 oz)	260	7	39	9
Chicken Fajita	1 (4.5 oz)	260	7	38	7
Chicken Parmesan	1 (4.5 oz)	280	7	43	5
Ham & Cheese	1 (4.5 oz)	280	7	40	7
Meatballs & Mozzarella	1 (4.5 oz)	290	7	44	8
Philly Steak & Cheese	1 (4.5 oz)	280	7	40	6
Sausage Egg & Cheese	1 (4.5 oz)	140	5	19	4
Steak Fajita	1 (4.5 oz)	260	7	39	10
Three Cheese & Chicken Quesadilla	1 (4.5 oz)	280	7	41	8
Turkey & Ham w/ Cheddar	1 (4.5 oz)	280	7	43	8
Turkey Broccoli & Cheese	1 (4.5 oz)	270	7	39	8
Madalena's Masterpiece					
Calzone Artichoke Parmesan	1 (10 oz)	570	29	51	6
Calzone Grilled Chicken	1 (10 oz)	520	22	43	5

FOOD	PORTION	CALS	FAT	CARB	SUGAR
Calzone Sausage Pepperoni	1 (10 oz)	640	36	48	6
Panini Garlic Chicken	1 (8 oz)	450	25	42	5
Panini Honey Ham	1 (8 oz)	520	25	46	7
Panini Turkey Pesto	1 (8 oz)	500	26	43	4
Panini Veggie	1 (8 oz)	480	26	43	5
Quesabake Mexican Sausage	1 (7 oz)	510	26	48	2
Quesabake Roasted Veggie	1 (7 oz)	460	24	47	tr
Smucker's					
Uncrustables Grilled Cheese	1 (1.8 oz)	150	6	17	3
Uncrustables Peanut Butter & Grape Jelly	1 (2 oz)	210	9	25	10
Uncrustables Peanut Butter & Strawberry Jam	1 (2 oz)	210	9	25	10
South Beach Diet					
Wrap Kit Deli Ham & Turkey	1 pkg	220	10	24	tr
Wrap Kit Grilled Chicken Caesar	1 pkg	230	10	24	tr
Wrap Kit Southwestern Style Chicken	1 pkg	240	10	26	2
Wrap Kits Turkey & Bacon Club	1 pkg	250	12	25	1
TAKE-OUT					
calzone cheese	1 (12 oz)	1020	54	86	26
crab cake w/ bun	1	308	8	36	4
croque monsieur	1 (12.4 oz)	765	46	43	9
fish fillet w/ tartar sauce	1	431	55	41	—
fish fillet w/ tartar sauce & cheese	1	524	29	48	—

FOOD	PORTION	CALS	FAT	CARB	SUGAR
fried egg	1	226	9	26	3
fried egg w/ cheese	1	340	19	26	—
gyro	1 (13.7 oz)	604	13	74	8
ham & egg	1	272	11	27	3
ham salad	1	323	15	28	3
ham w/ cheese	1	352	15	34	—
roast beef w/ cheese	1	402	18	27	—
roast beef plain	1	346	14	33	—

SAPODILLA

fresh	1	140	2	34	—

SAPOTES

fresh	1	301	1	76	—

SARDINES
CANNED

atlantic in oil w/ bone	1 can (3.2 oz)	192	11	0	0
atlantic in oil w/ bone	2	50	3	0	0
pacific in tomato sauce w/ bone	1	68	5	0	0
pacific in tomato sauce w/ bone	1 can (13 oz)	658	44	0	0

Beach Cliff

In Louisiana Hot Sauce	1 can (3.7 oz)	150	8	2	0
In Mustard Sauce	1 can (3.7 oz)	150	8	2	0
In Olive Oil	1 can (3.7 oz)	200	14	0	0
In Tomato Sauce	1 can (3.7 oz)	140	6	2	1
In Water	1 can (3.7 oz)	150	8	0	0
Small In Soybean Oil	1 can (3.7 oz)	200	12	1	0
W/ Hot Green Chilies	1 can (3.7 oz)	180	12	1	0

Brunswick

In Louisiana Hot Sauce	1 can (3.7 oz)	150	8	2	0
In Mustard Sauce	1 can (3.7 oz)	150	8	2	0
In Soybean Oil	1 can (3.7 oz)	110	12	1	0

FOOD	PORTION	CALS	FAT	CARB	SUGAR
In Spring Water	1 can (3.7 oz)	150	8	0	0
In Tomato Sauce	1 can (3.7 oz)	150	8	3	2
W/ Hot Tabasco Peppers	1 can (3.7 oz)	110	12	0	0
Bumble Bee					
In Hot Sauce	¼ cup	90	6	0	0
In Mustard	¼ cup	70	4	1	1
In Oil	1 can (3.7 oz)	130	9	0	0
In Water	1 can (3.7 oz)	120	7	0	0
Chicken Of The Sea					
In Hot Sauce	1 can (3.75 oz)	130	6	2	2
In Mustard Sauce	1 can (3.75 oz)	150	8	2	2
In Oil	1 can (3.75 oz)	190	14	2	0
In Tomato Sauce	1 can (3.75 oz)	130	6	2	2
In Water	1 can (3.75 oz)	100	4	2	0
Goya					
In Tomato Sauce	2 pieces (2.2 oz)	50	1	20	1
King Oscar					
In Olive Oil	1 can (3.75 oz)	150	11	0	0
Skinless Boneless In Soya Oil	3 pieces (1.9 oz)	120	7	0	0
Season					
Brisling In Water	1 can (3.75 oz)	145	10	0	0

SAUCE

JARRED

FOOD	PORTION	CALS	FAT	CARB	SUGAR
fish sauce chinese	1 tbsp	9	0	tr	—
fish sauce vietnamese nuoc mam	1 tbsp	6	0	1	—
hoisin	1 tbsp	35	1	7	—
morroccan tagine	½ cup (4 oz)	70	3	10	10
oyster	1 tbsp	8	0	2	—
A Taste Of Thai					
Chili Sauce Garlic Pepper	1 tsp	10	0	2	2
Chili Sauce Sweet Red	1 tsp	10	0	2	2

FOOD	PORTION	CALS	FAT	CARB	SUGAR
Peanut Satay	2 tbsp	80	5	9	5
A1					
Bold Steak Sauce	1 tbsp	20	0	5	4
Asian Gourmet					
Duck Sauce Peking Style	2 tbsp	40	0	13	11
Carb Options					
Alfredo	¼ cup	110	10	2	0
Asian Teriyaki Marinade	1 tbsp	5	1	1	0
Cheese	¼ cup	90	8	2	0
Garden Style	½ cup	80	5	7	4
Steak Sauce	1 tbsp	5	0	1	0
Consorzio					
Marinade Baja Lime	1 tbsp	60	6	3	0
Marinade California Teriyaki	1 tbsp	40	2	5	5
Marinade Dijon Peppercorn	1 tbsp	15	0	3	2
Marinade Jamaican Jerk	1 tbsp	10	0	3	2
Marinade Lemon Pepper	1 tbsp	60	6	1	1
Marinade Roasted Garlic	1 tbsp	35	2	5	4
Marinade Sesame Ginger	1 tbsp	25	1	4	4
Marinade Southwestern Chipotle	1 tbsp	30	2	4	2
Marinade Tropical Grill	1 tbsp	40	3	3	2
Del Monte					
Seafood Cocktail	¼ cup	100	0	24	22
Sloppy Joe Hickory Flavor	¼ cup	60	0	14	11
Sloppy Joe Original	¼ cup	50	0	11	9
Fage					
Tzatziki	2 tbsp	30	2	2	2
Gringo Billy's					
Chipotle Dipping & Grilling Sauce	1 tsp	5	0	1	0

FOOD	PORTION	CALS	FAT	CARB	SUGAR
Jok'n'Al					
Cocktail	¼ cup	29	0	6	2
Plum	1 tbsp	10	0	2	1
Kikkoman					
Teriyaki	1 tbsp	15	0	3	2
Lea & Perrins					
Worcestershire	1 tsp	5	0	1	1
Lee Kum Kee					
Plum Sauce	2 tbsp	100	0	26	23
Matouk's					
Calypso	1 tsp	0	0	0	0
Flambeau Sauce	1 tsp	0	0	0	0
Nando's					
Curry Coconut	¼ cup	71	5	6	3
Fresh Lemon	¼ cup	61	5	5	2
Marinade Lime & Cilantro	1 tbsp	27	2	2	1
Marinade Sundried Tomato	1 tbsp	15	1	1	1
Roasted Red	¼ cup	70	5	7	4
Sweet Apricot	¼ cup	51	0	12	7
Old El Paso					
Enchilada Mild	¼ cup	25	1	3	1
Steel's					
Sugar Free Cocktail w/ Dill & Lemon	¼ cup	36	0	1	1
Sugar Free Hoisin	2 tbsp	15	0	2	1
Sugar Free Mango Curry	1 tbsp	13	0	3	0
Sugar Free Peanut Sauce	1 tbsp	34	2	7	0
Sugar Free Sweet & Sour	2 tbsp	10	0	2	0
Ty Ling					
Duck	2 tbsp	70	0	19	11

FOOD	PORTION	CALS	FAT	CARB	SUGAR
Walden Farms					
Calorie Free Seafood Sauce	1 tbsp	0	0	0	0
Scampi Sauce Calorie Free	2 tbsp	0	0	0	0
MIX					
white as prep w/ milk	1 cup	241	13	21	—
A Taste Of Thai					
Pad Thai Sauce	2 tbsp	90	1	20	16
Peanut Sauce	¼ pkg	45	2	7	5
TAKE-OUT					
adobo fresco	2 tbsp	81	8	7	tr
bearnaise	1 oz	177	19	1	—
cucumber yogurt sauce	1½ tbsp	20	0	3	—
SAUERKRAUT					
Del Monte					
Bavarian Style	2 tbsp	15	0	4	3
Sauerkraut	2 tbsp	0	0	1	0
Silver Floss					
Sauerkraut	½ cup	20	0	5	1
SAUSAGE					
beef & pork	1 link (2.3 oz)	196	17	1	0
beef & pork w/ cheddar cheese	1 link (2.7 oz)	228	20	2	tr
bratwurst pork & beef	1 link (2.5 oz)	226	19	2	2
bratwurst pork cooked	1 link (2.5 oz)	226	19	2	2
chipolata	3.5 oz	342	32	1	1
chorizo	1 link (2.1 oz)	273	23	1	0
free range chicken breakfast	2 links (2.7 oz)	110	6	1	1
italian pork cooked	1 (2.4 oz)	230	18	3	1
knockwurst pork & beef	1 (2.5 oz)	221	20	2	0

FOOD	PORTION	CALS	FAT	CARB	SUGAR
polish kielbasa	2 oz	127	10	2	0
pork cooked	2 links (1.7 oz)	163	14	0	0
vienna canned	1 can (4 oz)	260	22	3	0
vienna canned	1 link (0.5 oz)	37	3	tr	0
zungenwurst (tongue)	3.5 oz	285	24	0	—
Armour					
Brown'N Serve Lite Original	3	120	8	3	1
Brown'N Serve Turkey	3 links	120	8	2	1
Hebrew National					
Knockwurst Beef	1 (3 oz)	260	24	1	0
Jennie-O					
Turkey Italian Sweet	1 link (3.9 oz)	160	10	0	0
Shady Brook					
Turkey Sweet Italian	1 (2.5 oz)	110	7	1	1

SAUSAGE DISHES
TAKE-OUT

FOOD	PORTION	CALS	FAT	CARB	SUGAR
italian sausage w/ peppers & onions	1 cup	210	11	14	—
sausage roll	1 (2.3 oz)	311	24	22	—

SAUSAGE SUBSTITUTES

FOOD	PORTION	CALS	FAT	CARB	SUGAR
meatless	1 patty (1.3 oz)	98	7	4	0
meatless	1 link (0.9 oz)	64	5	2	0
Lightlife					
Gimme Lean	2 oz	50	0	4	1
Smart Brats	1 (2 oz)	120	5	5	0
Smart Links Breakfast	2 (2 oz)	100	4	8	2
Smart Links Italian	1 (2 oz)	120	5	7	2
Smart Menu Breakfast Patty	1	45	2	3	0
Morningstar Farms					
Breakfast Links	2	60	2	2	0

FOOD	PORTION	CALS	FAT	CARB	SUGAR
Quorn					
Links	2 (1.6 oz)	70	3	2	0
SAVORY					
ground	1 tsp	4	tr	1	—
SCALLOP					
TAKE-OUT					
breaded & fried	2 lg	67	3	3	—
SCONE					
Finnegan's					
Irish Raisin	1 (2 oz)	170	4	31	5
King Arthur					
Cranberry Orange as prep	1	248	8	39	14
TAKE-OUT					
blueberry	1 (3 oz)	270	9	41	7
orange poppy	1 (3 oz)	260	6	47	12
plain	1 (3.5 oz)	362	14	54	—
raisin	1 (3 oz)	270	8	43	12
SCUP					
fresh baked	3 oz	115	3	0	0
SEA CUCUMBER					
dried	1 oz	74	tr	1	—
fresh	1 oz	20	tr	tr	—
SEA URCHIN					
canned	1 oz	39	1	3	—
fresh	1 oz	36	1	3	—
roe paste	1 tbsp	19	tr	3	—
SEAWEED					
agar dried	1 oz	87	tr	23	—
agar fresh	1 oz	tr	tr	2	—
hijiki dried	1 tbsp	9	0	2	—

FOOD	PORTION	CALS	FAT	CARB	SUGAR
irishmoss fresh	1 oz	14	tr	4	—
kelp fresh	1 oz	12	tr	3	—
kombu fresh	1 oz	12	tr	3	—
laver fresh	1 oz	10	tr	1	—
nori fresh	1 oz	10	tr	1	—
nori sheet dried	1 (8 x 8 in)	5	0	1	—
seahair dried	1 tbsp	13	0	3	—
spirulina dried	1 oz	83	2	7	—
spirulina fresh	1 oz	7	tr	1	—
tangle fresh	1 oz	12	tr	3	—
wakame fresh	1 oz	13	tr	3	—
SESAME					
seeds	1 tsp	16	2	tr	—
sesame butter	1 tbsp	95	8	4	—
sesame crunch candy	20 pieces (1.2 oz)	181	12	18	—
SESBANIA					
flower	1	1	0	tr	—
flowers cooked	1 cup	23	tr	5	—
SHAD					
american baked	3 oz	214	15	0	0
roe baked w/ butter & lemon	1 oz	36	1	tr	—
SHALLOTS					
Christopher Ranch					
Fresh	1 (1 oz)	20	0	4	2
Frieda's					
Fresh	1 tbsp (1 oz)	20	0	5	1
SHARK					
raw	3 oz	111	4	0	0

FOOD	PORTION	CALS	FAT	CARB	SUGAR
TAKE-OUT					
batter-dipped & fried	3 oz	194	12	5	–
SHEEPSHEAD FISH					
cooked	3 oz	107	1	0	0
SHELLFISH SUBSTITUTES					
crab imitation	1 cup (4.4 oz)	144	1	16	0
Chicken Of The Sea					
Imitation Crab	1 pkg (2.5 oz)	40	0	6	1
Louis Kemp					
Crab Delights	½ cup (3 oz)	80	0	11	0
Crab Delights Chunk Style	½ cup (3 oz)	80	0	11	0
Crab Delights Easy Shred	½ cup (3 oz)	80	0	13	3
Crab Delights Leg Style	½ cup (3 oz)	80	0	11	0
Lobster Delights Chunk or Salad Style	½ cup (3 oz)	80	0	12	4
Scallop Delights Bay Style	½ cup (3 oz)	80	0	12	0
TAKE-OUT					
crab salad	1 cup	395	26	21	1
SHERBET					
Breyers					
Orange	½ cup	120	2	26	19
Rainbow	½ cup	120	2	26	20
Hood					
Orange Burst	½ cup	120	1	27	20
SHRIMP					
CANNED					
chinese shrimp paste	1 tbsp	15	tr	1	–
Bumble Bee					
Broken Shrimp	¼ cup	40	0	0	1
Medium or Large or Jumbo	¼ cup	40	0	0	1
Small	¼ cup	40	0	0	1

FOOD	PORTION	CALS	FAT	CARB	SUGAR
Tiny	¼ cup	40	0	0	1
Chicken Of The Sea					
Tiny Small or Medium	½ can (2 oz)	45	1	1	1
FRESH					
cooked	4 large	22	tr	0	0
FROZEN					
Chicken Of The Sea					
Cooked Large Peeled Deveined Tail On	3 oz	80	1	0	0
Large Raw Cleaned Tail Off	4 oz	120	2	1	0
Margaritaville					
Calypso Coconut + Sauce	5 pieces	350	17	39	14
Island Lime	6 pieces	130	7	2	1
Jammin' Jerk	7 pieces	140	7	4	2
Paradise Cocktail + Sauce	5 pieces	85	0	6	5
Sunset Scampi	1 serv (½ pkg)	270	20	10	1
Surfside Skewers + Sauce	2 skewers	105	1	11	5
Phillips Seafood					
Breaded Shrimp	5 pieces	230	13	20	3
Buffalo Shrimp	5 pieces	260	13	26	7
Coconut Shrimp	5 pieces	330	20	27	8
Crab Stuffed Shrimp	3 pieces	160	10	1	1
TAKE-OUT					
breaded & fried	3 oz	206	10	10	–
jambalaya	¾ cup	188	5	26	–
shrimp newburg	1 serv (6.4 oz)	456	37	8	tr
shrimp w/ crab stuffing	5	158	8	5	tr
SMELT					
rainbow cooked	3 oz	106	3	0	0

FOOD	PORTION	CALS	FAT	CARB	SUGAR
SMOOTHIES					
Bolthouse Farms					
Strawberry Banana Fruit	8 oz	124	0	29	27
Jammin' Juice					
Mambo Mango	6 oz	92	0	25	24
Jammin' Nectars					
C-Beta Carrot	6 oz	96	0	23	21
Ginger Party	6 oz	6	0	19	17
Guanabana Limbo	6 oz	78	0	20	18
Pure Passion	6 oz	78	0	20	18
Razz-Ade	6 oz	89	0	21	20
Naked Juice					
Chocolate Karma	8 oz	190	3	31	24
Vanilla Chai	8 oz	170	3	27	19
Sambazon					
Acai Energy Mango Banana	8 oz	190	5	38	29
Acai Soy Energy	8 oz	210	6	25	19
Amazon Cherry	8 oz	156	0	16	15
Soy Blendz					
Mango Orange Dream	1 bottle (10 oz)	220	3	40	33
Mixed Berry Medley	1 bottle (10 oz)	210	3	38	31
Orange Citrus Splash	1 bottle (10 oz)	220	4	37	33
Strawberry Banana Blast	1 bottle (10 oz)	230	3	43	35
WholeSoy & Co.					
Organic Soy Peach	8 oz	210	3	34	29
Organic Soy Raspberry	8 oz	210	3	35	30
Organic Soy Strawberry	8 oz	210	3	34	29
SNACKS					
pork skins	1 oz	154	9	0	0
Baken-ets					
Fried Pork Skins	9 pieces	80	5	0	0

FOOD	PORTION	CALS	FAT	CARB	SUGAR
Fried Pork Skins Hot'n Spicy	9 pieces	80	5	tr	0
Fried Pork Skins Sweet & Tangy BBQ	9 pieces	80	5	1	0
Pork Cracklins	8 pieces	90	6	tr	0
Pork Cracklins Hot'n Spicy	8 pieces	80	5	tr	0
Bugles					
Baked Original	1⅓ cups	130	4	23	2
Chile Con Queso	1⅓ cups	160	9	18	1
Nacho	1½ cups	160	9	18	1
Original	1½ cups	160	9	18	1
Smokin'BBQ	1⅓ cups	150	8	19	2
Cheetos					
Asteriods Go Snack	¾ cup (1 oz)	160	10	15	1
Baked Crunchy	34 pieces (1 oz)	130	5	19	1
Crunchy	21 pieces (1 oz)	160	10	15	1
Natural White Cheddar	32 pieces (1 oz)	150	8	16	tr
Puffs	13 pieces (1 oz)	160	10	13	tr
Twisted	7 pieces (1 oz)	160	10	13	tr
Chester's					
Puffcorn Butter	3 cups	160	11	12	0
Puffcorn Cheese	3 cups	160	11	12	1
Chex Mix					
Cheddar	⅔ cup	140	5	21	2
Hot'N Spicy	⅔ cup	130	5	21	2
Nacho Fiesta	⅔ cup	120	4	22	2
Party Blend Bold	⅔ cup	140	6	20	2
Peanut Lovers	⅔ cup	140	6	19	2
Traditional	⅔ cup	130	4	22	2
Funyuns					
Mini Onion Rings	1 pkg	260	14	30	1

FOOD	PORTION	CALS	FAT	CARB	SUGAR
Glenny's					
Slim Carb Curls Cheddar Cheese	1 pkg (1 oz)	121	4	9	1
Go Snacks					
Onion Rings	13 pieces	140	7	18	tr
Good Sense					
Snack Mix Cajun Corn 'N Sesame	¼ cup	150	8	17	0
Trail Mix Dietary Snack Mix	¼ cup	130	6	14	7
Gram's Gourmet					
Crunchies Pork Rinds	⅛ pkg (0.5 oz)	70	5	0	0
Kangaroo					
Pita Snackers Crispy Cinnamon	10 pieces (1 oz)	90	2	19	2
Pita Snackers Sea Salt	10 pieces (1 oz)	90	2	18	1
Mauna Loa					
Tropical Nut & Fruit	¼ cup	180	8	23	14
Munchies					
Snack Mix Flamin' Hot	1 oz	140	6	17	tr
Snack Mix Kids	1 oz	130	4	20	5
Organic					
Trail Mix Tropical	⅓ cup	160	10	16	11
Organic Trails					
Trail Mix Summit Blend	¼ cup	150	8	19	14
Sabritones					
Chile & Lime	23 pieces	150	10	13	0
Tumaro's					
Organic Krispy Crunchy Puffs Cheddar	22	120	3	21	tr
Organic Krispy Crunchy Puffs Natural Corn	22	120	2	23	0
Organic Krispy Crunchy Puffs Ranch & Herb	22	130	4	20	2

FOOD	PORTION	CALS	FAT	CARB	SUGAR
Organic Krispy Crunchy Puffs Tangy BBQ	22	120	4	21	2
SNAIL					
TAKE-OUT					
escargot cooked	5	25	0	1	—
SNAKE					
fresh	3 oz	78	tr	3	—
SNAP BEANS					
FRESH					
Frieda's					
Purple Wax	⅔ cup	25	0	6	2
SNAPPER					
cooked	3 oz	109	1	0	0
SODA					
club	12 oz	0	0	0	0
shirley temple	1 serv	159	0	41	—
7 Up					
Diet	8 oz	0	0	0	0
Original	8 oz	100	0	26	26
AJ Stephans					
Birch Beer	1 bottle	170	0	45	43
Cream	1 bottle	170	0	45	43
Barq's					
Diet French Vanilla Creme	8 oz	1	0	tr	tr
Diet Red Creme	8 oz	4	0	0	0
Diet Root Beer	8 oz	1	0	tr	tr
Root Beer	8 oz	111	0	30	30
Carver's					
Ginger Ale	8 oz	94	0	24	24
Chronic 187					
Orange	1 bottle (12 oz)	300	0	77	75

FOOD	PORTION	CALS	FAT	CARB	SUGAR
Coca-Cola					
Blak	1 bottle (8 oz)	45	0	12	12
C2	8 oz	45	0	12	12
Zero	8 oz	0	0	0	0
Coke					
Cherry	8 oz	104	0	28	28
Diet	8 oz	1	0	tr	0
Diet Cherry	8 oz	1	0	tr	tr
Diet Vanilla	8 oz	1	0	tr	tr
Dr Pepper					
Original	1 can (12 oz)	150	0	40	40
Fresca					
Soda	8 oz	3	0	tr	tr
Hiball					
Club	1 bottle (10 oz)	5	0	0	0
Tonic Water	1 bottle (10 oz)	120	0	31	29
Inca Kola					
Diet	8 oz	1	0	tr	tr
Soda	8 oz	96	0	26	26
Jolt					
Blue	8 oz	120	0	32	32
Cola	8 oz	100	0	27	27
Ultra	8 oz	0	0	0	0
Kutztown					
Birch Beer	1 bottle (12 oz)	160	0	39	39
Sarsaparilla	1 bottle (12 oz)	150	0	38	28
Lucozade					
Soda	7 oz	136	0	36	—
Maine Root					
All Flavors	1 bottle (12 oz)	165	0	49	40
Mello Yellow					
Cherry	8 oz	118	0	32	32
Diet	8 oz	3	0	tr	tr

FOOD	PORTION	CALS	FAT	CARB	SUGAR
Mr. Pibb					
Diet	8 oz	1	0	tr	tr
Northern Neck					
Diet Ginger Ale	8 oz	4	0	0	0
Ginger Ale	8 oz	94	0	24	24
Orangina					
Sparkling Citrus	8 oz	90	0	23	21
Pepsi					
Edge	1 can (12 oz)	70	0	20	20
Schweppes					
Ginger Ale	8 oz	120	0	34	32
Sprite					
Diet Zero	8 oz	0	0	0	0
Soda	8 oz	96	0	26	26
Stewart's					
Diet Cream	1 bottle (12 oz)	0	0	0	0
Sunkist					
Diet Orange	8 oz	0	0	0	0
Orange	8 oz	130	0	35	35
Tab					
Soda	8 oz	1	0	tr	tr
Uno Mas					
All Flavors	1 can (12 oz)	130	0	31	31
Virgil's					
Micro Brewed Root Beer	1 bottle (12 oz)	160	0	42	42
SOLE					
cooked	3 oz	99	1	0	0
TAKE-OUT					
breaded & fried	3.2 oz	211	11	15	–

FOOD	PORTION	CALS	FAT	CARB	SUGAR
SOUP					
CANNED					
Butterball					
Chicken Broth Reduced Sodium 99% Fat Free	1 cup	10	0	2	0
Campbell's					
98% Fat Free Cream Of Mushroom	1 cup	70	3	9	1
98% Fat Free Cream Of Chicken as prep	1 cup	70	3	10	1
Cheddar Cheese	1 cup	110	5	12	2
Chicken Broth	½ cup	20	1	1	1
Chunky Beef Barley	1 cup	160	3	22	4
Chunky Chicken & Dumplings	1 cup	190	8	18	2
Chunky Chicken Corn Chowder	1 cup	230	13	21	4
Chunky Chili Roadhouse Beef & Bean	1 cup	220	8	25	7
Chunky Classic Chicken Noodle	1 cup	120	3	16	3
Chunky New England Clam Chowder	1 cup	240	13	23	1
Chunky Old Fashioned Vegetable Beef	1 cup	130	3	18	2
Chunky Sirloin Burger w/ Country Vegetables	1 cup	180	7	20	4
Chunky Vegetable	1 cup	130	4	22	5
Classics Minestrone	1 cup	90	1	17	3
Classics Old Fashioned Vegetable	1 cup	90	2	16	3
Classics Vegetarian Vegetable as prep	1 cup	90	1	18	6

FOOD	PORTION	CALS	FAT	CARB	SUGAR
Cream Of Chicken	1 cup	120	8	10	1
Cream Of Chicken w/ Herbs	1 cup	90	4	10	2
Double Noodle	1 cup	90	2	17	1
Healthy Request Cream Of Chicken as prep	1 cup	80	3	12	2
Kitchen Classics Bean With Bacon	1 cup	180	4	28	4
Kitchen Classics Chicken Noodle	1 cup	980	1	13	1
Kitchen Classics Chicken w/ White & Wild Rice	1 cup	100	1	18	1
Kitchen Classics Lentil	1 cup	120	1	23	1
Select Chicken Rice	1 cup	100	1	17	2
Select Chicken w/ Egg Noodles	1 cup	90	2	12	2
Select Creamy Potato w/ Roasted Garlic	1 cup	180	10	20	3
Select Italian Style Wedding	1 cup	110	3	16	3
Select Mexican Chicken Tortilla	1 cup	150	3	22	1
Select Roasted Chicken w/ Long Grain & Wild Rice	1 cup	130	1	17	2
Soup At Hand Chicken & Stars	1 pkg	70	2	11	1
Soup At Hand Chicken w/ Mini Noodles	1 pkg (10.75 oz)	80	2	12	2
Soup At Hand Cream Of Broccoli	1 pkg (10.75 oz)	160	8	16	3
Soup At Hand Creamy Chicken	1 pkg (10.75 oz)	130	8	13	1

FOOD	PORTION	CALS	FAT	CARB	SUGAR
Soup At Hand Creamy Tomato	1 pkg	180	4	34	16
Soup At Hand Vegetable Medley	1 pkg (10.75 oz)	110	2	20	8
Soup At Hand Velvety Potato	1 pkg (10.75 oz)	160	7	21	5
College Inn					
Beef Broth 99% Fat Free	1 cup	20	1	0	0
Beef Broth Fat Free Lower Sodium	1 cup	15	0	0	0
Chicken Broth Light & Fat Free	1 cup	5	0	0	0
Gold's					
Borscht Low Calorie	1 cup	20	0	5	5
Borscht Unsalted	1 cup	70	0	17	16
Hungarian Cabbage	6 oz	70	0	18	14
Healthy Choice					
Bean & Ham	1 cup	170	3	29	4
Beef & Potato	1 cup	110	1	19	3
Chicken & Dumplings	1 cup	130	2	22	0
Chicken & Pasta	1 cup	110	2	18	3
Chicken Corn Chowder	1 cup	140	2	26	5
Chicken Fiesta	1 cup	100	2	17	0
Chicken w/ Rice	1 cup	90	3	12	tr
Chicken w/ Roasted Garlic	1 cup	120	2	19	4
Chili Beef	1 cup	170	2	31	5
Clam Chowder	1 cup	110	2	21	2
Country Vegetable	1 cup	100	1	22	5
Creamy Tomato	1 cup	100	2	22	13
Garden Vegetable	1 cup	120	1	25	6
Hearty Chicken	1 cup	120	2	20	2
Italian Bean & Pasta	1 cup	100	2	18	2

FOOD	PORTION	CALS	FAT	CARB	SUGAR
Old Fashioned Chicken Noodle	1 cup	110	2	16	tr
Roasted Italian Style Chicken	1 cup	120	2	18	4
Split Pea w/ Ham	1 cup	170	3	30	4
Turkey w/ Rice	1 cup	90	2	16	2
Vegetable Beef	1 cup	130	1	24	5
Vegetable Clam Chowder	1 cup	230	1	16	3
Zesty Gumbo	1 cup	100	2	16	2
Manischewitz					
Clear Chicken Condensed	½ cup	15	1	2	0
Pacific Foods					
Beef Broth	1 cup	20	0	1	0
Creamy Butternut Squash	1 cup	90	2	17	4
Creamy Roasted Carrot	1 cup	100	1	18	5
Creamy Roasted Red Pepper & Tomato	1 cup	100	2	16	10
Hearty Beef Barley	1 cup	110	2	16	2
Hearty Chicken Noodle	1 cup	80	1	12	1
Hearty Chicken Tortilla	1 cup	130	2	22	5
Hearty Roasted Red Pepper & Corn Chowder	1 cup	210	12	21	2
Organic Creamy Tomato	1 cup	100	2	16	10
Organic French Onion	1 cup	35	0	6	1
Organic Vegetarian Broth	1 cup	15	0	3	1
Progresso					
99% Fat Free Beef Barley	1 cup	130	2	20	3
Carb Monitor Chicken Vegetable	1 cup	70	2	7	2
Chicken Rice w/ Vegetable	1 cup	100	2	15	1
Rich & Hearty Chicken & Homestyle Noodles	1 cup	110	3	14	2

FOOD	PORTION	CALS	FAT	CARB	SUGAR
Traditional Beef Barley	1 cup	150	5	18	3
Traditional Chicken & Herb Dumplings	1 cup	110	3	15	1
Traditional Chicken Noodle	1 cup	100	2	13	1
Traditional Hearty Chicken & Rotini	1 cup	100	2	14	1
Turkey Noodle	1 cup	90	2	11	1
Vegetable Classics French Onion	1 cup	50	2	8	3
Vegetable Classics Green Split Pea	1 cup	170	3	28	6
Vegetable Classics Hearty Tomato	1 cup	110	1	23	9
Vegetable Classics Lentil	1 cup	150	2	28	1
Vegetable Classics Macaroni & Bean	1 cup	160	4	25	1
Vegetable Classics Minestrone	1 cup	110	2	19	2
Vegetable Classics Tomato Rotini	1 cup	140	1	30	12
Vegetable Classics Vegetable	1 cup	80	1	16	3
Rienzi					
Chicken & Rice	1 cup	110	3	17	2
Italian Wedding Bell	1 cup	130	7	12	2
Snow's					
Clam Chowder	1 cup	200	15	13	3
Swanson					
Beef Broth 100% Fat Free Lower Sodium	1 cup	15	0	1	1
Chicken Broth 99% Fat Free	1 cup	15	1	1	1

FOOD	PORTION	CALS	FAT	CARB	SUGAR
Wolfgang Puck					
Chicken Parmesan w/ Pasta	1 cup	300	12	15	2
Hearty Lentil & Vegetable	1 cup	170	3	29	2
FROZEN					
Phillips Seafood					
Cream Of Crab	1 cup	310	25	12	6
Shrimp Bisque	1 cup	280	18	18	11
MIX					
beef broth cube	1 cube	6	tr	1	—
chicken broth cube	1 cube (4.8 g)	9	tr	1	—
A Taste Of Thai					
Coconut Ginger	2 tsp	15	1	2	2
Alpine Aire					
Low Carb Bay Shrimp Bisque	1 pkg	150	11	6	1
Low Carb Beefy Vegetable	1 pkg	100	4	7	1
Low Carb Broccoli Cheddar	1 pkg	140	10	6	1
Low Carb Mushroom & Chicken w/ Roasted Garlic	1 pkg	130	8	7	2
Azumaya					
Asian Style Thin Noodle	1 cup	120	0	24	2
Asian Style Wide Noodle	1 cup	120	0	24	2
Fantastic					
Noodle Bowls Mandarin Broccoli	1 pkg (2.2 oz)	220	0	40	2
MiniCarb					
Miso w/ Tofu & Shitake	1 pkg	33	1	5	2
Szechuan Beef	1 pkg	24	1	4	0
Thai Coconut Cream	1 pkg	100	6	9	0

FOOD	PORTION	CALS	FAT	CARB	SUGAR
Miso-Cup					
Golden Vegetable as prep	1 cup	30	1	3	1
Miso Reduced Sodium as prep	1 cup	25	1	3	tr
Organic Miso as prep	1 cup	35	1	4	tr
Savory Seaweed as prep	1 cup	30	1	3	tr
Nueva Cocina					
Frijoles Negros Con Chipotle Chile	1 cup	140	1	27	2
Sopa De Calabaza	1 cup	180	8	25	7
Sopa De Frijoles Colorados	1 cup	140	1	27	2
Sopa De Frijoles Negros	1 cup	140	0	27	2
Sopa De Maiz	1 cup	150	7	28	13
Sopa De Tortilla	1 cup	140	4	34	5
Rapunzel					
Cubes Vegetable Bouillon No Salt Added	½ cube	25	2	0	0
Cubes Vegetable Bouillon w/ Sea Salt	½ cube	15	1	0	0
Cubes Vegetable Bouillon w/ Sea Salt & Herbs	½ cube	15	2	0	0
Simply Asia					
Soy Noodle Bowl	1 pkg	70	0	10	3
Slim-Fast					
Creamy Broccoli	1 pkg	210	5	30	13
Creamy Chicken	1 pkg	220	5	33	15
Creamy Potato Cheddar & Chive	1 pkg	220	5	35	15
TAKE-OUT					
beef stew soup	1 cup (8.8 oz)	221	5	20	—
black bean turtle soup	1 cup	241	1	45	—
broccoli cheese	1 cup	165	9	15	7

FOOD	PORTION	CALS	FAT	CARB	SUGAR
corn & cheese chowder	¾ cup	215	12	21	—
egg drop	1 cup	73	4	1	tr
gazpacho	1 cup	46	tr	5	—
greek lemon	¾ cup	63	2	7	—
hot & sour	1 serv (14 oz)	173	8	8	1
matzo ball soup	1 cup	118	5	10	tr
onion soup gratinee	1 serv	492	27	38	6
sopa de feijao portuguese bean & sausage	1 cup	220	7	30	5
thai lemon grass	1 bowl	100	4	5	—
vietnamese pho beef noodle	1 serv (7.8 oz)	480	12	78	2
wonton soup	1 cup	205	3	26	—
zupa koprowa polish dill soup	1 bowl	54	2	6	—

SOUR CREAM
Breakstone's
Sour Cream	2 tbsp (1 oz)	60	5	1	1

Cabot
Light	2 tbsp	35	3	2	0
Sour Cream	2 tbsp	50	5	1	0

Crowley
Sour Cream	2 tbsp	60	5	1	1

Hood
Fat Free	2 tbsp	20	0	4	2
Low Fat	2 tbsp	35	2	3	2
Sour Cream	2 tbsp	60	5	2	1

SOURSOP
fresh cut up	1 cup	150	1	38	—

SOY
lecithin	1 tbsp	104	14	0	0

FOOD	PORTION	CALS	FAT	CARB	SUGAR
Fearn					
Granules	¼ cup	110	1	13	5
Powder	¼ cup	100	5	7	0
Good Sense					
Soynuts Honey Roasted	⅓ cup	140	6	11	4
Soynuts Roasted & Salted	⅓ cup	140	7	10	0
Soynuts Roasted w/o Salt	⅓ cup	140	7	10	0
SOYBEANS					
dried cooked	1 cup	298	15	17	–
dry roasted	½ cup	387	19	28	–
green cooked	½ cup	127	6	10	–
roasted	½ cup	405	22	29	–
sprouts raw	½ cup	43	2	3	–
sprouts steamed	½ cup	38	2	3	–
sprouts stir fried	1 cup	125	7	9	–
Arrowhead					
Organic not prep	¼ cup	180	8	14	3
Eden					
Organic Black	½ cup (4.6 oz)	120	6	8	1
Frieda's					
Edamame	½ cup (2.6 oz)	100	3	10	2
SOY SAUCE					
shoyu	1 tbsp	9	tr	2	–
soy sauce	1 tbsp	7	tr	1	–
tamari	1 tbsp	11	tr	1	–
SPAGHETTI SAUCE					
JARRED					
Barilla					
Boscaiola Mushrooms & Garlic	½ cup	90	3	11	7
Restaurant Creations Cheese & Tomatoes	¼ cup	110	8	5	1

FOOD	PORTION	CALS	FAT	CARB	SUGAR
Restaurant Creations Garlic Herbs & Tomatoes	¼ cup	100	8	6	3
Restaurant Creations Pesto & Tomatoes	¼ cup	150	12	7	2
Catelli					
Garden Select Country Mushroom	½ cup	80	2	13	7
Garden Select Diced Tomatoes & Basil	½ cup	80	2	13	8
Garden Select Fine Herbs	½ cup	80	2	13	8
Garden Select Garlic & Onion	½ cup	80	2	13	7
Garden Select Parmesan & Romano	½ cup	80	3	12	7
Garden Select Zucchini Primavera	½ cup	80	2	15	9
Classico					
Italian Sausage	½ cup	90	2	13	8
Tomato & Basil	½ cup	60	1	11	6
Del Monte					
Chunky Garlic & Herb	½ cup	60	2	11	9
Chunky Italian Herb	½ cup	60	1	12	8
Tomato & Basil	½ cup	70	1	16	11
With Four Cheese	½ cup	70	2	15	10
With Garlic & Onion	½ cup	80	1	16	10
With Green Peppers & Mushrooms	½ cup	80	1	16	10
With Meat	½ cup	60	1	14	9
With Mushrooms	½ cup	60	1	14	9
Francesco Rinaldi					
Chunky Garden Tomato Garlic & Onion	½ cup (4.4 oz)	70	3	12	11

FOOD	PORTION	CALS	FAT	CARB	SUGAR
Hunt's					
Basil Garlic & Oregano	¼ cup	15	0	3	2
Cheese & Garlic	½ cup	50	1	9	7
Chunky Vegetable	½ cup	50	1	11	8
Diced In Tomato Sauce	½ cup	30	0	7	4
Family Favorites Lasagna	¼ cup	30	0	6	5
Four Cheese	½ cup	50	1	10	7
Italian Sausage	½ cup	60	2	10	7
Light	½ cup	45	0	9	6
Meat	½ cup	68	1	11	7
No Added Sugar	½ cup	45	1	9	6
Roasted Garlic & Onion	½ cup	50	1	10	7
Traditional	½ cup	50	1	10	7
With Mushrooms	½ cup	50	1	10	7
Newman's Own					
Sockarooni	½ cup	60	2	9	7
Ragu					
Chunky Garden Style Tomato Garlic & Onion	½ cup (4.5 oz)	110	3	18	13
Tuttorosso					
Pasta Sauce Meat	½ cup	90	3	15	9
Walden Farms					
Alfredo Sauce Calorie Free	¼ cup	0	0	0	0
Marinara Calorie Free	⅓ cup	0	0	0	0
REFRIGERATED					
Buitoni					
Alfredo	¼ cup	140	12	5	2
Alfredo Light	¼ cup	80	5	5	2
Alfredo Portabello Mushroom	¼ cup	100	8	5	2
Marinara	½ cup	80	3	11	7
Marinara Roasted Garlic	½ cup	60	2	9	6
Pesto	¼ cup	330	27	11	4

FOOD	PORTION	CALS	FAT	CARB	SUGAR
Pesto w/ Basil	¼ cup	300	26	9	4
Pesto w/ Basil Reduced Fat	¼ cup	230	18	9	5
Pesto w/ Sun Dried Tomatoes	¼ cup	210	18	9	4
Tomato Herb Parmesan	½ cup	120	8	9	7
TAKE-OUT					
bolognese	5 oz	195	15	4	—

SPANISH FOOD
FROZEN
Amy's
Burrito Especial	1 (6 oz)	260	6	45	4

El Monterey
Quesadllas Chicken Breast & Cheese	1 (5 oz)	280	13	21	1

Healthy Choice
Chicken Enchiladas	1 pkg	360	7	59	3
Enchilada Chicken	1 pkg	300	7	46	4

Jose Ole
Burrito Chicken	1 (5 oz)	260	4	48	1

Lean Cuisine
One Dish Favorites Chicken Enchilada	1 pkg (9 oz)	280	5	49	7

TAKE-OUT
burrito w/ beans & cheese	2 (6.5 oz)	377	12	55	—
burrito w/ beef	2 (7.7 oz)	523	21	59	—
chimichanga w/ beef & cheese	1 (6.4 oz)	443	23	39	—
enchilada w/ cheese & beef	1 (6.7 oz)	324	18	30	—
enchirito w/ cheese beef & beans	1 (6.8 oz)	344	16	34	—
frijoles w/ cheese	1 cup (5.9 oz)	226	8	29	—
nachos w/ cheese	6 to 8 (4 oz)	345	19	36	—

FOOD	PORTION	CALS	FAT	CARB	SUGAR
tostada w/ beans & cheese	1 (5.1 oz)	223	10	27	–
tostada w/ beef & cheese	1 (5.7 oz)	315	16	23	–

SPINACH
CANNED
Del Monte
| Whole Leaf | ½ cup | 30 | 0 | 4 | 0 |

FRESH
baby raw	2 cups	20	0	5	0
cooked	½ cup	21	tr	3	–
raw chopped	½ cup	6	tr	1	–

Fresh Express
| Baby Spinach | 3 cups | 20 | 0 | 3 | 0 |
| Spicy Spinach | 3 cups (3 oz) | 10 | 0 | 6 | 0 |

Ready Pac
| Baby | 2 cups | 20 | 0 | 5 | 0 |
| Microwave Spinach as prep | ½ cup | 20 | 0 | 3 | 0 |

FROZEN
Green Giant
| Creamed Low Fat Sauce | ½ cup | 80 | 3 | 9 | 5 |

Taverna
| Spinach Pie | 1 piece (4.8 oz) | 190 | 6 | 24 | 4 |

TAKE-OUT
| indian saag | 1 serv | 28 | 2 | 2 | – |
| spanakopita spinach pie | 1 cup (6 oz) | 196 | 3 | 35 | 4 |

SPOT
| baked | 3 oz | 134 | 5 | 0 | 0 |

SPROUTS
kidney bean	½ cup	27	tr	4	–
lentil sprouts	½ cup	40	tr	8	–
mung bean	½ cup	16	tr	3	–

FOOD	PORTION	CALS	FAT	CARB	SUGAR
pea	½ cup	77	tr	17	—
radish	½ cup	8	tr	1	—
Brassica					
Broccoli Sprouts	½ cup (1 oz)	16	0	2	0
TAKE-OUT					
mung bean stir fried	½ cup	31	tr	7	—

SQUAB

FOOD	PORTION	CALS	FAT	CARB	SUGAR
boneless baked	3.5 oz	175	3	0	0
breast w/o skin raw	1 (3.5 oz)	135	5	0	0

SQUASH

FRESH

FOOD	PORTION	CALS	FAT	CARB	SUGAR
acorn cooked mashed	½ cup	41	tr	11	—
acorn cubed baked	½ cup	57	tr	15	—
butternut baked	½ cup	41	tr	11	—
hubbard baked	½ cup	51	tr	11	—
hubbard cooked mashed	½ cup	35	tr	8	—
scallop sliced cooked	½ cup	14	tr	3	—
spaghetti cooked	½ cup	23	tr	5	—
Frieda's					
Acorn	¾ cup (3 oz)	35	0	9	3
Baby Crookneck	⅔ cup (3 oz)	15	0	3	2
Baby Scallop	⅔ cup (3 oz)	15	0	3	2
Eight Ball	2 (4.4 oz)	18	0	4	1
Hubbard	¾ cup (3 oz)	35	0	7	3
Mini Pumpkin	¾ cup (3 oz)	20	0	6	4
Spaghetti	¾ cup (3 oz)	30	0	6	3
Star Spangled	⅔ cup (3 oz)	20	0	3	2
Turban	¾ cup (3 oz)	30	0	7	3
Martin Farms					
Butternut Fresh Cut	½ cup	40	0	10	5
TAKE-OUT					
fritter	1 (0.8 oz)	81	5	8	1

FOOD	PORTION	CALS	FAT	CARB	SUGAR
SQUID					
fried	3 oz	149	6	7	–
Margaritaville					
Captain's Calamari Strips + Sauce	⅓ pkg	330	20	28	3
SQUIRREL					
roasted	3 oz	147	4	0	0
STARFRUIT					
fresh	1	42	tr	10	–
Frieda's					
Dried	⅓ cup (1.4 oz)	120	0	29	26
STRAWBERRIES					
DRIED					
Frieda's					
Dried	½ cup (1.4 oz)	150	0	34	29
FRESH					
strawberries	1 cup	45	1	10	–
FROZEN					
unsweetened	1 cup	52	tr	14	–
STRAWBERRY JUICE					
Adina					
California Kiss Hibiscus Strawberry	8 oz	80	0	21	18
Ceres					
Strawberry	8 oz	115	0	28	24
Giant Berry Farms					
Just Strawberries	1 bottle (12 oz)	140	0	33	19
Hi-C					
Blast	8 oz	120	0	32	31

FOOD	PORTION	CALS	FAT	CARB	SUGAR
STUFFING/DRESSING					
Pepperidge Farm					
Herb Seasoned	¾ cup (1.5 oz)	170	2	33	2
TAKE-OUT					
bread	1 cup	352	17	44	5
cornbread	½ cup	179	9	22	0
oyster	1 cup	304	18	29	3
sausage	½ cup	292	11	40	–
STURGEON					
cooked	3 oz	115	4	0	0
smoked	1 oz	48	1	0	0
SUCKER					
white baked	3 oz	101	3	0	0
SUGAR					
brown packed	1 cup (7.7 oz)	828	0	214	214
brown unpacked	1 cup (5.1 oz)	547	0	141	140
brown organic	1 tsp	17	0	4	4
cinnamon sugar	1 tsp	16	tr	4	4
maple	1 piece (1 oz)	99	tr	25	24
powdered	1 tbsp (0.3 oz)	31	0	8	8
powdered unsifted	1 cup (4.2 oz)	467	tr	119	115
raw	1 pkg (5 g)	19	0	5	5
sugarcane stem	3 oz	54	0	14	–
white	1 cup (7 oz)	773	0	200	200
white	1 packet (3 g)	12	0	3	3
white	1 tsp (4 g)	15	0	4	4
Domino					
Dark Brown	1 tsp	15	0	4	4
Gluco Burst					
Arctic Cherry	1 pkg (1.3 oz)	70	0	16	15
SUGAR APPLE					
fresh	1	146	tr	37	–

FOOD	PORTION	CALS	FAT	CARB	SUGAR
SUGAR SUBSTITUTES					
Equal					
Flavor Sticks	1 pkg	0	0	tr	tr
Packet	1 pkg	0	0	tr	tr
Spoonful	1 tsp	0	0	tr	tr
Sugar Lite	1 tsp	8	0	2	2
Fran Gare's					
Miracle Sweet	1 tsp	10	0	5	0
Keto					
Sweet	½ tsp	0	0	0	0
Lo Han					
Sweet	2 scoops	2	0	2	0
SomerSweet					
Sweetener	¼ tsp	0	0	tr	0
Splenda					
Sugar Blend For Baking	½ tsp	10	0	2	2
Sweetener	1 pkg	0	0	tr	tr
Steel's					
Brown	1 tsp	10	0	1	0
Sugar Substitute	1 tsp	10	0	1	0
Stevita					
Spoonable	⅓ tsp	0	0	0	0
Sugar Twin					
Packets	1	0	0	tr	—
Spoonable Brown	1 tsp	0	0	0	0
Spoonable White	1 tsp	0	0	0	0
SweetLeaf					
SteviaPlus	1 pkg	0	0	0	0
Whey Low					
Gold	1 tsp	4	0	4	4
Granular	1 tsp	4	0	4	4
Powder	1 tsp	4	0	4	4

FOOD	PORTION	CALS	FAT	CARB	SUGAR
SUNCHOKE					
Frieda's					
Sunchoke	½ cup (3 oz)	70	0	14	0
SUNFISH					
pumpkinseed baked	3 oz	97	1	0	0
SUNFLOWER					
seeds dry roasted w/ salt	¼ cup	185	15	9	–
seeds w/ hulls dried	¼ cup	66	6	2	tr
David					
Kernels Original	¼ cup	200	17	5	1
Seeds BBQ	¼ cup	190	15	5	1
Seeds BBQ Sizzlin	¼ cup	190	16	6	1
Seeds Jalapeno	¼ cup	190	15	5	1
Seeds Nacho Cheese	¼ cup	180	15	6	1
Seeds Original	¼ cup	190	15	5	1
Seeds Ranch	¼ cup	190	15	6	1
Seeds Reduced Sodium	¼ cup	190	15	5	1
Frito Lay					
Seeds	3 tbsp	180	15	5	tr
Good Sense					
Nuts Honey Roasted	¼ cup	190	15	7	2
Nuts Raw	¼ cup	170	15	6	0
Nuts Roasted & Salted	¼ cup	190	15	5	1
Seeds In Shell Roasted & Salted	½ cup	150	9	13	0
Sunflower Nuts Roasted w/o Salt	¼ cup	190	16	5	1
SunGold					
SunButter	2 tbsp	200	16	7	3
SUSHI					
TAKE-OUT					
california roll	1 piece (0.8 oz)	28	1	4	tr

FOOD	PORTION	CALS	FAT	CARB	SUGAR
fresh salmon rolls	4 pieces	250	7	37	5
sashimi	1 serv (6 oz)	198	7	4	1
tuna roll	1 piece (0.7 oz)	23	tr	3	tr
vegetable roll	1 piece (1.2 oz)	27	1	5	tr
vinegared ginger	⅓ cup (1.6 oz)	48	tr	12	4
wasabi	2 tsp (0.3 oz)	5	tr	1	—
yellowtail roll	1 piece (0.6 oz)	25	1	3	tr

SWAMP CABBAGE

chopped cooked	½ cup	10	tr	2	—

SWEETBREAD (PANCREAS)

beef braised	3 oz	230	15	0	0
lamb braised	3 oz	199	13	0	0
veal braised	3 oz	218	12	0	0

SWEET POTATO

baked w/ skin	1 (3 ½ oz)	118	tr	28	—
canned in syrup	½ cup	106	tr	25	—
leaves cooked	½ cup	11	tr	2	—
mashed	½ cup	172	tr	40	—
Princella					
In Light Syrup	⅔ cup	160	0	39	20
Royal Prince					
Orange Pineapple	½ cup	160	0	38	24
TAKE-OUT					
candied	3.5 oz	144	3	29	—
pudding	1 cup	215	6	37	14

SWISS CHARD

cooked	½ cup	18	tr	4	—
Frieda's					
Bright Lights	1 cup (3 oz)	15	0	3	1

SWORDFISH

cooked	3 oz	132	4	0	0

FOOD	PORTION	CALS	FAT	CARB	SUGAR
SYRUP					
corn dark & light	¼ cup	240	tr	65	65
maple	1 cup (11.1 oz)	824	1	212	191
maple	1 tbsp	52	0	13	12
rose hip	1 oz	9	0	2	2
sorghum	1 cup (11.6 oz)	957	0	247	247
sorghum	1 tbsp (0.7 oz)	61	0	16	16
sugar syrup	¼ cup	76	0	20	20
Cary's					
Maple	¼ cup	210	0	53	50
DaVinci Gourmet					
Sugar Free All Flavors	1 tbsp	0	0	0	0
Estee					
Blueberry	¼ cup	30	0	8	0
Karo					
Corn Syrup Dark	1 tbsp	120	0	31	11
Corn Syrup Light	2 tbsp	120	0	31	12
Nesquik					
Strawberry Calcium Fortified	2 tbsp	100	0	27	25
Smucker's					
Blackberry	¼ cup	210	0	52	52
Blueberry	¼ cup	210	0	52	52
Boysenberry	¼ cup	210	0	52	52
Red Raspberry	¼ cup	210	0	52	52
Strawberry	¼ cup	210	0	52	52
Sundae Syrup 3 Musketeers	2 tbsp	110	2	23	18
Sundae Syrup Butterscotch	2 tbsp	100	0	25	20
Sundae Syrup Caramel	2 tbsp	100	0	25	20
Sundae Syrup Strawberry	2 tbsp	110	0	26	23

FOOD	PORTION	CALS	FAT	CARB	SUGAR
Spectrum					
Balsamic Organic	1 tbsp	35	0	9	9
TAMARILLOS					
Frieda's					
Gold or Red	2 (4.2 oz)	40	0	9	2
TAMARIND					
fresh	1	5	tr	1	–
fresh cut up	1 cup	287	1	75	–
TANGERINE					
FRESH					
Sunkist					
Fresh	1 (3.8 oz)	50	1	15	12
TANGERINE JUICE					
Italian Volcano					
Organic	1 serv (6.75 oz)	94	1	20	19
Naked Juice					
Tangerine Scream	8 oz	110	0	25	25
TAPIOCA					
pearl dry	½ cup (2.7 oz)	272	tr	67	–
TARO					
chips	10 (0.8 oz)	115	6	16	–
leaves cooked	½ cup	18	tr	3	–
shoots sliced cooked	½ cup	10	tr	2	–
sliced cooked	½ cup (2.3 oz)	94	tr	23	–
Frieda's					
Taro Root	⅔ cup (3 oz)	90	0	22	1
TARPON					
fresh	3 oz	87	2	0	0
TARRAGON					
ground	1 tsp	5	tr	1	–

FOOD	PORTION	CALS	FAT	CARB	SUGAR
TEA/HERBAL TEA					
HERBAL					
chamomile brewed	1 cup	2	tr	tr	0
Tetley					
Chamomile	1 cup	0	0	0	0
Orange & Peach	1 cup	0	0	0	0
Peppermint	1 cup	0	0	tr	0
REGULAR					
Celestial Seasonings					
Green Tea Blueberry Breeze	1 cup	0	0	0	0
Green Tea Raspberry Garden as prep	1 cup	0	0	0	0
Honey Darjeeling as prep	1 cup	0	0	0	0
Teahouse Chai Original India Spice	1 cup	0	0	0	0
DaVinci Gourmet					
Sugar Free Tea Concentrate Green	2 tbsp	0	0	0	0
Sugar Free Tea Concentrate Lemon	2 tbsp	0	0	0	0
Sugar Free Tea Concentrate Spiced Chai	1.5 tbsp	0	0	0	0
Lipton					
100% Natural	1 teabag	0	0	0	0
Brisk Tea as prep	1 teabag	0	0	0	0
Decaffeinated Brisk Tea as prep	1 serv	0	0	0	0
Low Carb Creations					
Chai as prep	1 cup	25	2	3	tr
Oregon					
Chai Latte Cider	½ cup	110	0	26	25
Chai Latte Java	½ cup	42	0	10	10

FOOD	PORTION	CALS	FAT	CARB	SUGAR
Chai Latte Kashmir Green Tea	½ cup	81	1	19	18
Chai Latte Nog	½ cup	90	0	15	14
Chai Latte The Original	½ cup	78	0	19	18
Red Rose					
Decaffeinated	1 cup	0	0	0	0
Salada					
Original Blend Black Tea	1 tea bag	0	0	0	0
Tea Tech					
Instant Green Tea All Flavors	1 tube	0	0	tr	0
XtraGreen Tea Mix All Flavors	1 tube	0	0	tr	0
Tetley					
British Blend Round Teabags	1 cup	0	0	0	0
Chai Black Tea	1 cup	0	0	tr	0
Decaffeinated Tea Bag as prep	1	0	0	0	0
Earl Grey	1 cup	0	0	0	0
English Breakfast	1 cup	0	0	tr	0
Honey Lemon Green Tea	1 cup	0	0	0	0

TEMPEH
Lightlife

FOOD	PORTION	CALS	FAT	CARB	SUGAR
Garden Veggie	1 serv (4 oz)	230	10	14	0
Organic Flax	1 serv (4 oz)	230	10	14	0
Organic Grilles Lemon	1 patty (2.7 oz)	140	6	11	2
Organic Grilles Tamari	1 patty (2.7 oz)	130	5	9	2
Organic Soy	1 serv (4 oz)	210	9	14	0
Organic Three Grain	1 serv (4 oz)	240	9	21	0
Organic Wild Rice	1 serv (4 oz)	280	11	14	0

FOOD	PORTION	CALS	FAT	CARB	SUGAR
THYME					
ground	1 tsp	4	tr	1	–
TILAPIA					
Beacon Light					
Farm Raised Fillets	3 oz	85	1	1	0
TILEFISH					
cooked	3 oz	125	4	0	0
TOFU					
fresh fried	1 piece (0.5 oz)	35	3	1	–
Azumaya					
Extra Firm	1 serv (2.8 oz)	70	4	2	0
Firm	1 serv (2.8 oz)	70	4	2	0
Lite Silken	1 serv (3.2 oz)	40	1	3	0
Lite Extra Firm	1 serv (2.8 oz)	60	2	3	0
Seasoned Oriental Spice	1 serv (3 oz)	90	5	3	tr
Seasoned Zesty Garlic & Onion	1 serv (3 oz)	90	5	3	tr
Silken	1 serv (3.2 oz)	40	2	1	0
Nasoya					
Chinese Spice	¼ pkg (3 oz)	90	5	3	tr
Extra Firm	⅕ pkg (2.8 oz)	80	4	2	0
Firm	⅕ pkg (2.8 oz)	70	3	2	0
Garlic & Onion	¼ pkg (3 oz)	90	5	3	tr
Lite Firm	⅕ pkg (2.8 oz)	40	2	0	0
Lite Silken	⅕ pkg (3.2 oz)	30	1	0	0
Seasoned Ginger Sesame	½ pkg (5.5 oz)	210	6	27	20
Seasoned Sweet & Sour	½ pkg (5.5 oz)	190	4	26	20
Seasoned Teriyaki	½ pkg (5.5 oz)	190	4	24	20
Seasoned Thai Peanut	½ pkg (5.5 oz)	240	9	24	18
Silken	⅕ pkg (3.2 oz)	45	3	2	tr
Soft	⅕ pkg (2.8 oz)	60	3	1	0

FOOD	PORTION	CALS	FAT	CARB	SUGAR
TofuMate Breakfast Scramble	¼ pkg	15	0	3	0
TofuMate Eggless Salad	¼ pkg	15	0	4	0
TofuMate Mandarin Stirfry	¼ pkg	25	0	6	4
TofuMate Mediterranean Herb	¼ pkg	15	0	3	1
TofuMate Szechwan Stirfry	¼ pkg	25	0	4	0
TofuMate Texas Taco	¼ pkg	15	0	3	0
TAKE-OUT					
soy sauce marinated & grilled	1 serv (4 oz)	181	11	6	–

TOMATILLO

fresh	1 (1.2 oz)	11	tr	2	–

TOMATO
CANNED
Cento

Paste	2 tbsp	30	0	6	3
Puree	¼ cup	25	0	5	3

Contadina

Crushed w/ Italian Herbs	¼ cup	20	0	3	2
Petite Cut Diced	½ cup	25	0	6	4

Del Monte

Chunky Pasta Style	½ cup	45	0	11	8
Diced	½ cup	25	0	6	4
Diced No Salt Added	½ cup	25	0	6	4
Diced w/ Basil Garlic & Oregano	½ cup	50	0	11	8
Diced w/ Green Pepper & Onion	½ cup	40	0	9	7
Diced Zesty Chili Style	½ cup	30	0	8	6

FOOD	PORTION	CALS	FAT	CARB	SUGAR
Diced Zesty w/ Mild Green Chilies	½ cup	30	0	6	3
Petite Cut	½ cup	25	0	6	4
Petite Cut Garlic & Olive Oil	½ cup	45	1	10	7
Sauce	¼ cup	20	0	4	4
Stewed Cajun Recipe	½ cup	35	0	9	7
Stewed Italian Recipe	½ cup	30	0	8	6
Stewed Mexican Recipe	½ cup	35	0	9	7
Stewed No Salt Added	½ cup	35	0	9	7
Stewed Original	½ cup	35	0	9	7
Wedges	½ cup	35	0	9	7
Hunt's					
Crushed	½ cup	30	0	7	5
Diced Original	½ cup	20	0	5	4
Diced w/ Basil Garlic & Oregano	½ cup	25	0	6	5
Diced w/ Green Pepper Celery & Onions	½ cup	45	0	10	8
Diced w/ Mild Green Chilies	½ cup	30	0	6	5
Diced w/ Roasted Garlic	½ cup	30	0	6	5
Diced w/ Sweet Onion	½ cup	45	0	10	7
Family Favorites Meatloaf	¼ cup	30	0	7	4
Paste	2 tbsp	25	0	6	4
Paste No Salt Added	2 tbsp	30	0	6	4
Paste w/ Basil Garlic & Oregano	2 tbsp	25	0	6	4
Petite Diced	½ cup	20	0	5	3
Petite Diced w/ Mushrooms	½ cup	40	1	6	5
Puree	½ cup	30	0	7	4
Sauce	¼ cup	15	0	3	2

FOOD	PORTION	CALS	FAT	CARB	SUGAR
Sauce Garlic & Herb	½ cup	40	1	8	5
Sauce No Salt Added	2 tbsp	30	0	6	4
Sauce Roasted Garlic	¼ cup	15	0	3	2
Stewed	½ cup	35	0	8	6
Stewed No Salt Added	½ cup	40	0	9	6
Whole No Salt Added	¼ cup	20	0	4	3
Whole No Salt Added	4 oz	20	0	4	3
Redpack					
Chunky Style In Puree	½ cup	30	0	6	2
Crushed In Puree	¼ cup	20	0	4	2
Paste	2 tbsp	0	0	6	3
Rienzi					
Paste	2 tbsp	25	0	5	4
Ro-Tel					
Diced In Sauce	½ cup	40	0	8	7
Mexican Festival	½ cup	30	0	6	3
Original	½ cup	20	0	4	3
Tuttorosso					
Puree	¼ cup	20	0	4	3
DRIED					
sun dried	1 piece	5	tr	1	—
sun dried in oil	1 piece (3 g)	6	tr	1	—
Frieda's					
Red Chopped	⅓ cup (1.1 oz)	100	1	19	11
FRESH					
bruschetta	¼ cup	50	3	6	4
grape tomatoes	20	30	0	6	4
green	1	30	tr	6	—
red	1 (4.5 oz)	26	tr	6	—
Eurofresh					
Tomatoes On The Vine	1 med (5.2 oz)	35	1	7	4
Frieda's					
Baby Roma	⅔ cup (3 oz)	120	0	4	2

FOOD	PORTION	CALS	FAT	CARB	SUGAR
Tear Drop	⅔ cup (3 oz)	20	0	4	2
TAKE-OUT					
bruschetta on toasted italian bread	1 slice	106	3	18	2
stewed	1 cup	80	3	13	–

TOMATO JUICE
Campbell's
Juice	8 oz	50	0	10	7

Del Monte
Juice	8 oz	50	0	10	7

Luvli Juices
Smashing Tomato	1 bottle (10 oz)	125	1	28	24
Spicy Tomato	1 bottle (10 oz)	125	1	28	24

TONGUE
beef simmered	3 oz	241	19	0	0
lamb braised	3 oz	234	17	0	0
pork braised	3 oz	230	16	0	0
veal braised	3 oz	172	9	0	0

TORTILLA
Alvarado Street Bakery
Sprouted Wheat Burrito Size	1 (2.2 oz)	170	4	30	0

CarbOle
Low-Carb	1 (2 oz)	100	4	14	0

Food For Life
Sprouted Corn	2 (1.7 oz)	120	1	25	0

La Tortilla Factory
Low Carb Whole Wheat	1 lg	100	3	21	1
Low Carb Whole Wheat	1 reg	60	2	12	0

Manny's
Burrito Tortilla	1 (2.1 oz)	180	5	30	1
Fajita Tortilla	1 (2 oz)	170	5	28	1

FOOD	PORTION	CALS	FAT	CARB	SUGAR
Fat Free	1 (1 oz)	65	0	14	0
Low Carb	1 (1.7 oz)	140	7	13	0
Soft Taco Tortilla	1 (1 oz)	80	2	14	tr
Tortilla Wrap Tomato Basil	1 (1.4 oz)	100	2	19	0
White Corn Gluten Free	1 (2 oz)	60	1	11	0
Whole Wheat	1 (2 oz)	170	4	27	1
Super Bakery					
Organic	1 (2.5 oz)	210	5	35	0
Tumaro's					
Low In Carbs Garden Vegetable	1 (8 inch)	130	4	18	tr
Low In Carbs Green Onion	1 (8 inch)	130	4	17	tr
Low In Carbs Multi-grain	1 (8 inch)	146	4	18	1
Low In Carbs Salsa	1 (8 inch)	130	4	18	tr
TREE FERN					
chopped cooked	½ cup	28	tr	8	—
TRITICALE					
dry	½ cup (3.4 oz)	323	2	69	—
TROUT					
baked	3 oz	162	7	0	0
rainbow cooked	3 oz	129	4	0	0
seatrout baked	3 oz	113	4	0	0
TRUFFLES					
fresh	0.5 oz	4	tr	9	—
TUNA					
CANNED					
light in oil	3 oz	169	7	0	0
light in water	3 oz	99	1	0	0
white in oil	3 oz	158	7	0	0
white in water	3 oz	116	2	0	0

FOOD	PORTION	CALS	FAT	CARB	SUGAR
Bumble Bee					
Chunk Light In Oil	¼ cup	110	6	0	0
Chunk Light In Water	2 oz	60	1	0	0
Chunk Light Touch Of Lemon In Water	¼ cup	60	1	0	0
Chunk White In Oil	¼ cup	100	5	0	0
Chunk White In Water	¼ cup	60	1	0	0
Chunk White In Water Very Low Sodium	¼ cup	70	1	0	0
Light In Oil	¼ cup	110	6	0	0
Solid White In Oil	¼ cup	90	3	0	0
Solid White In Water	2 oz	70	1	0	0
Tonno In Olive Oil	¼ cup	120	6	0	0
Chicken Of The Sea					
Albacore In Spring Water	2 oz	80	4	0	0
Chunk Light In Oil	2 oz	110	6	0	0
Chunk Light In Water	¼ cup (2 oz)	60	1	0	0
Chunk White In Spring Water	½ can	60	1	0	0
Chunk White Low Sodium In Spring Water	1 can (3 oz)	80	1	0	0
Premium Albacore Pouch	2 oz	60	1	0	0
Coral					
Light In Water	¼ cup	60	1	0	0
StarKist					
Solid White Albacore In Water	¼ cup	70	1	0	0
FRESH					
bluefin cooked	3 oz	157	5	0	0
bluefin raw	3 oz	122	4	0	0
skipjack baked	3 oz	112	1	0	0
yellowfin baked	3 oz	118	1	0	0

FOOD	PORTION	CALS	FAT	CARB	SUGAR
SHELF-STABLE					
Bumble Bee					
Steak Entrees Ginger & Soy	1 pkg (4 oz)	170	3	3	3
Steak Entrees Lemon & Cracked Pepper	1 pkg (4 oz)	160	1	0	0
Steak Entrees Mesquite Grilled	1 pkg (4 oz)	150	2	0	0
TUNA DISHES					
MIX					
Chicken Of The Sea					
Salad Kit	1 serv (3.5 oz)	380	24	18	5
Tuna Salad Kit Single Mayo & Onion	1 pkg	380	24	18	5
TAKE-OUT					
tuna salad	1 cup	383	19	19	–
TURBOT					
european baked	3 oz	104	3	0	0
TURKEY					
FRESH					
back w/ skin roasted	½ back (9 oz)	637	38	0	0
breast w/ skin roasted	4 oz	212	8	0	0
dark meat w/ skin roasted	3.6 oz	230	12	0	0
dark meat w/o skin roasted	1 cup (5 oz)	262	10	0	0
dark meat w/o skin roasted	3 oz	170	7	0	0
ground cooked	3 oz	188	11	0	0
leg w/ skin roasted	2.5 oz	147	7	0	0
leg w/ skin roasted	1 (1.2 lbs)	1133	54	0	0
light meat w/ skin roasted	from ½ turkey (2.3 lbs)	2069	87	0	0

FOOD	PORTION	CALS	FAT	CARB	SUGAR
light meat w/ skin roasted	4.7 oz	268	11	0	0
light meat w/o skin roasted	4 oz	183	4	0	0
neck simmered	1 (5.3 oz)	274	11	0	0
skin roasted	1 oz	141	13	0	0
skin roasted	from ½ turkey (9 oz)	1096	98	0	0
w/ skin roasted	8.4 oz	498	23	0	0
w/ skin roasted	½ turkey (4 lbs)	3857	181	0	0
w/ skin neck & giblets roasted	½ turkey (8.8 lbs)	4123	190	1	—
w/o skin roasted	1 cup (5 oz)	238	7	0	0
w/o skin roasted	7.3 oz	354	10	0	0
wing w/ skin roasted	1 (6.5 oz)	426	23	0	0
Jennie-O					
Ground	4 oz	160	8	0	0
Shady Brook					
Cutlets	4 oz	110	1	0	0
Ground	4 oz	160	8	0	0
Tenderloin Rotisserie	4 oz	130	4	5	1
READY-TO-EAT					
bologna	1 slice (1 oz)	59	4	1	1
breast	1 slice (0.75 oz)	23	tr	0	0
prebasted breast w/ skin roasted	1 breast (3.8 lbs)	2175	60	0	0
prebasted breast w/ skin roasted	½ breast (1.9 lbs)	1087	30	0	0
prebasted thigh w/ skin roasted	1 thigh (11 oz)	494	27	0	0
salami cooked beef	1 slice (0.9 oz)	67	6	tr	tr
turkey loaf breast meat	1 pkg (6 oz)	187	3	0	0
turkey loaf breast meat	2 slices (1.5 oz)	47	1	0	0

FOOD	PORTION	CALS	FAT	CARB	SUGAR
turkey salad sandwich spread	¼ cup	104	7	4	0
Healthy Choice					
Smoked Breast	4 slices (1.8 oz)	60	2	2	0
Hebrew National					
98% Fat Free Smoked Breast	5 slices (2 oz)	60	1	0	0
Oscar Mayer					
Smoked Turkey Breast	2 oz	60	1	2	0
Smoked White	3 slices (3 oz)	90	3	2	tr
Turkey Bologna	3 slices (3 oz)	160	12	4	1
Turkey Cotto Salami	3 slices (3 oz)	130	8	tr	tr
TURKEY DISHES					
FROZEN					
Banquet					
Homestyle Gravy & Sliced Turkey	2 slices + gravy	130	9	3	1
READY-TO-EAT					
Jennie-O					
Stuffed Breast Cheddar Cheese & Broccoli	1 serv (6 oz)	240	9	3	1
Stuffed Turkey Breast Pepper Cheese & Rice	1 piece (6 oz)	250	7	13	1
Turkey Breast Roast In Homestyle Gravy	1 serv (5 oz)	110	1	3	1
TAKE-OUT					
boneless breast w/ cranberry apple stuffing	1 serv (5 oz)	260	9	10	2
TURKEY SUBSTITUTES					
Lightlife					
Smart Deli Roast Turkey	4 slices (2 oz)	80	0	4	0

FOOD	PORTION	CALS	FAT	CARB	SUGAR
TURMERIC					
ground	1 tsp	8	tr	1	—
TURNIPS					
canned greens	½ cup	17	tr	3	—
cooked mashed	½ cup (4.2 oz)	47	tr	10	—
TURTLE					
raw	3.5 oz	85	1	0	0
TUSK FISH					
raw	3.5 oz	79	tr	0	0
VANILLA					
vanilla extract	1 tsp	17	0	0	0
Steel's					
Sugar Free	1 tbsp	24	0	6	0
VEAL					
breast braised	3 oz	226	14	0	0
chop cooked	1 med (6.5 oz)	230	13	0	0
chop breaded fried	1 med (6.5 oz)	290	12	13	0
cubed braised	3 oz	160	4	0	0
cutlet cooked	3 oz	141	4	0	0
ground broiled	3 oz	146	6	0	0
leg roasted	3 oz	136	4	0	0
loin roasted	3 oz	184	10	0	0
patty breaded fried	1 (2.8 oz)	211	13	7	1
shank braised	3 oz	162	5	0	0
VEAL DISHES					
TAKE-OUT					
cordon bleu	1 serv (8 oz)	490	35	4	2
parmigiana	1 serv (6.4 oz)	362	21	15	3
scallopini	1 slice + sauce (3.4 oz)	238	17	2	1
stew	1 serv (8.8 oz)	192	6	18	4

FOOD	PORTION	CALS	FAT	CARB	SUGAR
veal marengo	1 serv (8.8 oz)	274	9	7	3
veal marsala	1 slice + sauce (3.4 oz)	268	19	6	2
veal paprikash	1 serv (8.6 oz)	280	12	5	1
veal picatta	1 piece + sauce (3.5 oz)	154	9	2	tr

VEGETABLE JUICE
V8
| Lemon Twist | 1 bottle (12 oz) | 70 | 0 | 14 | 11 |

VEGETABLES MIXED
CANNED
Del Monte
Mixed	½ cup	40	0	8	3
Mixed Vegetables w/ Potatoes	½ cup	45	0	10	3
Peas And Carrots	½ cup	60	0	11	4
Savory Sides Homestyle Vegetable Medley	½ cup	70	3	11	3
Savory Sides Rio Grande Vegetables	½ cup	70	0	14	3
Veg-All
| Original Mixed | ½ cup | 40 | 0 | 8 | 2 |
FRESH
River Ranch
Broccoli & Carrots	1 cup	25	0	5	3
Broccoli & Cauliflower	1 cup	25	0	4	2
Stir Fry Blend	1 cup	30	0	5	3
Vegetable Medley	1 cup	25	0	6	3
FROZEN
Birds Eye
| Baby Pea & Vegetable Blend | ¾ cup | 40 | 0 | 7 | 3 |

FOOD	PORTION	CALS	FAT	CARB	SUGAR
Szechuan Vegetables In A Sesame Sauce	1 cup	60	2	9	6
Green Giant					
Seasoned Broccoli & Carrots w/ Garlic & Herbs	½ cup	45	1	8	2
Lean Cuisine					
Cafe Classics Roasted Potatoes w/ Broccoli & Cheddar Cheese Sauce	1 pkg (10.25 oz)	230	5	35	8
Pictsweet					
Peas & Carrots	⅔ cup	50	0	9	4
TAKE-OUT					
buddha's delight	1 serv (16 oz)	174	5	17	8
curry	1 serv (7.7 oz)	398	33	22	—
gyoza potstickers vegetable	8 (4.9 oz)	210	4	34	7
pakoras	1 (2 oz)	108	5	12	—
ratatouille	1 serv (3.5 oz)	96	7	7	7
samosa	2 (4 oz)	170	6	22	2
succotash	½ cup	111	1	23	—
tapenade grilled vegetables	¼ cup	40	3	4	2
VENISON					
roasted	4 oz	215	4	0	0
VINEGAR					
balsamic of modena	1 tbsp (0.5 oz)	10	0	3	3
cider	1 tbsp	tr	0	1	—
Heinz					
White	2 tbsp	2	0	0	0
Spectrum					
Apple Cider Organic	1 tbsp	7	0	2	0
Balsamic Organic	1 tbsp	6	0	2	0

FOOD	PORTION	CALS	FAT	CARB	SUGAR
Brown Rice Organic	1 tbsp	10	0	2	0
Golden Balsamic Organic	1 tbsp	6	0	2	2
Red Wine Organic	1 tbsp	0	0	0	0
White Organic	1 tbsp	2	0	tr	0
White Wine Organic	1 tbsp	0	0	0	0

WAFFLES

FROZEN

plain	1 4 in sq (1.2 oz)	88	3	14	–

EnviroKidz

Organic Gorilla Banana	2 (2.7 oz)	230	8	34	9

READY-TO-EAT

Gol D Lite

Low Carb Belgian	1 (0.9 oz)	100	5	15	0
Low Carb Belgian Chocolate Covered	1 (1.1 oz)	130	8	18	0

Kashi

GoLean Blueberry	2	170	3	33	4
GoLean Original	2	170	3	33	4

Thomas'

Homestyle	1 (1.6 oz)	140	5	19	7

TAKE-OUT

plain	1 (7 in diam)	218	11	25	–

WALNUTS

halves	14 (1 oz)	190	19	4	1

Waymouth Organic

Raw Walnuts	¼ cup	210	20	3	0

Sweet Delights

Walnut Roasters	⅓ pkg (1 oz)	210	20	3	0

WATER

ice cubes	3	0	0	0	0
tap water	8 oz	0	0	0	0

FOOD	PORTION	CALS	FAT	CARB	SUGAR
Absopure					
Natural Spring	8 fl oz	0	0	0	0
Blu Italy					
Sparkling Lemon	8 oz	0	0	0	0
Calabria					
Mineral	8 oz	0	0	0	0
Clearly Canadian					
Sparkling All Flavors	8 oz	45	0	10	10
Dasani					
Purfied Water	8 oz	0	0	0	0
w/ Lemon	8 oz	2	0	0	0
w/ Raspberry	8 oz	1	0	0	0
Evamor					
Artesian Water	8 fl oz	0	0	0	0
Fiji					
Natural Artesian	1 bottle (16.9 oz)	0	0	0	0
FlavH20					
All Flavors	1 can (12.3 oz)	80	0	21	20
Glaceau Vitamin Water					
Balance Cran Grapefruit	8 oz	50	0	13	12
Defense	8 oz	50	0	13	13
Endurance Peach Mango	8 oz	50	0	13	13
Energy Tropical Citrus	8 oz	40	0	9	8
Essential Orange Orange	8 oz	40	0	9	8
Focus Kiwi Strawberry	8 oz	40	0	9	8
Formula 50	8 oz	50	0	13	13
Multi-V Lemonade	8 oz	40	0	9	8
Perform Lemon Lime	8 oz	50	0	13	13
Power-C Dragonfruit	8 oz	40	0	9	8
Rescue Green Tea	8 oz	40	0	9	8
Revive Fruit Punch	8 oz	50	0	13	12
Stress-B Lemon Lime	8 oz	40	0	9	8

FOOD	PORTION	CALS	FAT	CARB	SUGAR
Hint					
Flavored Water All Flavors	1 bottle (15 oz)	0	0	0	0
Metromint					
Peppermint Water	8 oz	0	0	0	0
Multi Vitamin Enhanced Water					
All Flavors	8 oz	50	0	12	12
No Carb All Flavors	8 oz	0	0	0	0
O Waters					
All Flavors	8 oz	0	0	0	0
Paradiso					
Slightly Sparkling	8 oz	0	0	0	0
Pellegrino					
Mineral Water	8 oz	0	0	0	0
Pink2O					
Fortified	1 bottle (20 oz)	0	0	0	0
Propel					
Fitness Water All Flavors	1 bottle (23.7 oz)	30	0	7	6
Rapid					
Hydra-Cell Water	1 bottle (16.9 oz)	0	0	0	0
San Benedetto					
Nautral Mineral Water	1 liter	0	0	0	0
Sanfaustino					
Mineral	8 oz	0	0	0	0
Speedo Sportswater					
All Flavors	8 oz	10	0	3	2
Stacker 2					
Protein Water All Flavors	1 bottle (19.44 oz)	80	0	1	0
Sulinka					
Sparkling Mineral	8 oz	0	0	0	0
Tao Tea					
Lychee Water	8 oz	67	0	21	21

FOOD	PORTION	CALS	FAT	CARB	SUGAR
Thorpedo					
Ultra Low GI Energy Water	8 oz	45	0	11	10
Trinity					
Energize	8 oz	50	0	12	12
Multi-Essential	8 oz	50	0	12	12
Revive	8 oz	50	0	12	12
Strength	8 oz	50	0	12	12
Think	8 oz	50	0	12	12
Vasa					
Natural Spring	8 oz	0	0	0	0
VitaZest					
All Flavors	8 oz	0	0	0	0
Volvic					
Natural Lemon	8 oz	0	0	1	1
Natural Orange	8 oz	30	0	7	7
Voss					
Artesian	8 oz	0	0	0	0
W20 For Women					
All Flavors	8 oz	40	0	10	10
Water+					
Energy Fruit Punch	8 oz	45	0	12	12
Fitness + Lemon	8 oz	45	0	12	12
Focus Mixed Berry	8 oz	45	0	12	12
Lean Peach	8 oz	40	0	12	12
Recovery Strawberry Kiwi	8 oz	45	0	12	12
Ultra C Orange	8 oz	45	0	12	12
Wateroos					
All Flavors	1 box (8 oz)	0	0	0	0

WATER CHESTNUTS

FOOD	PORTION	CALS	FAT	CARB	SUGAR
fresh sliced	½ cup	66	tr	15	–

FOOD	PORTION	CALS	FAT	CARB	SUGAR
WATERCRESS					
garden fresh	½ cup	8	tr	1	—
Frieda's					
Watercress	1 cup	10	0	1	0
WATERMELON					
cut up	1 cup	50	1	11	—
wedge	1/16	152	2	35	—
Dulcinea					
Fresh Mini Seedless	2 cups	88	0	27	25
Frieda's					
Yellow Seedless	½ cup (3 oz)	25	0	6	6
Sundia					
Fresh	2 cups	80	0	27	25
WATERMELON JUICE					
Snapple					
What-A-Melon	8 oz	90	0	25	23
Sundia					
100% Natural	8 oz	110	1	27	24
WAX BEANS					
CANNED					
Del Monte					
Wax Beans	½ cup	20	0	4	2
WHALE					
raw	3.5 oz	134	3	0	0
WHEAT					
Bob's Red Mill					
Vital Wheat Gluten	¼ cup	120	1	6	0
Near East					
Pilaf Mix Wheat as prep	1 cup	220	5	40	2
Taboule Salad Mix as prep	⅔ cup	110	3	21	1

FOOD	PORTION	CALS	FAT	CARB	SUGAR
NOW					
Wheat Gluten Flour	¼ cup	125	0	5	0
WHEAT GERM					
plain toasted	¼ cup (1 oz)	108	3	14	–
Hodgson Mill					
Untoasted	2 tbsp	55	1	7	0
Mother's					
Toasted	2 tbsp	50	1	6	1
WHEY					
whey cheese	1 oz	126	8	9	0
WHIPPED TOPPINGS					
Cabot					
Whipped Cream	2 tbsp	30	2	2	1
Estee					
Whipped Topping as prep	1 serv	10	1	1	0
Hood					
Light Sugar Free Whipped Cream	2 tbsp	10	1	tr	0
Whipped Light Cream	2 tbsp	20	2	tr	tr
Reddiwip					
Chocolate	2 tbsp	15	1	1	tr
Extra Creamy	2 tbsp	15	2	tr	tr
Fat Free	2 tbsp	5	0	1	1
Original	2 tbsp	15	1	tr	tr
WHITE BEANS					
canned	1 cup	306	1	58	–
dried regular cooked	1 cup	249	1	45	–
WHITEFISH					
baked	3 oz	146	6	0	0
smoked	1 oz	39	tr	0	0

FOOD	PORTION	CALS	FAT	CARB	SUGAR
WHITING					
cooked	3 oz	98	1	0	0
WILD RICE					
cooked	1 cup (5.7 oz)	166	1	35	—
Gourmet House					
Cracked not prep	¼ cup	170	0	35	0
Hand Harvested not prep	¼ cup	170	0	35	0
Quick Cooking not prep	½ cup	170	0	25	0
White & Wild not prep	¼ cup	170	0	35	1
Wild & Rice Garden Blend not prep	¼ cup	190	1	40	1
WINE					
cooking	1 oz	15	0	2	tr
dessert dry	1 glass (4 oz)	179	0	14	1
haiku	1 serv	93	0	3	—
japanese plum	3 oz	139	tr	16	—
japanese sake	1 oz	33	0	2	—
kir	1 serv	78	0	3	—
madeira	3.5 oz	169	0	10	10
port	3.5 oz	156	0	11	11
red	1 glass (4 oz)	85	0	2	—
rosé	1 glass (4 oz)	84	0	2	—
sake screwdriver	1 serv	175	tr	23	—
sangria	1 serv	88	tr	6	—
sangria blanco	1 serv	155	tr	24	—
sherry	2 oz	84	0	5	—
sweet dessert	1 glass (4 oz)	189	0	16	9
vermouth dry	3.5 oz	105	0	1	—
vermouth sweet	3.5 oz	167	0	12	—
wassail wine	1 serv	142	tr	22	—
white	1 glass (4 oz)	80	0	1	—

FOOD	PORTION	CALS	FAT	CARB	SUGAR
wine cooler	1 serv	218	tr	8	—
wine spritzer	1 serv	60	0	1	—

XANTHAN GUM
Bob's Red Mill
| Xanthan Gum | 1 tbsp | 8 | 0 | 9 | 0 |

YAM
CANNED
Bruce
| In Syrup | ⅔ cup | 150 | 1 | 36 | 23 |
FRESH
| yam cubed cooked | ½ cup | 79 | tr | 19 | — |
Frieda's
| Name | ¾ cup | 100 | 0 | 24 | 0 |

YEAST
baker's compressed	1 cake (0.6 oz)	18	tr	3	—
baker's dry	1 pkg (¼ oz)	21	tr	3	—
baker's dry	1 tbsp	35	1	5	—
brewer's dry	1 tbsp	25	tr	3	—

YELLOW BEANS
| fresh cooked w/o salt | ½ cup | 22 | tr | 5 | — |
| fresh raw | ½ cup | 17 | tr | 4 | — |

YELLOWTAIL
| baked | 3 oz | 159 | 6 | 0 | 0 |

YOGURT
Cabot
Non Fat	8 oz	100	0	19	13
Non Fat French Vanilla	8 oz	130	0	24	19
Non Fat Raspberry	8 oz	130	0	24	19
Dannon
| Light'N Fit w/ Fiber Blueberry | 4 oz | 70 | 0 | 13 | 8 |

FOOD	PORTION	CALS	FAT	CARB	SUGAR
Fage					
Sheep & Goat's Milk	1 pkg (7 oz)	190	12	10	10
Stonyfield Farm					
Kids' Lowfat BaNilla	1 pkg (4 oz)	110	1	21	18
Light Black Cherry	1 pkg (6 oz)	100	0	28	17
Light Blueberry	1 pkg (4 oz)	100	0	28	17
Light Peach	1 pkg (6 oz)	100	0	28	17
Light Strawberry	1 pkg (4 oz)	100	0	28	17
Nonfat French Vanilla	1 pkg	90	0	18	16
Nonfat Strawberry	1 pkg	140	0	26	24
O'Soy Chocolate	1 pkg (6 oz)	160	3	28	22
O'Soy Peach	1 pkg (4 oz)	100	2	16	13
Squeezers Lowfat Strawberry	1 tube (2 oz)	60	1	11	9
Whole Milk French Vanilla	1 pkg (6 oz)	190	6	27	24
Total					
Greek Yogurt 0% Fat	1 pkg (5.3 oz)	80	0	6	6
Greek Yogurt 2% Fat	1 pkg (7 oz)	130	4	8	8
Greek Yogurt Classic	1 pkg (7 oz)	180	20	6	6
Greek Yogurt Light	1 pkg (5.3 oz)	130	8	5	5
Honey	1 pkg (3.5 oz)	250	12	28	28
WholeSoy & Co.					
Organic Soy Apricot Mango	1 pkg (6 oz)	160	3	30	19
Organic Soy Lemon	1 pkg (6 oz)	160	3	29	18
Organic Soy Plain	1 pkg (6 oz)	150	3	27	12
Organic Soy Raspberry	1 pkg (6 oz)	170	3	32	19
Organic Soy Vanilla	1 pkg (6 oz)	150	3	28	12
Yoplait					
Healthy Heart All Flavors	1 pkg (6 oz)	180	2	35	27

YOGURT DRINKS

FOOD	PORTION	CALS	FAT	CARB	SUGAR
Dannon					
DanActive	1 bottle (3.5 oz)	90	2	15	15

FOOD	PORTION	CALS	FAT	CARB	SUGAR
Stonyfield Farm					
Kids' Juice Smoothie Orange Strawberry Banana Wave	1 bottle (6 oz)	160	2	29	26
Smoothie Light Strawberry	1 bottle (10 oz)	130	0	40	19
Smoothie Lowfat Strawberry	1 bottle (10 oz)	250	3	46	41
YOGURT FROZEN					
vanilla soft serve	½ cup (4 fl oz)	114	4	17	16
Dannon					
Light'N Fit w/ Fiber Strawberry	4 oz	70	0	13	8
Edy's					
Black Cherry Vanilla Swirl	½ cup	90	0	19	14
Caramel Praline Crunch	½ cup	100	0	23	17
Chocolate	½ cup	90	0	19	12
Strawberry	½ cup	100	0	22	15
Vanilla	½ cup	90	0	19	13
Vanilla Chocolate Swirl	½ cup	90	0	19	13
Hood					
Fat Free Old Fashioned Vanilla	½ cup	110	0	24	15
Fat Free Strawberry	½ cup	100	0	23	15
Vanilla Swiss Almond	½ cup	150	5	25	17
WholeSoy & Co.					
Organic All Flavors	½ cup	120	1	25	19
ZUCCHINI					
baby raw	1 (0.5 oz)	3	tr	1	–
raw sliced	½ cup	9	tr	2	–
sliced cooked	½ cup	14	tr	4	–

FOOD	PORTION	CALS	FAT	CARB	SUGAR
Frieda's					
Baby	⅔ cup (3 oz)	20	0	3	2
TAKE-OUT					
breaded & fried	6 slices (3 oz)	141	11	10	3
indian paalkora	1 serv	46	2	7	–

PART TWO

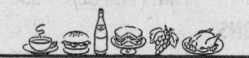

Restaurant Chains

A Cup of Joe to Go?

Coffee, a complicated chemical compound, has both positive and negative effects on diabetes.

The good news: coffee drinkers seem to be at lower risk for type 2 diabetes.

The bad news: caffeine makes your body less able to use insulin for a few hours after drinking coffee.

Welcome to the wonderful world of science, which always presents more puzzles for researchers to solve.

FOOD	PORTION	CALS	FAT	CARB	SUGAR
A&W					
BEVERAGES					
Root Beer Float	1 sm (14.4 oz)	330	5	70	57
MAIN MENU SELECTIONS					
Cheese Curds	1 serv	570	40	27	3
Cheese Dog	1	320	20	25	4
Cheeseburger	1	470	24	40	10
Cheeseburger Deluxe	1	510	28	41	9
Cheeseburger Deluxe Bacon	1	570	33	41	10
Cheeseburger Deluxe Bacon Double	1	800	48	47	10
Cheeseburger Deluxe Double	1	720	42	46	10
Coney Chili Dog	1	310	18	24	5
Coney Chili Dog Cheese	1	350	21	27	5
Fries	1 lg	430	18	61	1
Fries Cheese	1 serv	380	19	50	0
Fries Chili	1 serv	370	16	49	2
Fries Chili & Cheese	1 serv	400	19	51	2
Fries Kids	1 serv	310	13	45	0
Hamburger	1	430	22	31	6
Hamburger Deluxe	1	460	26	37	9
Hot Dog Plain	1	280	17	22	4
Onion Rings	1 serv	350	17	45	3
Sandwich Crispy Chicken	1	580	25	57	8
Sandwich Grilled Chicken	1	430	15	37	10
Sauce BBQ	1 serv (1 oz)	40	0	10	6
Sauce Honey Mustard	1 serv (1 oz)	100	6	12	6
Sauce Ranch	1 serv (1 oz)	160	17	2	1
Sauce Sweet & Sour	1 serv (1 oz)	45	0	12	7

FOOD	PORTION	CALS	FAT	CARB	SUGAR
ARBY'S					
BEVERAGES					
Chocolate Shake	1 (14 oz)	480	16	84	—
Hot Chocolate	1 serv (8.6 oz)	110	1	23	—
Jamocha Shake	1 (14 oz)	470	15	82	—
Strawberry Shake	1 (14 oz)	500	13	87	—
Vanilla Shake	1 (14 oz)	470	15	83	—
BREAKFAST SELECTIONS					
Add Egg	1 serv (2 oz)	110	9	2	—
Add Swiss Cheese Slice	1 slice (0.5 oz)	45	3	0	—
Biscuit w/ Bacon	1 (3.2 oz)	320	21	27	—
Biscuit w/ Butter	1 (2.9 oz)	280	17	27	—
Biscuit w/ Ham	1 (4.3 oz)	330	20	28	—
Biscuit w/ Sausage	1 (4.2)	460	33	27	—
Croissant w/ Bacon	1 (2.5 oz)	300	20	28	—
Croissant w/ Ham	1 (3.7 oz)	310	19	29	—
Croissant w/ Sausage	1 (3.6 oz)	420	32	28	—
French Toast Syrup	1 serv (0.5 oz)	130	0	32	—
Sourdough w/ Bacon	1 (5 oz)	380	7	29	—
Sourdough w/ Ham	1 (4 oz)	220	7	30	—
Sourdough w/ Sausage	1 (4 oz)	330	19	29	—
Toastix w/o Syrup	1 serv (4.4 oz)	370	17	48	—
DESSERTS					
Apple Turnover Iced	1 (4.5 oz)	420	16	65	—
Cherry Turnover Iced	1 (4.5 oz)	410	16	63	—
MAIN MENU SELECTIONS					
Arby's Sauce	1 serv (0.5 oz)	15	0	4	—
Au Jus Sauce	1 serv (3 oz)	5	1	1	—
Baked Potato Broccoli'N Cheddar	1 (14 oz)	540	24	71	—
Baked Potato Deluxe	1 (13 oz)	650	34	67	—
Baked Potato w/ Butter & Sour Cream	1 (11.2 oz)	500	24	65	—

FOOD	PORTION	CALS	FAT	CARB	SUGAR
BBQ Dipping Sauce	1 serv (1 oz)	40	0	10	—
Bronco Berry Sauce	1 serv (1.5 oz)	90	0	23	—
Chicken Finger 4-Pak	1 serv (6.77 oz)	640	38	42	—
Chicken Finger Snack w/ Curly Fries	1 serv (6.4 oz)	580	32	55	—
Curly Fries	1 lg (7 oz)	620	30	78	—
Curly Fries	1 med (4.5 oz)	400	20	50	—
Curly Fries	1 sm (3.8 oz)	310	15	39	—
Curly Fries Cheddar	1 serv (6 oz)	460	24	54	—
German Mustard	1 pkg (0.25 oz)	5	0	0	—
Homestyle Fries	1 lg (7.5 oz)	560	24	79	—
Homestyle Fries	1 med (5 oz)	370	16	53	—
Homestyle Fries	1 sm (4 oz)	300	13	42	—
Homestyle Fries Child-Size	1 serv (3 oz)	220	10	32	—
Honey Mustard	1 serv (1 oz)	130	12	5	—
Horsey Sauce	1 pkg (0.5 oz)	60	5	3	—
Jalapeno Bites	1 serv (4 oz)	330	21	30	—
Ketchup	1 pkg (0.3 oz)	10	0	2	—
Marinara Sauce	1 serv (1.5 oz)	35	1	4	—
Mayonnaise	1 pkg (0.4 oz)	90	10	0	—
Mayonnaise Light Cholesterol Free	1 pkg (0.4 oz)	20	2	1	—
Mozzarella Sticks	4 (4.8 oz)	470	29	34	—
Onion Petals	1 serv (4 oz)	410	24	43	—
Potato Cakes	2 (3.5 oz)	250	16	26	—
Sandwich Chicken Bacon 'N Swiss	1 (7.4 oz)	610	33	49	—
Sandwich Chicken Breast Fillet	1 (7.2 oz)	540	30	47	—
Sandwich Chicken Cordon Bleu	1 (8.4 oz)	630	35	47	—

FOOD	PORTION	CALS	FAT	CARB	SUGAR
Sandwich Grilled Chicken Deluxe	1 (8.7 oz)	450	22	37	—
Sandwich Hot Ham 'N Swiss	1 (5.9 oz)	340	13	35	—
Sandwich Market Fresh Roast Beef & Swiss	1 (12.5 oz)	810	42	73	—
Sandwich Market Fresh Roast Beef Ranch & Bacon	1 (13.5 oz)	880	44	74	—
Sandwich Market Fresh Roast Chicken Caesar	1 (12.7 oz)	820	38	75	—
Sandwich Market Fresh Roast Ham & Swiss	1 (12.5 oz)	730	34	74	—
Sandwich Market Fresh Roast Turkey & Swiss	1 (12.5 oz)	760	33	75	—
Sandwich Market Fresh Ultimate BLT	1 (10.5 oz)	820	49	72	—
Sandwich Roast Beef Arby-Q	1 (6.4 oz)	360	14	40	—
Sandwich Roast Beef Beef 'N Cheddar	1 (6.9 oz)	480	24	43	—
Sandwich Roast Beef Big Montana	1 (11 oz)	630	32	41	—
Sandwich Roast Beef Giant	1 (7.9 oz)	480	23	41	—
Sandwich Roast Beef Junior	1 (4.4 oz)	310	13	34	—
Sandwich Roast Beef Melt w/ Cheddar	1 (5.2 oz)	340	15	36	—
Sandwich Roast Beef Regular	1 (5.4 oz)	350	16	34	—
Sandwich Roast Beef Super	1 (8.5 oz)	470	23	47	—

FOOD	PORTION	CALS	FAT	CARB	SUGAR
Sandwich Roast Chicken Club	1 (8.4 oz)	520	28	38	—
Sub Sandwich French Dip	1 (10 oz)	440	18	42	—
Sub Sandwich Hot Ham'N Swiss	1 (9.7 oz)	530	27	45	—
Sub Sandwich Italian	1 (11 oz)	780	53	49	—
Sub Sandwich Philly Beef'N Swiss	1 (10.8 oz)	700	42	46	—
Sub Sandwich Roast Beef	1 (11.6 oz)	760	48	47	—
Sub Sandwich Turkey	1 (10.6 oz)	630	37	51	—
Tangy Southwest Sauce	1 serv (1.5 oz)	250	26	3	—
SALAD DRESSINGS					
Bleu Cheese	1 serv (2 oz)	300	31	3	—
Buttermilk Ranch	1 serv (2 oz)	290	30	3	—
Buttermilk Ranch Light	1 serv (2 oz)	100	6	12	—
Caesar	1 serv (2 oz)	310	34	1	—
Honey French	1 serv (2 oz)	290	24	18	—
Italian Reduced Calorie	1 serv (2 oz)	25	1	3	—
Italian Parmesan	1 serv (2 oz)	240	24	4	—
Thousand Island	1 serv (2 oz)	290	28	9	—
SALADS					
Caesar Side Salad	1 (5 oz)	45	2	4	—
Caesar Salad w/o Dressing	1 serv (8 oz)	90	4	8	—
Chicken Finger w/o Dressing	1 serv (13 oz)	570	34	39	—
Croutons Seasoned	1 serv (0.25 oz)	30	1	5	—
Croutons Cheese & Garlic	1 serv (0.63 oz)	100	6	10	—
Garden Salad	1 (12.3 oz)	70	1	14	—
Grilled Chicken	1 serv (16.3 oz)	210	5	14	—
Grilled Chicken Caesar w/o Dressing	1 serv (12 oz)	230	8	8	—
Roast Chicken	1 serv (14.8 oz)	160	3	15	—

FOOD	PORTION	CALS	FAT	CARB	SUGAR
Side Salad	1 (5.7 oz)	25	0	5	—
Turkey Club Salad w/o Dressing	1 serv (12 oz)	350	21	9	—

AU BON PAIN
BAKED SELECTIONS

FOOD	PORTION	CALS	FAT	CARB	SUGAR
Bagel Cinnamon Crisp	1 (6 oz)	540	7	123	44
Baguette	1 loaf (10.6 oz)	680	3	136	2
Bread Stick	1 (2.3 oz)	200	3	37	3
Cinnamon Roll	1 (4 oz)	300	5	60	25
Cookie Chocolate Chip	1 (2 oz)	230	7	39	23
Cookie Chocolate Chunk Macadamia	1 (2 oz)	250	13	31	17
Cookie Gingerbread Man w/ Raisins & Icing	1 (2.7 oz)	280	7	52	28
Cookie Oatmeal Raisin	1 (2 oz)	210	6	38	13
Cookie Peanut Butter	1 (2 oz)	240	12	21	16
Cookie Shortbread	1 (2.3 oz)	240	7	44	12
Cookie Walnut Raisin	1 (2 oz)	250	13	31	17
Cookie English Toffee	1 (2 oz)	230	7	38	22
Creme De Fleur	1 serv (5.55 oz)	470	19	69	23
Croissant Almond	1 (4.7 oz)	480	25	58	18
Croissant Apple	1 (3.5 oz)	200	3	40	16
Croissant Chocolate	1 (3.1 oz)	330	10	53	23
Croissant Cinnamon Raisin	1 (3.8 oz)	300	5	60	13
Croissant Raspberry Cheese	1 (3.6 oz)	290	9	47	17
Croissant Sweet Cheese	1 (3.6 oz)	320	12	46	15
Danish Cranberry	1 (4.5 oz)	350	9	59	25
Danish Lemon	1 (4.3 oz)	340	9	59	23
Danish Sweet Cheese	1 (4.2 oz)	390	16	55	21
Focaccia	1 piece (5.4 oz)	430	16	61	2
Four Grain Bread	1 serv (4.7 oz)	400	4	74	2

FOOD	PORTION	CALS	FAT	CARB	SUGAR
French Roll	1 (4.2 oz)	260	1	53	0
French Roll Roast Beef	1 (11 oz)	540	19	58	1
Hearth Roll	1 (3 oz)	210	2	38	1
Holiday Cookie w/ Icing & Sprinkles	1 (1.6 oz)	150	3	31	14
Loaf Multigrain	1 slice (1.8 oz)	130	1	24	0
Muffin Banana Walnut	1 (5.4 oz)	430	21	57	27
Muffin Blueberry	1 (5.6 oz)	470	15	79	44
Muffin Bran Raisin	1 (5.5 oz)	400	12	77	31
Muffin Carrot	1 (5.8 oz)	520	25	67	38
Muffin Corn	1 (5.7 oz)	390	16	56	26
Muffin Cranberry Walnut	1 (5.4 oz)	500	27	57	26
Muffin Low Fat 3 Berry	1 (4.4 oz)	270	3	58	29
Muffin Low Fat Chocolate Cake	1 (4.2 oz)	470	0	117	113
Muffin Milk Chocolate Chunk	1 (5.3 oz)	530	23	77	42
Muffin Pumpkin	1 (6 oz)	510	18	74	38
Parisienne Loaf	1 loaf (19 oz)	1210	5	244	2
Petit Pain	1 (2.9 oz)	180	1	37	0
Roll Braided w/ Topping	1 (10 oz)	430	14	63	8
Roll Pecan	1 (6 oz)	620	24	94	40
Sandwich Loaf Country White	1 serv (1.75 oz)	110	1	23	0
Sandwich Loaf Tomato Herb	1 serv (1.75 oz)	120	1	27	0
Scone Chocolate Walnut	1 (4 oz)	420	19	56	27
Scone Cranberry Orange Almond	1 (4 oz)	400	15	60	26
Scone Maple Oat Pecan Date	1 (4 oz)	410	17	58	27
Scone Orange	1 (4.2 oz)	370	13	56	11

FOOD	PORTION	CALS	FAT	CARB	SUGAR
Shortbread Heart ½ Chocolate	1 (2.7 oz)	290	10	51	13
Shortbread Heart w/ Red Sugar	1 (2.5 oz)	270	7	51	19
Sourdough Bagel Asiago Cheese	1 (4.8 oz)	340	5	57	5
Sourdough Bagel Cheddar Scallion	1 (4.1 oz)	310	5	51	5
Sourdough Bagel Cinnamon Crisp	1 (4.6 oz)	360	5	52	13
Sourdough Bagel Cinnamon Raisin	1 (4.5 oz)	300	1	65	4
Sourdough Bagel Cranberry Nut	1 (4.7 oz)	400	7	73	15
Sourdough Bagel Double Cheddar Jalpeno	1 serv (4.1 oz)	320	6	50	5
Sourdough Bagel Dutch Apple	1 (4.7 oz)	380	3	80	22
Sourdough Bagel Everything	1 (4.4 oz)	330	3	54	5
Sourdough Bagel Focaccia	1 (4.1 oz)	320	5	61	5
Sourdough Bagel Honey 9 Grain	1 (4.8 oz)	310	2	66	5
Sourdough Bagel Onion	1 (4.4 oz)	320	1	67	8
Sourdough Bagel Plain	1 (4 oz)	300	1	61	5
Sourdough Bagel Poppy Seed	1 (4.4 oz)	330	3	64	5
Sourdough Bagel Sesame	1 (4.4 oz)	340	4	64	5
Sourdough Bagel Wild Blueberry	1 (4.1 oz)	280	1	58	7
Streudal Cherry	1 serv (4 oz)	380	23	37	–
Streudel Apple	1 serv (4.35 oz)	400	23	48	18

FOOD	PORTION	CALS	FAT	CARB	SUGAR
SALADS					
Caesar w/o Dressing	1 serv (7.8 oz)	240	12	19	2
Chef's	1 serv (10.3 oz)	290	15	11	7
Chicken Caesar	1 serv (10.2 oz)	380	18	19	2
Chicken Oriental	1 serv (8.6 oz)	220	6	16	8
Chicken Pesto Salad	1 serv (8 oz)	400	23	7	2
Garden	1 serv (9.3 oz)	160	5	26	5
Garden Side	1 serv (5.1 oz)	90	2	14	3
Gorgonzola & Walnut	1 serv (5 oz)	330	28	8	3
Mozzarella & Red Pepper Salad	1 serv (10.5 oz)	360	25	10	6
Tuna	1 serv (13.2 oz)	440	24	28	7
SANDWICHES AND FILLINGS					
Club Hot Roasted Turkey	1 (11.7 oz)	630	28	53	3
Cream Cheese Plain	1 serv (2 oz)	190	10	0	0
Cream Cheese Reduced Fat Honey Walnut	1 serv (2 oz)	150	10	10	10
Cream Cheese Reduced Fat Sundried Tomato	1 serv (2 oz)	140	12	3	2
Cream Cheese Reduced Fat Veggie	1 serv (2 oz)	140	12	3	1
Croissant Spinach & Cheese	1 (3.6 oz)	220	9	29	4
Croque Madame	1 (11 oz)	570	22	53	5
Croque Monsieur	1 (11 oz)	590	25	53	5
Egg On A Bagel	1 serv (7.1 oz)	500	5	64	6
Egg On A Bagel w/ Bacon	1 serv (7.6 oz)	580	12	84	6
Egg On A Bagel w/ Cheese	1 serv (7.85 oz)	590	12	84	6
Egg On A Bagel w/ Cheese & Bacon	1 serv (8.35 oz)	670	19	84	6
Focaccia Chicken & Mozzarella	1 serv (13.75 oz)	800	14	73	4

FOOD	PORTION	CALS	FAT	CARB	SUGAR
Focaccia Chicken Tarragon w/ Field Greens	1 (12.5 oz)	870	47	54	3
Focaccia Garden Vegetable Goat Cheese w/ Artichoke Spread	1 (14.25 oz)	570	21	75	5
Focaccia Hickory Smoked Ham & Brie	1 (13.3 oz)	620	27	72	5
Focaccia Smoked Turkey & Swiss w/ Cilantro	1 (13.25 oz)	810	40	68	4
Fo-Ca-Cha-Cha Chicken	1 serv (11.15 oz)	730	17	75	5
French Roll Ham	1 (11 oz)	390	16	58	3
French Roll Hot Grilled Chicken	1 (11 oz)	620	23	57	1
French Roll Hot Roast Turkey	1 (11 oz)	500	15	59	1
French Roll Tuna	1 (10.6 oz)	550	21	58	3
Hot Croissant Spinach & Cheese	1 (4 oz)	290	9	39	5
Pane Bagniate	1 (12 oz)	670	28	71	6
Sandwich Arizona Chicken	1 (12 oz)	600	15	56	2
Sandwich Cheese	1 (7.2 oz)	590	26	54	0
Sandwich Fresh Mozzarella Tomato & Pesto	1 (11 oz)	790	43	60	4
Sandwich Honey Dijon Chicken	1 (13.6 oz)	750	24	65	11
Sandwich Thai Chicken	1 (11.4 oz)	550	12	62	4
Wrap Chicken Caesar	1 (10.5 oz)	640	26	61	2
Wrap Fields & Feta	1 (13.5 oz)	620	19	100	6
Wrap Honey Smoked Turkey	1 (15 oz)	520	7	85	14

FOOD	PORTION	CALS	FAT	CARB	SUGAR
Wrap Roast Beef & Brie	1 (14 oz)	570	28	64	3
SOUPS					
Autumn Pumpkin	1 serv (8 oz)	170	9	18	2
Black Bean	1 serv (8 oz)	180	1	33	2
Chicken Florentine	1 serv (8 oz)	140	8	14	2
Chicken Noodle	1 serv (8 oz)	100	2	12	2
Clam Chowder	1 serv (8 oz)	220	15	16	1
Corn & Green Chili Bisque	1 serv (8 oz)	200	10	21	4
Corn Chowder	1 serv (8 oz)	270	15	28	4
Curried Rice & Lentil	1 serv (8 oz)	140	2	24	2
French Moroccan Tomato Lentil	1 serv (8 oz)	130	2	22	4
Garden Vegetable	1 serv (8 oz)	50	1	8	3
Low Sodium Mediterranean Pepper	1 serv (12 oz)	280	6	44	4
Low Sodium Southwest Vegetable	1 serv (12 oz)	220	5	34	4
Old Fashioned Tomato	1 serv (8 oz)	140	6	19	11
Pasta E Fagioli	1 serv (8 oz)	240	7	36	3
Potato Cheese	1 serv (8 oz)	190	10	21	2
Potato Leek	1 serv (8 oz)	200	13	18	2
Red Beans & Rice	1 serv (8 oz)	200	5	31	2
Soup Bread Bowl	1 (9.25 oz)	600	3	118	3
Southern Black Eyed Pea	1 serv (8 oz)	320	2	56	4
Split Pea	1 serv (8 oz)	160	1	27	2
Tomato Florentine	1 serv (8 oz)	120	3	17	5
Tuscan Vegetable	1 serv (8 oz)	140	4	22	2
Vegetable Beef Barley	1 serv (8 oz)	110	3	14	2
Vegetarian Chili	1 serv (8 oz)	170	2	31	3
Vegetarian Lentil	1 serv (8 oz)	120	1	21	2
Wild Mushroom Bisque	1 serv (8 oz)	140	7	16	3

FOOD	PORTION	CALS	FAT	CARB	SUGAR
AUNTIE ANNE'S					
BEVERAGES					
Dutch Ice Blue Raspberry	1 (14 oz)	165	0	38	35
Dutch Ice Grape	1 (14 oz)	180	0	43	41
Dutch Ice Kiwi Banana	1 (14 oz)	190	0	44	41
Dutch Ice Lemonade	1 (14 oz)	315	0	77	77
Dutch Ice Mocha	1 (14 oz)	400	10	74	52
Dutch Ice Orange Creme	1 (14 oz)	280	0	64	59
Dutch Ice Pina Colada	1 (14 oz)	220	0	53	50
Dutch Ice Strawberry	1 (14 oz)	220	0	50	48
Dutch Ice Wild Cherry	1 (14 oz)	210	0	48	45
Dutch Shake Chocolate	1 (14 oz)	580	27	75	67
Dutch Shake Coffee	1 (14 oz)	590	27	77	70
Dutch Shake Strawberry	1 (14 oz)	610	27	78	74
Dutch Shake Vanilla	1 (14 oz)	510	27	58	54
Dutch Smoothie Blue Raspberry	1 (14 oz)	230	8	34	33
Dutch Smoothie Grape	1 (14 oz)	230	8	36	35
Dutch Smoothie Kiwi Banana	1 (14 oz)	240	8	38	35
Dutch Smoothie Lemonade	1 (14 oz)	300	8	53	51
Dutch Smoothie Mocha	1 (14 oz)	330	13	50	39
Dutch Smoothie Orange Creme	1 (14 oz)	280	8	46	44
Dutch Smoothie Pina Colada	1 (14 oz)	260	8	44	41
Dutch Smoothie Strawberry	1 (14 oz)	250	8	40	39
Dutch Smoothie Wild Cherry	1 (14 oz)	250	8	41	39

FOOD	PORTION	CALS	FAT	CARB	SUGAR
DIPPING SAUCES					
Caramel Dip	1 serv (1.5 oz)	135	3	27	21
Cheese Sauce	1 serv (1.25 oz)	100	8	4	3
Chocolate Dip	1 serv (1.25 oz)	130	4	24	12
Cream Cheese Light	1 serv (1.25 oz)	70	6	1	1
Cream Cheese Strawberry	1 serv (1.25 oz)	110	10	4	3
Hot Salsa Cheese	1 serv (1.25 oz)	100	8	4	4
Marinara Sauce	1 serv (1.25 oz)	10	0	4	2
Sweet Mustard	1 serv (1.25 oz)	60	2	8	8
PRETZELS					
Almond	1	400	8	72	15
Almond w/o Butter	1	350	2	72	15
Cinnamon Raisin w/o Butter	1	350	2	74	16
Cinnamon Sugar	1	450	9	83	26
Garlic	1	350	5	68	9
Garlic w/o Butter	1	320	1	66	9
Glazin' Raisin	1	510	4	107	38
Glazin' Raisin w/o Butter	1	470	1	104	37
Jalapeno	1	310	5	59	9
Jalapeno w/o Butter	1	270	1	58	8
Maple Crumb	1	550	6	112	42
Maple Crumb w/o Butter	1	520	3	112	42
Original	1	370	4	72	10
Original w/o Butter	1	340	1	72	10
Parmesan Herb	1	440	13	72	10
Parmesan Herb w/o Butter	1	390	5	74	10
Sesame	1	410	12	64	9
Sesame w/o Butter	1	350	6	63	9
Sour Cream & Onion	1	340	5	66	10
Sour Cream & Onion w/o Butter	1	310	1	66	9

FOOD	PORTION	CALS	FAT	CARB	SUGAR
Stixs	4	247	3	48	7
Stixs w/o Butter	4	227	1	48	7
Whole Wheat	1	370	5	72	10
Whole Wheat w/o Butter	1	350	2	72	10

BAJA FRESH
MAIN MENU SELECTIONS

FOOD	PORTION	CALS	FAT	CARB	SUGAR
Baja Burrito Chicken	1 serv	820	35	75	—
Baja Burrito Steak	1 serv	920	42	75	—
Black Beans	1 serv	360	3	61	—
Burrito Bean & Cheese Chicken	1 serv	1000	33	104	—
Burrito Bean & Cheese Steak	1 serv	1100	41	104	—
Burrito Bean & Cheese Vegetarian	1 serv	870	31	104	—
Burrito Dos Manos Chicken	1 full serv	1480	40	202	—
Burrito Dos Manos Steak	1 full serv	1580	48	202	—
Burrito Mexicano Chicken	1 serv	830	13	124	—
Burrito Mexicano Steak	1 serv	920	20	124	—
Burrito Ultimo Chicken	1 serv	860	30	90	—
Burrito Ultimo Steak	1 serv	950	37	90	—
Cebollitas	1 serv	40	2	5	—
Chips & Salsa Baja	1 serv	1100	50	134	—
Enchiladas Cheese	1 serv	850	37	92	—
Enchiladas Chicken	1 serv	780	25	91	—
Enchiladas Steak	1 serv	890	33	94	—
Enchiladas Verde Cheese	1 serv	840	35	91	—
Enchiladas Verde Chicken	1 serv	770	23	91	—
Enchiladas Verde Vegetarian	1 serv	720	22	100	—
Fajitas Chicken Corn Tortillas	1 serv	1200	29	164	—

FOOD	PORTION	CALS	FAT	CARB	SUGAR
Fajitas Chicken Flour Tortillas	1 serv	1360	37	176	—
Fajitas Steak Corn Tortillas	1 serv	1360	42	164	—
Fajitas Steak Flour Tortillas	1 serv	1530	50	176	—
Grilled Vegetarian	1 serv	770	27	100	—
Mini Quesa-Dita Cheese	1 serv	620	20	81	—
Mini Quesa-Dita Chicken	1 serv	670	21	81	—
Mini Quesa-Dita Steak	1 serv	700	23	81	—
Mini Tosta-Dita Chicken	1 serv	570	17	67	—
Mini Tosta-Dita Steak	1 serv	630	22	67	—
Nachos Cheese	1 serv	1880	103	166	—
Nachos Chicken	1 serv	2010	105	166	—
Nachos Steak	1 serv	2100	113	166	—
Pinto Beans	1 serv	320	1	56	—
Quesadilla	1 serv	1180	70	92	—
Quesadilla Cheese	1 serv	1130	69	80	—
Quesadilla Chicken	1 serv	1260	71	80	—
Quesadilla Steak	1 serv	1350	79	80	—
Rice	1 serv	280	4	55	—
Taco Baja Style Chicken	1 serv	190	5	26	—
Taco Baja Style Steak	1 serv	220	7	26	—
Taco Baja Style Wild Gulf Shrimp	1 serv	190	5	26	—
Taco Chilito Chicken	1 serv	320	10	38	—
Taco Chilito Steak	1 serv	340	12	38	—
Taco Fish	1 serv	270	13	31	—
Taco Mahi Mahi	1 serv	260	10	32	—
Taquitos Chicken w/ Beans	1 serv	750	36	64	—
Taquitos Chicken w/ Rice	1 serv	710	36	64	—
Taquitos Steak w/ Beans	1 serv	820	42	69	—
Taquitos Steak w/ Rice	1 serv	790	42	67	—
Tostada Chicken	1 serv	1140	52	102	—
Tostada Steak	1 serv	1230	60	102	—

FOOD	PORTION	CALS	FAT	CARB	SUGAR
Tostada Vegetarian	1 serv	1010	50	102	—
SALAD DRESSINGS					
Fat Free Salsa Verde	1 serv (2.6 oz)	15	0	3	—
Guacamole	2 oz	70	6	5	—
Olive Oil Vinaigrette	1 serv (2.6 oz)	230	25	1	—
Pico De Gallo	1 serv	50	1	12	—
Pronto Guacamole	1 serv	550	30	61	—
Ranch	1 serv (2.6 oz)	220	19	6	—
Salsa Baja	1 serv	70	3	7	—
Salsa Roja	1 serv	70	1	13	—
Salsa Verde	1 serv	50	0	11	—
Sour Cream	1 oz	60	5	2	—
SALADS					
Baja Ensalada Chicken	1 serv	310	18	17	—
Baja Ensalada Fish	1 serv	360	15	27	—
Baja Ensalada Steak	1 serv	460	18	17	—
Side Salad	1 serv	70	3	10	—

BASKIN-ROBBINS

FOOD	PORTION	CALS	FAT	CARB	SUGAR
FROZEN YOGURT					
Cafe Mocha Truly Free Soft Serve	1 reg	140	1	27	11
Chocolate Nonfat Soft Serve	1 reg	190	1	39	36
Lowfat Maui Brownie Madness	1 reg	250	9	34	—
ICE CREAM					
Cappuccino Blast w/ Whipped Cream	1 reg	340	16	44	43
Chocolate	1 reg	270	16	31	29
Chocolate Chip	1 reg	270	17	26	25
Espresso'n Cream Lowfat	1 reg	180	3	31	29
Jamoca Almond Fudge	1 reg	280	16	30	29

FOOD	PORTION	CALS	FAT	CARB	SUGAR
Peach Crumb Pie No Sugar Added	1 reg	180	5	27	7
Pralines'n Cream	1 reg	280	15	33	32
Shake Chocolate	16 oz	750	43	80	69
Shake Vanilla	16 oz	630	35	69	61
Smoothie Very Strawberry w/ Soft Serve Ice Cream	1 reg	320	1	70	47
Thin Mint No Sugar Added	1 reg	160	4	27	7
Vanilla	1 reg	270	16	24	23
ICES					
Daiquiri Ice	1 reg	130	0	33	32
Sherbet Rainbow	1 reg	160	2	34	32
Sorbet Peachy Keen	1 reg	110	0	29	26

BEAR ROCK CAFE
BAKED SELECTIONS

FOOD	PORTION	CALS	FAT	CARB	SUGAR
Almond French Horn	1	491	23	68	38
Bear Claw	1	260	6	43	11
Cinnamon Roll w/ Cream Cheese Icing	1	540	26	68	34
English Muffin	1	120	1	25	1
Pecan Sticky Bun	1	555	33	52	26
SALAD DRESSINGS					
Balsamic Vinaigrette	1 serv (1.5 oz)	156	17	1	1
Blue Cheese	1 serv (1.5 oz)	230	25	2	2
Caesar	1 serv (1.5 oz)	198	21	3	3
Creamy Italian	1 serv (1.5 oz)	180	18	4	3
Fat Free Ranch	1 serv (1.5 oz)	40	0	11	4
Fat Free Vidalia Onion	1 serv (1.5 oz)	56	tr	12	11
Honey Mustard	1 serv (1.5 oz)	184	16	10	10
Oil & Vinegar	1 serv (1.5 oz)	250	28	1	1
Ranch	1 serv (1.5 oz)	213	23	3	1
Red Wine Vinaigrette	1 serv (1.5 oz)	198	21	4	3
Sesame Oriental	1 serv (1.5 oz)	128	6	17	13

FOOD	PORTION	CALS	FAT	CARB	SUGAR
Sweet Vidalia Onion	1 serv (1.5 oz)	170	13	14	14
Thousand Island	1 serv (1.5 oz)	184	18	6	4
SALADS					
Almond Citrus Chicken w/o Dressing	1 serv	443	25	26	18
BLT Chicken w/o Dressing	1 serv	394	22	9	6
BLT w/o Dressing	1 lg	285	19	7	6
BLT w/o Dressing	1 sm	146	10	4	4
Caesar Chicken w/ Dressing	1 serv	580	43	12	9
Caesar w/ Dressing	1 lg	451	40	11	9
Caesar w/ Dressing	1 sm	236	20	7	5
Dusk Mountain Blackened Chicken w/o Dressing	1 serv	304	19	13	7
Fruit Salad	1 serv (4 oz)	61	tr	15	14
Lodge	1 sm	55	5	7	4
Lodge w/o Dressing	1 lg	82	7	12	6
Low Carb BLT	1 serv	721	63	13	9
Low Carb Side Salad w/ Dressing	1 serv	316	31	10	6
Low Carb w/ Chicken w/ Dressing	1 serv	567	49	14	8
Low Fat Grilled Chicken w/o Dressing	1 serv	151	4	9	5
Mount Fuji w/ Dressing	1 serv	554	31	62	33
SANDWICHES					
Bagel & Cream Cheese	1	378	11	59	4
Bear Cristo	1	310	32	48	15
BLT	1	585	42	34	5
Coop's Chicken Salad Croissant	1	439	31	46	12
Fajita Chicken	1	659	40	47	2
Fireside Jack	1	699	42	53	12

FOOD	PORTION	CALS	FAT	CARB	SUGAR
Garden	1	390	24	35	7
Giant Panda Wrap	1	556	23	68	21
Grilled Cheese	1	480	32	29	2
Ham & Swiss On Rye	1	394	13	38	10
Hoot Owl	1	641	42	32	3
Italian Asiago Focaccia	1	901	60	60	6
Low Carb Wrap	1	308	11	28	5
Low Fat Ham	1	309	7	39	11
Low Fat Turkey	1	280	3	35	6
Mountain Bird	1	691	38	51	11
Peanut Butter & Jelly	1	387	15	53	23
Reuben's Peak	1	540	23	49	3
Rising Sunflower	1	591	41	34	7
Roast Turkey & Bacon	1	522	30	31	2
Rockside Focaccia	1	958	52	57	2
Sasquash	1	408	26	41	12
The Early Bear Bagel + Bacon	1	530	21	59	3
The Early Bear English Muffin + Bacon	1	344	19	26	1
The Early Bear English Muffin + Sausage	1	514	34	25	1
The Moose	1	976	54	54	17
Turkey On Whole Wheat	1	602	41	36	6
SOUPS					
Aztec Black Bean	1 serv	162	1	28	5
Baked Potato Mountain Chowder	1 serv	352	16	42	5
Chicken & Dumpling	1 serv	249	7	28	6
Chicken Gumbo	1 serv	123	3	10	5
Chicken Noodle	1 serv	165	3	25	6
Chicken w/ Wild Rice	1 serv	313	16	29	3

FOOD	PORTION	CALS	FAT	CARB	SUGAR
Cream Of Broccoli w/ Cheddar	1 serv	264	17	21	0
French Onion	1 serv	121	5	17	9
Grande Chili	1 serv	351	12	36	10
In Bread Bowl Aztec Black Bean	1 serv	545	3	105	8
In Bread Bowl Baked Potato Mountain Chowder	1 serv	735	17	119	7
In Bread Bowl Chicken & Dumplings	1 serv	632	9	104	8
In Bread Bowl Chicken Gumbo	1 serv	506	4	86	8
In Bread Bowl Chicken Noodle	1 serv	548	5	101	8
In Bread Bowl Chicken w/ Wild Rice	1 serv	696	18	105	5
In Bread Bowl Cream Of Broccoli w/ Cheddar	1 serv	647	18	97	2
In Bread Bowl French Onion	1 serv	504	7	93	11
In Bread Bowl Grande Chili	1 serv	734	14	113	12
In Bread Bowl New England Clam Chowder	1 serv	653	9	113	16
In Bread Bowl Normandy Vegetable Cheddar	1 serv	728	22	102	14
In Bread Bowl Tomato Florentine	1 serv	533	4	104	14
New England Clam Chowder	1 serv	270	8	36	14
Normandy Vegetable Cheddar	1 serv	345	21	26	12
Tomato Florentine	1 serv	150	2	27	12

FOOD	PORTION	CALS	FAT	CARB	SUGAR
BEN & JERRY'S					
Sugar Cone	1	48	tr	10	3
FROZEN YOGURT					
Black Raspberry Low Fat	½ cup	140	2	28	21
Cherry Garcia	½ cup	170	3	32	27
Chocolate Fudge Brownie	½ cup	190	3	36	31
Half Baked	½ cup	210	4	30	29
Phish Food	½ cup	230	5	42	30
ICE CREAM					
Brownie Batter	½ cup	310	18	32	26
Butter Pecan	½ cup	290	21	20	18
Cherry Garcia	½ cup	250	15	26	23
Chocolate Chip Cookie Dough	½ cup	280	16	31	24
Chocolate Chocolate Cookie	½ cup	280	14	34	26
Chocolate For A Change	½ cup	270	17	36	23
Chocolate Fudge Brownie	½ cup	280	14	33	29
Chubby Hubby	½ cup	330	21	32	24
Chunky Monkey	½ cup	300	19	30	26
Coffee For A Change	½ cup	240	15	21	19
Coffee Heath Bar Crunch	½ cup	310	18	32	25
Everything But The	½ cup	320	19	30	27
Fudge Central	½ cup	300	18	31	27
Half Baked	½ cup	280	14	34	31
Karamel Sutra	½ cup	290	15	33	27
Makin' Whoopie Pie	½ cup	270	14	33	24
Mint Chocolate Cookie	½ cup	270	16	26	22
New York Super Fudge Chunk	½ cup	270	20	30	25
Oatmeal Cookie Chunk	½ cup	280	16	32	23
One Sweet Whirled	½ cup	280	15	33	27

FOOD	PORTION	CALS	FAT	CARB	SUGAR
Organic Chocolate Fudge Brownie	½ cup	260	13	30	25
Organic Strawberry	½ cup	200	12	20	17
Organic Sweet Cream & Cookies	½ cup	240	15	23	18
Organic Vanilla	½ cup	220	14	18	16
Peanut Butter Cup	½ cup	380	26	29	25
Peanut Butter Me Up	½ cup	330	21	28	24
Phish Food	½ cup	280	13	38	23
Pistachio Pistachio	½ cup	280	19	21	18
Uncanny Cashew	½ cup	290	19	27	22
Vanilla Almond	1 bar (3.7 oz)	340	23	30	22
Vanilla Heath Bar Crunch	½ cup	300	19	29	27
Vanilla For A Change	½ cup	240	16	21	19
SORBETS					
Berry Berry Extraordinary	½ cup	100	0	25	22
Mango Lime	½ cup	100	0	27	22
Strawberry Kiwi	½ cup	100	0	27	22
BIG APPLE BAGELS					
BAGELS					
Apple Cinnamon	1	332	2	70	6
Banana Nut	1	340	2	68	4
Blueberry	1	330	2	68	2
Cheddar Herb	1	352	6	60	2
Chocolate Chip	1	348	2	68	4
Cinnamon Raisin	1	336	2	70	2
Cinnamon Sugar	1	175	2	74	2
Cranberry Walnut	1	352	2	72	6
Egg	1	328	2	66	2
Everything	1	336	2	68	2
Garlic	1	330	2	68	2
Honey Oat	1	320	2	68	2
Jalapeno	1	350	6	30	2

FOOD	PORTION	CALS	FAT	CARB	SUGAR
Onion	1	336	2	70	2
Pizza Bagel	1	481	6	85	3
Plain	1	334	2	68	2
Poppy	1	344	2	68	2
Pumpernickel	1	332	2	68	2
Salt	1	324	2	33	2
Sesame	1	358	4	66	2
Spinach	1	356	2	72	2
Strawberry	1	342	2	72	4
Tomato Basil	1	322	2	66	2
Vegetable	1	318	2	66	2
Wheat	1	330	2	34	2
SANDWICHES					
All American Duo	1	762	28	78	1
Big Apple Club	1	797	37	75	2
Breakfast BLT	1	704	31	83	5
Chicken Caesar	1	611	19	78	3
Classic Turkey	1	552	14	74	1
Enchilada Bagellata	1	522	11	84	3
Grilled Chicken	1	571	17	77	3
Holey Guacamole	1	476	5	76	2
Kick-N Roast Beef	1	579	15	79	1
Lox & Cream Cheese	1	602	21	78	3
Mediterranean Veg-Out	1	506	9	90	3
Morning Classic	1	486	11	73	2
Northern Omelette	1	699	31	73	2
Roma Italian	1	764	34	76	1
Toasted Cafe Chicken Melt	1	815	32	80	6
Toasted Deli Style Turkey	1	732	25	76	3
Toasted Roast Beef Parmesan Grinder	1	583	15	76	4
Toasted Spicy Italian Sub	1	770	34	77	1

FOOD	PORTION	CALS	FAT	CARB	SUGAR
Toasted Tuna Melt	1	641	23	75	2
Turkey Club	1	782	34	75	2

BILLY'S BURGER HUT
BEVERAGES
Shake Chocolate	1 (20 oz)	420	10	63	50
Shake Vanilla	1 (20 oz)	320	10	49	44

MAIN MENU SELECTIONS
Big Billy's Roast Beef Sub	1	843	54	62	12
Billyburger	1	426	22	35	6
Billyburger w/ Cheese	1	498	35	35	8
Billy's Best Red Potato Salad	1 serv	190	9	12	4
Billy's Biggest Burger ½ Pounder w/ Everything	1	852	58	61	15
Billy's Famous 7 Layer Salad	1 serv	558	49	18	9
Billy's Seafood Sandwich	1	399	18	43	9
Caesar Side Salad	1 serv	360	28	12	1
Chili w/ Cheese & Onion	1 serv	380	12	35	8
Cowboy Cobb Salad	1 serv	735	45	25	10
Cowboy Coleslaw	1 serv	180	9	11	4
French Fries	1 reg	230	12	25	7
Onion Rings	1 serv	250	10	37	6
Super Billy Burger w/ Bacon	1	663	41	39	9

BLIMPIE
COOKIES
Chocolate Chunk	1	200	10	26	16
Macadamia White Chunk	1	210	10	26	15
Oatmeal Raisin	1	190	8	27	16
Peanut Butter	1	220	12	23	14
Sugar	1	330	17	24	24

FOOD	PORTION	CALS	FAT	CARB	SUGAR
SALAD DRESSINGS AND TOPPINGS					
Caesar Dressing	1 serv (1.5 oz)	208	22	2	1
Cracked Peppercorn Dressing	1 serv (1.5 oz)	237	25	2	2
Frank's Red Hot Buffalo Sauce	1 serv (1 oz)	13	tr	2	1
French's Honey Mustard	1 tbsp	5	0	1	1
GourMayo Chipotle Chili	1 tbsp	50	5	1	0
GourMayo Sun Dried Tomato	1 tbsp	50	5	1	0
GourMayo Wasabi Horseradish	1 tbsp	50	5	1	0
Guacamole	1 serv (1.5 oz)	194	18	7	6
Oil & Vinegar	1 serv	36	4	1	0
Pesto Dressing	1 serv (1 oz)	132	13	1	0
SALADS					
Antipasto	1 reg serv	244	13	10	6
Chef	1 reg serv	212	9	9	5
Chili Ole	1 reg serv	480	27	42	2
Grilled Chicken w/ Caesar Dressing	1 reg serv	347	27	9	5
Grilled Chicken w/o Dressing	1 serv	139	5	7	4
Roast Beef 'N Blue	1 reg serv	390	16	29	0
Seafood	1 reg serv	122	4	16	5
Tuna	1 reg serv	261	20	8	3
Zesto Pesto Turkey	1 reg serv	370	19	31	1
SANDWICHES					
6 Inch Hot Sub BLT	1	588	32	49	8
6 Inch Hot Sub Buffalo Chicken	1	400	13	50	7
6 Inch Hot Sub Buffalo Chicken w/o Cheese	1	320	7	50	7
6 Inch Hot Sub ChiliMax	1	511	13	71	10

FOOD	PORTION	CALS	FAT	CARB	SUGAR
6 Inch Hot Sub Grilled Chicken	1	373	9	50	8
6 Inch Hot Sub Meatball	1	572	27	55	12
6 Inch Hot Sub MexiMelt	1	425	9	65	9
6 Inch Hot Sub Pastrami	1	507	17	53	11
6 Inch Hot Sub Steak & Onion Melt	1	440	16	49	9
6 Inch Hot Sub VegiMax	1	395	7	60	8
6 Inch Sub Blimpie Best	1	476	16	52	10
6 Inch Sub Club	1	440	12	51	9
6 Inch Sub Ham & Cheese	1	436	13	52	10
6 Inch Sub Roast Beef	1	468	14	49	7
6 Inch Sub Roast Beef w/o Cheese	1	388	8	49	7
6 Inch Sub Seafood	1	355	8	58	9
6 Inch Sub Tuna	1	493	23	51	7
6 inch Sub Turkey	1	424	11	49	7
6 Inch Sub Turkey w/o Cheese	1	344	5	49	7
Cheddar	1 slice	52	5	0	0
Grilled Subs Beef Turkey & Cheddar	1	600	31	49	9
Grilled Subs Cuban	1	462	12	50	9
Grilled Subs Pastrami	1	462	14	52	11
Grilled Subs Reuben	1	630	33	55	15
Provolone	1 slice	80	6	0	0
Swiss	1 slice	80	6	0	0
Wraps Beef & Cheddar	1	714	37	57	5
Wraps Chicken Caesar	1	646	35	56	6
Wraps Southwestern	1	674	35	54	4
Wraps Steak & Onions	1	716	37	64	7
Wraps Ultimate BLT	1	831	50	60	7
Wraps Zesty Italian	1	638	33	74	13

FOOD	PORTION	CALS	FAT	CARB	SUGAR
SIDE ORDERS					
Cole Slaw	1 serv (5 oz)	180	13	13	13
Macaroni Salad	1 serv (5 oz)	360	25	25	6
Mustard Potato Salad	1 serv (5 oz)	160	5	21	13
Potato Chips Cheddar & Sour Cream	1 bag	210	11	25	0
Potato Chips Jalapeno	1 bag	210	11	25	0
Potato Chips Lea & Perrins Barbecue	1 bag	210	10	25	2
Potato Chips Regular	1 bag	210	11	25	0
Potato Chips Romano & Garlic	1 bag	210	11	25	0
Potato Chips Sour Cream & Onion	1 bag	210	11	25	1
Potato Salad	1 serv (5 oz)	270	19	19	10
SOUPS					
Chicken w/ White & Wild Rice	1 serv (8 oz)	230	12	21	2
Cream Of Broccoli & Cheese	1 serv (8 oz)	190	12	15	5
Cream Of Potato	1 serv (8 oz)	190	9	24	3
Garden Vegetable	1 serv (8 oz)	80	1	14	5
Grande Chili w/ Beans & Beef	1 serv (8 oz)	250	7	30	7
Homestyle Chicken Noodle	1 serv (8 oz)	120	3	18	4
Tomato Basil w/ Raviolini	1 serv (8 oz)	110	1	22	5
Vegetable Beef	1 serv (8 oz)	80	2	13	3

BOB EVANS
BAKED SELECTIONS

FOOD	PORTION	CALS	FAT	CARB	SUGAR
Biscuit	1	277	12	36	6
Bread Apple Walnut	1 slice	142	6	21	11
Bread Banana Nut	1 slice	186	7	30	18

FOOD	PORTION	CALS	FAT	CARB	SUGAR
Bread Garlic	1 slice	218	16	16	1
Bread Sourdough	1	130	1	26	0
Bun Kaiser	1	167	2	30	3
Bun Mini	1	105	1	20	3
English Muffin	1	139	1	28	2
Roll Cinnamon Swirl Frosted	1	607	26	82	36
Roll Cinnamon Swirl Unfrosted	1	510	23	65	20
Roll Dinner	1	201	5	34	6
Texas Toast	1 slice	120	1	12	1
BREAKFAST SELECTIONS					
Bacon	1 piece	36	4	0	0
Belgian Waffle	1	351	10	58	17
Canadian Bacon	1 piece	21	1	0	0
Country Biscuit Breakfast	1 serv	841	41	71	22
Egg Hardboiled	1	60	4	1	0
Egg Over Easy	1	93	7	1	1
Eggs Scrambled	1 serv	170	11	2	0
Eggs Benedict	1 serv	514	23	37	7
French Toast	1 slice	135	2	14	4
Fruit Cup	1 serv	164	1	42	36
Grits	1 serv	187	7	29	0
Ham Smoked	1 slice	66	2	2	1
Home Fries	1 serv	193	7	28	14
Hotcake Blueberry	1	192	5	33	12
Hotcake Buttermilk	1	176	5	29	9
Hotcake Cinnamon	1	166	5	28	8
Hotcake Multigrain	1	208	6	34	10
Lite Sausage Breakfast	1 serv	479	21	50	24
Mush	1 serv	73	1	14	0
Oatmeal Plain	1 serv	185	3	34	1
Omelette Border	1	847	60	60	4

FOOD	PORTION	CALS	FAT	CARB	SUGAR
Omelette Cheese	1	457	40	3	0
Omelette Farmer's Market	1	634	49	11	3
Omelette Garden Harvest	1 serv	437	33	13	4
Omelette Ham & Cheese	1 serv	486	39	2	0
Omelette Sausage & Cheese	1 serv	729	51	2	0
Omelette Southwestern Chicken	1 serv	641	51	5	2
Omelette Western	1 serv	503	39	6	3
Pot Roast Hash Breakfast	1 serv	698	41	36	19
Sausage	1 link	117	13	0	0
Sausage Lite	1 link	100	7	0	0
Skillet Chicken Cordon Bleu	1 serv	880	56	35	16
Skillet Sunshine	1 serv	754	48	35	16
Strawberry Yogurt	1 serv	145	1	28	26
CHILDREN'S MENU SELECTIONS					
Colorful Cool Cakes	1 serv	542	17	87	30
Garden Salad	1 kid serv	41	2	3	1
Hot Diggety Dog Plain	1	446	33	23	1
L'il Homesteader	1 serv	414	25	34	13
Mac & Cheese	1 serv	330	12	45	9
Mini Cheeseburger	1 serv	252	14	20	3
Pizza Pizzazz	1 serv	520	20	58	5
Plenty O Pancakes	1 serv	515	17	81	26
Quesadilla Chicken	1 serv	542	31	39	1
Smiley Face Potatoes	1 serv	335	13	49	1
Spaghetti & Meatballs	1 serv	523	21	57	8
Sundae Fudge Blast	1 serv	254	10	37	28
Sundae Oreo Cookies 'n' Cream	1 serv	315	13	64	34
Sundae Rainbow	1 serv	320	14	46	24
Sundae Reese's I'm Smiling	1 serv	325	15	42	32

FOOD	PORTION	CALS	FAT	CARB	SUGAR
DESSERTS					
A La Mode Vanilla Ice Cream	1 serv	159	8	19	15
Cake Hershey's Hot Fudge	1 slice	688	25	94	71
Cake Pineapple Upside Down	1 slice	500	25	67	52
Oreo Cheesecake	1 slice	625	38	61	42
Peach Cobbler	1 serv	499	25	64	27
Pie Apple Dumpling	1 slice	682	30	100	56
Pie Banana Cream	1 slice	456	25	52	37
Pie Coconut Cream	1 slice	461	23	57	41
Pie French Silk	1 slice	653	44	59	44
Pie Lemon Meringue	1 slice	536	18	89	65
Pie Reese's Peanut Butter Cup	1 slice	1130	60	129	60
Pie Strawberry Supreme	1 slice	589	39	59	39
Pie No Sugar Added Apple	1 slice	483	28	52	0
Sundae Fudge	1	501	19	78	56
Sundae Reese's	1 serv	769	35	104	79
MAIN MENU SELECTIONS					
Applesauce	1 serv	101	0	26	20
Baked Potato Loaded	1	427	18	56	7
Baked Potato Plain	1	207	0	54	6
Broccoli Florets	1 serv	156	1	8	3
Broccoli Florets Cheddar	1 serv	230	9	14	4
Carrots Glazed	1 serv	188	8	29	20
Catfish Grilled New Orleans	1 piece	255	19	4	1
Cheeseburger Bacon Plain	1	1005	76	31	3
Cheeseburger Plain	1	691	46	31	3
Chicken Quesadilla	1 serv	502	36	50	6
Chicken & Broccoli Alfredo	1 serv	826	29	90	7
Chicken Fried	1 piece	291	30	9	1

FOOD	PORTION	CALS	FAT	CARB	SUGAR
Chicken Grilled	1 piece	229	10	0	0
Chicken Pot Pie	1 serv	758	49	46	10
Chicken Tenders Grilled	1 piece	103	7	0	0
Chicken-N-Noodle	1 serv	407	22	32	4
Coleslaw	1 serv	198	13	18	16
Corn Buttered	1 serv	225	14	26	2
Cottage Cheese	1 serv	122	5	4	4
Country Fried Steak w/ Gravy	1 serv	535	37	31	2
Country Fried Steak w/o Gravy	1 serv	481	33	26	0
Dressing Bread & Celery	1 serv	362	20	36	4
Fish Market Halibut	1 piece	209	12	13	0
French Fries	1 serv	217	7	35	0
Green Beans w/ Ham	1 serv	83	3	8	4
Grilled Garden Vegetables	1 serv	290	23	17	8
Hamburger Patty	1	388	30	0	0
Hamburger Plain	1	585	36	30	3
Hamburger Shroomin' Onion Plain	1	695	44	32	4
Home Fries	1 serv	193	7	28	14
Mashed Potatoes	1 serv	171	6	15	1
Meat Loaf	1 serv	626	44	14	7
Mushrooms Grilled	1 serv	152	12	10	0
Onion Rings	1 serv	460	27	49	6
Open Faced Roast Beef Dinner	1 serv	633	29	31	8
Pork Chop Dinner	1 serv	466	28	2	2
Pork Chop Dinner w/ Garlic Herb Butter	1 serv	624	39	16	3
Pork Chop Dinner w/ Wildfire Barbecue Sauce	1 serv	645	35	29	17
Rice Pilaf	1 serv	163	3	32	3

FOOD	PORTION	CALS	FAT	CARB	SUGAR
Salmon	1 serv	334	18	0	0
Salmon w/ Garlic Herb Butter	1 serv	491	29	14	1
Salmon w/ Wildfire Barbecue Sauce	1 serv	512	25	27	15
Sandwich Bob's BLT	1	795	54	55	2
Sandwich Chicken Salad	1	694	43	55	7
Sandwich Fish Market Haddock	1	570	25	65	0
Sandwich Fried Chicken	1	508	23	39	17
Sandwich Fried Chicken Club	1	994	70	40	18
Sandwich Grilled Cheese	1	391	17	25	4
Sandwich Grilled Chicken	1	447	18	30	3
Sandwich Grilled Chicken Club	1	993	70	32	4
Sandwich Pot Roast	1	728	35	68	11
Sandwich Turkey Bacon Melt	1	872	52	55	1
Seniors Chicken & Broccoli Alfredo	1 serv	513	21	49	4
Seniors Chicken Pot Pie	1 serv	758	49	46	10
Seniors Spaghetti & Meatballs	1 serv	617	29	59	8
Seniors Steak Tips & Noodles	1 serv	550	25	46	3
Seniors Stir-Fry Grilled Chicken	1 serv	479	18	54	19
Spaghetti & Marinara Sauce	1 serv	619	7	104	14
Spaghetti w/ Meatballs	1 serv	1087	45	116	16
Steak Monterey	1 serv	584	41	7	2
Steak Tips & Noodles	1 serv	985	37	90	5

FOOD	PORTION	CALS	FAT	CARB	SUGAR
Stir-Fry Grilled Chicken	1 serv	728	28	31	83
Stir-Fry Grilled Shrimp	1 serv	713	17	98	39
Stir-Fry Vegetable	1 serv	497	7	98	39
T-Bone Steak Plain	1 serv	1335	92	7	2
T-Bone Steak w/ Garlic Herb Butter	1 serv	1492	102	21	4
Turkey & Dressing	1 serv	542	24	41	5
SALAD DRESSINGS AND TOPPINGS					
Dressing Bleu Cheese	1 serv (1.5 oz)	220	23	3	1
Dressing Colonial	1 serv (1.5 oz)	232	21	12	12
Dressing French	1 serv (1.5 oz)	219	21	10	8
Dressing Honey Mustard	1 serv (1.5 oz)	192	18	8	7
Dressing Hot Bacon	1 serv (1.5 oz)	106	3	18	17
Dressing Lite Italian	1 serv (1.5 oz)	82	7	4	3
Dressing Oriental	1 serv (1.5 oz)	194	16	12	12
Dressing Ranch	1 serv (1.5 oz)	156	16	1	1
Dressing Ranch Lite	1 serv (1.5 oz)	103	10	2	1
Dressing Raspberry Vinaigrette	1 serv (1.5 oz)	155	13	12	12
Dressing Thousand Island	1 serv (1.5 oz)	212	20	7	7
Dressing Wildfire Ranch	1 serv (1.5 oz)	212	9	9	1
Gravy Chicken	1 serv (3 oz)	29	1	4	1
Gravy Country	1 serv (3 oz)	54	4	6	2
Gravy Sausage	1 serv (7 oz)	244	12	14	1
Syrup	1 serv (3 oz)	213	0	55	44
Syrup Sugar Free	1 serv (3 oz)	47	0	11	0
Topping Oregon Berry	1 serv (3 oz)	49	0	12	5
Topping Strawberry	1 serv (3 oz)	50	0	12	10
Whipped Topping	1 serv	69	5	5	5
SALADS					
Chicken Salad Plate	1 serv	789	46	78	65
Cobb Salad w/ Grilled Chicken	1 serv	778	54	14	7

FOOD	PORTION	CALS	FAT	CARB	SUGAR
Country Spinach w/ Grilled Chicken	1 serv	532	38	11	4
Frisco Salad w/ Fried Chicken	1 serv	672	40	39	7
Frisco Salad w/ Grilled Chicken	1 serv	599	40	13	7
Fruit & Yogurt	1 serv	414	2	96	83
Raspberry Grilled Chicken	1 serv	637	42	18	13
Specialty Side	1 serv	174	9	16	3
Wildfire Fried Chicken Salad	1 serv	806	31	100	22
Wildfire Grilled Chicken Salad	1 serv	733	30	74	22
SOUPS					
Bean	1 cup	125	3	16	0
Cheddar Baked Potato	1 cup	307	18	25	7
Vegetable Beef	1 cup	198	5	13	6
BOJANGLES					
Biscuit	1	243	12	29	—
Biscuit + Bacon	1	290	17	26	—
Biscuit + Bacon Egg Cheese	1	550	42	27	—
Biscuit + Cajun Filet	1	454	21	46	—
Biscuit + Country Ham	1	270	15	26	—
Biscuit + Egg	1	400	30	26	—
Biscuit + Sausage	1	350	23	26	—
Biscuit + Smoked Sausage	1	380	26	27	—
Biscuit + Steak	1	649	49	37	—
Botato Rounds	1 serv	235	11	31	—
Buffalo Bites	1 serv	180	5	5	—
Cajun Pintos	1 serv	110	0	18	—
Cajun Spiced Breast	1 serv	278	17	12	—
Cajun Spiced Leg	1 serv	284	19	11	—

FOOD	PORTION	CALS	FAT	CARB	SUGAR
Cajun Spiced Thigh	1 serv	310	23	11	—
Cajun Spiced Wing	1 serv	355	25	11	—
Chicken Supremes	1 serv	337	16	26	—
Corn On The Cob	1 serv	140	2	34	—
Dirty Rice	1 serv	166	6	24	—
Green Beans	1 serv	25	0	5	—
Macaroni & Cheese	1 serv	198	14	12	—
Marinated Cole Slaw	1 serv	136	3	26	—
Potatoes w/o Gravy	1 serv	80	1	16	—
Sandwich Cajun Filet w/o Mayo	1	337	11	41	—
Sandwich Cajun Filet w/ Mayo	1	437	22	41	—
Sandwich Grilled Filet w/ Mayo	1	335	16	25	—
Sandwich Grilled Filet w/o Mayo	1 serv	235	5	25	—
Seasoned Fries	1 serv	344	19	39	—
Southern Style Breast	1 serv	261	16	12	—
Southern Style Leg	1 serv	254	15	11	—
Southern Style Thigh	1 serv	308	21	14	—
Southern Style Wing	1 serv	337	21	19	—
Sweet Biscuit Bo Berry	1	220	10	29	—
Sweet Biscuit Cinnamon	1	320	18	37	—

BOSTON MARKET
DESSERTS

FOOD	PORTION	CALS	FAT	CARB	SUGAR
Apple Pie	1 slice	550	31	66	36
Brownie Caramel Pecan	1	900	47	114	88
Brownie Chocolate	1	580	23	88	65
Chocolate Cake	1 serv	290	32	86	68
Chocolate Mania	1 serv	290	16	37	29
Cookie Chocolate Chip	1	390	19	51	28
Cookie Oatmeal Scotchie	1	390	20	47	24

FOOD	PORTION	CALS	FAT	CARB	SUGAR
Cornbread	1 piece	120	4	21	8
Strawberry Bliss	1 serv	100	11	16	11
MAIN MENU SELECTIONS					
½ Spicy Tuscan Rotisserie Chicken	1 serv	630	34	8	5
½ Sweet Garlic Rotisserie Chicken w/ Skin	1 serv	590	33	4	4
¼ Dark Spicy Tuscan Rotisserie Chicken	1 serv	340	22	4	2
¼ Dark Sweet Rotisserie Chicken No Skin	1 serv	190	10	1	1
¼ Dark Sweet Rotisserie Chicken w/ Skin	1 serv	320	21	2	2
¼ White Spicy Tuscan Rotisserie Chicken	1 serv	200	5	4	1
¼ White Sweet Garlic Rotisserie Chicken No Skin Or Wing	1 serv	170	4	2	1
¼ White Sweet Rotisserie Chicken w/ Skin & Wing	1 serv	280	12	2	2
Butternut Squash	1 serv	150	6	25	12
Carver Meatloaf w/ Cheese	1	1070	55	102	21
Carver Chicken w/ Cheese & Sauce	1	670	33	68	13
Carver Turkey w/ Cheese & Sauce	1	690	29	58	13
Coleslaw	1 serv	310	22	29	17
Cranberry	1 serv	120	2	25	22
Creamed Spinach	1 serv	260	20	11	2
Cripsy Baked Country Chicken w/ Gravy	1 serv	440	23	33	1
Garlic Dill New Potatoes	1 serv	130	3	25	2

FOOD	PORTION	CALS	FAT	CARB	SUGAR
Green Bean Casserole	1 serv	80	5	9	3
Green Beans	1 serv	70	4	6	1
Homestyle Mashed Potatoes & Gravy	1 serv	230	9	32	4
Honey Glazed Ham	1 serv	210	8	10	10
Hot Cinnamon Apples	1 serv	250	5	56	49
Macaroni & Cheese	1 serv	280	11	33	8
Mashed Potatoes	1 serv	210	9	30	4
Meatloaf Double Sauced Angus	1 serv	510	34	22	4
Meatloaf Double Sauced Angus & Beef Gravy	1 serv	580	39	27	4
Meatloaf Double Sauced Angus & Chunky Tomato	1 serv	550	34	30	10
Pot Pie Pastry Topped	1	750	46	57	4
Poultry Gravy	1 serv	15	1	2	0
Roasted Sirloin	5 oz	270	10	0	0
Rotisserie Turkey Hand Carved	1 serv	170	1	3	3
Savory Stuffing	1 serv	190	8	27	5
Seasonal Fruit Salad	1 serv	70	0	16	15
Squash Casserole	1 serv	330	24	20	8
Steamed Vegetable Medley	1 serv	30	0	6	2
Sweet Corn	1 serv	180	4	30	13
Sweet Potato Casserole	1 serv	280	13	39	23
SALADS					
Asian Rotisserie Chicken Salad No Dressing or Noodles	1 serv	270	5	22	14
Asian Rotisserie Chicken Salad w/ Dressing & Noodles	1 serv	540	15	57	45

FOOD	PORTION	CALS	FAT	CARB	SUGAR
Caesar	1 entree	470	40	17	3
Caesar Rotisserie Chicken	1 serv	640	44	19	4
Caesar Side Salad	1 serv	300	26	13	2
Southwest Chicken Salad	1 serv	750	49	40	16
SOUPS					
Chicken Tortilla + Toppings	1 serv	170	8	18	2
Hearty Chicken Noodle	1 cup	101	5	8	1
Tortilla Soup No Toppings	1 serv	80	5	7	2

BREWSTER'S COFFEE

FOOD	PORTION	CALS	FAT	CARB	SUGAR
Americano	1 serv (16 oz)	12	0	2	0
Black Forest Coffee	1 serv (16 oz)	198	5	37	29
Cafe Caramello	1 serv (16 oz)	212	8	31	26
Cappuccino 2% Milk	1 serv (16 oz)	195	7	20	0
Cappuccino Fat Free Milk	1 serv (16 oz)	133	1	18	0
Italiano 2% Milk	1 serv (16 oz)	131	5	13	0
Italiano Fat Free Milk	1 serv (16 oz)	89	1	12	0
Jittery Monkey 2% Milk	1 serv (16 oz)	482	11	82	52
Jittery Monkey Fat Free Milk	1 serv (16 oz)	429	6	80	52
Latte 2% Milk	1 serv (16 oz)	212	7	22	0
Latte Cinnamon Toast 2% Milk	1 serv	299	7	45	26
Latte Cinnamon Toast Fat Free Milk	1 serv (16 oz)	240	1	44	26
Latte Creme Caramel 2% Milk	1 serv (16 oz)	303	7	47	27
Latte Creme Caramel Fat Free Milk	1 serv (16 oz)	244	1	45	27
Latte Fat Free Milk	1 serv (16 oz)	145	1	20	0
Latte Oregon Chai Tea 2% Milk	1 serv (16 oz)	274	5	48	34
Latte Oregon Chai Tea Fat Free Milk	1 serv (16 oz)	231	1	47	34

FOOD	PORTION	CALS	FAT	CARB	SUGAR
Latte Raspberry Cheesecake 2% Milk	1 serv (16 oz)	319	7	51	30
Latte Raspberry Cheesecake Fat Free Milk	1 serv (16 oz)	259	1	50	30
Mocha w/ Whipped Cream 2% Milk	1 serv (16 oz)	454	12	71	39
Mocha w/ Whipped Cream Fat Free Milk	1 serv (16 oz)	392	6	70	39

BRUEGGER'S BAGELS

BAGELS

FOOD	PORTION	CALS	FAT	CARB	SUGAR
Blueberry	1	330	2	68	14
Chocolate Chip	1	310	5	69	19
Cinnamon Raisin	1	320	2	68	16
Cinnamon Sugar	1	340	2	71	15
Everything	1	310	2	62	8
Garlic	1	310	2	62	7
Honey Grain	1	330	3	64	10
Jalapeno Bagel	1	310	2	63	7
Onion	1	310	2	62	8
Orange Cranberry	1	330	2	68	17
Plain	1	300	2	61	7
Poppy Seed	1	310	3	61	7
Pumpernickel	1	320	3	64	11
Rosemary Olive Oil	1	350	6	62	10
Salt	1	300	2	61	7
Sesame	1	320	2	61	7
Sun Dried Tomato	1	320	2	65	11

DESSERTS

FOOD	PORTION	CALS	FAT	CARB	SUGAR
Blondies	1	370	23	42	29
Brownie Chocolate Chunk	1	330	19	39	26
Brownie Mint	1	300	17	34	27
Bruegger Bar	1	420	24	47	31
Cappuccino Bar	1	420	25	45	32

FOOD	PORTION	CALS	FAT	CARB	SUGAR
Luscious Lemon Bar	1	350	20	39	24
Oatmeal Cranberry Mountains	1	430	24	49	22
Raspberry Sammies	1	270	13	36	18
SANDWICH FILLINGS					
Atlantic Smoked Salmon	2 oz	90	3	tr	tr
Cream Cheese Bacon Scallion	2 tbsp	100	8	4	1
Cream Cheese Chive	2 tbsp	100	9	2	1
Cream Cheese Garden Veggie	2 tbsp	90	8	3	2
Cream Cheese Garden Veggie Light	2 tbsp	60	4	2	1
Cream Cheese Herb Garlic Light	2 tbsp	70	5	3	2
Cream Cheese Honey Walnut	2 tbsp	110	8	5	2
Cream Cheese Jalapeno	2 tbsp	100	9	3	2
Cream Cheese Light Strawberry	2 tbsp	70	4	4	3
Cream Cheese Olive Pimento	2 tbsp	100	9	2	1
Cream Cheese Plain	2 tbsp	90	8	4	1
Cream Cheese Plain Light	2 tbsp	70	5	3	2
Cream Cheese Smoked Salmon	2 tbsp	100	9	2	1
Cream Cheese Wildberry	2 tbsp	100	9	4	2
Hummus	2 tbsp	60	4	4	0
Tuna Salad	1 serv (2.5 oz)	180	14	6	4
SANDWICHES					
Atlantic Smoked Salmon	1	470	12	66	10
Chicken Breast	1	440	6	62	7
Chicken Fajita	1	500	12	74	15

FOOD	PORTION	CALS	FAT	CARB	SUGAR
Chicken Salad w/ Mayo	1	460	12	67	11
Deli-Style Ham w/ Honey Mustard	1	440	5	77	21
Egg Cheese	1	480	15	66	10
Egg Cheese Sausage	1	680	33	66	11
Egg Cheese Bacon	1	560	22	66	10
Egg Cheese Ham	1	520	17	66	10
Garden Veggie	1	390	3	80	15
Herby Turkey	1	530	14	73	11
Leonardo Da Veggie	1	460	11	69	11
Santa Fe Turkey	1	480	10	71	13
Turkey w/ Mayo	1	480	14	65	10

BURGER KING
BEVERAGES

FOOD	PORTION	CALS	FAT	CARB	SUGAR
Shake Strawberry	1 sm	620	32	71	61
Shake Vanilla	1 sm	560	32	56	46

BREAKFAST SELECTIONS

FOOD	PORTION	CALS	FAT	CARB	SUGAR
Croissan'wich Bacon Egg & Cheese	1	360	22	25	4
Croissan'wich Egg & Cheese	1	320	19	24	3
Croissan'wich Ham Egg & Cheese	1	360	20	25	3
Croissan'wich Sausage Egg & Cheese	1	520	39	24	4
Croissan'wich w/ Sausage & Cheese	1	420	31	23	4
French Toast Sticks	5 pieces	390	20	46	11
Hash Browns	1 lg	390	25	38	0
Hash Browns	1 sm	230	15	23	0
Sourdough Breakfast Sandwich Bacon Egg & Cheese	1	380	22	30	3

FOOD	PORTION	CALS	FAT	CARB	SUGAR
Sourdough Breakfast Sandwich Ham Egg & Cheese	1	380	20	30	3
Sourdough Breakfast Sandwich Sausage Egg & Cheese	1	540	39	30	3
DESSERTS					
Chocolate Chip Cookies	2	440	16	68	32
Hershey Sundae Pie	1	300	18	31	23
MAIN MENU SELECTIONS					
Bacon Cheeseburger	1	400	20	32	6
Bacon Double Cheeseburger	1	580	34	32	6
Baguette Santa Fe Fire Grilled Chicken	1	350	5	47	4
Baguette Savory Mustard Fire Grilled Chicken	1	350	5	47	5
Baguette Smokey BBQ Fire Grilled Chicken	1	350	5	48	5
Baja BBQ Sauce	1 serv	14	tr	3	2
BK Veggie Burger	1	340	10	47	8
Cheeseburger	1	360	17	31	6
Chicken Tenders	8 pieces	340	19	20	0
Chicken Tenders	5 pieces	210	12	13	0
Chili	1 serv	190	8	17	5
Dipping Sauce Sweet And Sour	1 serv	40	0	10	5
Double Cheeseburger	1	540	31	32	6
Double Hamburger	1	450	24	31	6
Double Whopper	1	980	62	52	11
Double Whopper w/ Cheese	1	1070	70	53	11
Dutch Apple Pie	1 serv	340	14	52	23

FOOD	PORTION	CALS	FAT	CARB	SUGAR
French Fries No Salt Added	1 lg	500	25	63	tr
French Fries No Salt Added	1 sm	230	11	29	0
French Fries Salted	1 lg	500	25	63	tr
French Fries Salted	1 sm	230	11	29	0
Hamburger	1	310	14	31	6
Onion Rings	1 lg	480	23	60	7
Onion Rings	1 sm	180	9	22	3
Sandwich BK Fish Filet	1	520	30	44	4
Sandwich Grilled Chicken Caesar Club	1	540	27	40	5
Sandwich Original Chicken	1	560	28	52	5
Sandwich Whopper	1	580	26	48	7
Whopper	1	710	43	52	11
Whopper w/ Cheese	1	800	50	53	11
Whopper Jr.	1	390	22	32	6
Whopper Jr. w/ Cheese	1	440	26	32	6
SALAD DRESSINGS AND TOPPINGS					
Breakfast Syrup	1 serv	80	0	21	14
Dipping Sauce Barbecue	1 serv	35	0	9	7
Dipping Sauce Honey	1 serv	90	0	23	22
Dipping Sauce Honey Mustard	1 serv	90	6	9	4
Dipping Sauce Ranch	1 serv	140	15	tr	tr
Dipping Sauce Zesty Onion Ring	1 serv	150	15	3	2
Dressing Kraft Catalina	1 serv	180	16	10	9
Dressing Kraft Fat Free Ranch	1 serv	60	0	6	1
Dressing Kraft Ranch	1 serv	220	23	2	2

FOOD	PORTION	CALS	FAT	CARB	SUGAR
Dressing Light Done Right Light Italian	1 serv	50	5	4	3
Dressing Signature Creamy Caesar	1 serv	140	13	4	2
Fire Roasted Sauce	1 serv	9	tr	2	tr
Grape Jam	1 serv	30	0	7	6
Peppers & Onions Flame Roasted	1 serv	18	tr	3	2
Savory Mustard Sauce	1 serv	21	tr	4	3
Strawberry Jam	1 serv	30	0	7	6
SALADS					
Chicken Caesar & Croutons w/o Dressing	1 serv	230	7	5	3
Side Salad w/o Dressing	1 serv	25	0	5	3

BURGERVILLE
BEVERAGES

FOOD	PORTION	CALS	FAT	CARB	SUGAR
Milkshake Black Forest	1 (16 oz)	600	20	103	–
Milkshake Blackberry	1 (16 oz)	610	25	95	–
Milkshake Caramel Apple	1 (16 oz)	540	26	69	–
Milkshake Chocolate	1 (16 oz)	520	23	73	–
Milkshake Fresh Strawberry	1 (16 oz)	560	21	88	–
Milkshake Mocha Perk	1 (16 oz)	590	25	83	–
Milkshake Pumpkin	1 (16 oz)	460	22	60	–
Milkshake Vanilla	1 (16 oz)	500	20	74	–
Smoothies Chocolate Monkey	1 (16 oz)	470	1	105	–
Smoothies Fresh Blackberry	1 (16 oz)	420	0	94	–
Smoothies Fresh Raspberry	1 (16 oz)	470	0	103	–
Smoothies Fresh Strawberry	1 (16 oz)	390	0	86	–

FOOD	PORTION	CALS	FAT	CARB	SUGAR
Smoothies Strawberry Splash	1 (16 oz)	310	1	70	—
Smoothies Triple Berry Blast	1 (16 oz)	360	0	77	—
BREAKFAST SELECTIONS					
American Cheese	2 slices	90	7	0	0
Bagel Bacon Egg	1	450	11	64	—
Bagel Cheese	1	290	6	53	—
Bagel Ham Egg	1	450	8	65	—
Bagel Plain	1	310	1	63	—
Bagel Sausage Egg	1	640	29	65	—
Biscuit Bacon Egg	1	400	23	32	—
Biscuit Ham Egg	1	400	20	33	—
Biscuit Sausage Egg	1	590	41	33	—
Tillamook Cheese	1 slice	120	10	1	—
MAIN MENU SELECTIONS					
Cheeseburger	1	370	20	29	—
Cheeseburger Double Beef	1	470	27	29	—
Cheeseburger Pepper Bacon	1	680	45	28	—
Cheeseburger Tillamook	1	630	40	32	—
Cheeseburger Walla Walla Onion	1	679	44	39	—
Chicken Strips	5 pieces	550	30	36	—
Colossal	1	530	30	31	—
French Fries	1 kid size	220	12	24	—
French Fries	1 reg	390	22	44	—
Gardenburger	1	460	19	53	—
Gardenburger Spicy Black Bean	1	550	32	45	—
Halibut	3 pieces	230	14	10	—
Hamburger	1	320	16	29	—

FOOD	PORTION	CALS	FAT	CARB	SUGAR
Onion Rings Walla Walla	3 pieces	485	29	50	—
Roasted Turkey Salad w/o Hazelnuts	1 serv	375	19	22	—
Rogue River Blue Cheese Bacon Burger	1	510	56	29	—
Sandwich Crispy Chicken	1	450	18	55	—
Sandwich Deluxe Crispy Chicken	1	610	30	56	—
Sandwich Grilled Chicken	1	350	3	45	—
Sandwich Halibut	1	490	30	35	—
Sandwich Turkey Club	1	490	32	27	—
Side Salad w/o Dressing	1 serv	70	4	5	—
Smoked Salmon Salad w/o Hazelnuts	1 serv	370	18	21	—
Sweet Potato Fries	1 serv	530	29	60	—
Turkey Burger	1	470	21	32	—
CAPTAIN D'S SEAFOOD					
Baked Chicken Dinner	1 serv	350	5	49	4
Baked Fish Dinner	1 serv	390	5	49	4
Baked Potato	1 serv	190	0	44	3
Baked Salmon Dinner	1 serv	470	8	58	12
Carb Counter Chicken Dinner	1 serv	320	15	19	8
Carb Counter Fish Dinner	1 serv	350	15	19	8
Cole Slaw	1 serv	150	6	22	0
Corn On The Cob	1 serv	150	3	34	8
Fresh Steamed Broccoli	1 serv	25	1	5	2
Green Beans	1 serv	90	3	15	4
Rice Pilaf	1 serv	160	1	35	2
Shrimp Scampi Dinner	1 serv	370	5	50	4
Side Salad w/o Dressing	1	30	1	6	3
Tuscan Style Vegetables	1 serv	30	0	7	3

FOOD	PORTION	CALS	FAT	CARB	SUGAR

CARIBOU COFFEE

FOOD	PORTION	CALS	FAT	CARB	SUGAR
Black Forest Mocha	1 med	553	19	83	73
Black Forest Wild Drink	1 med	553	19	86	73
Cappuccino	1 med (16 oz)	113	1	15	13
Cappuccino 2%	1 med (16 oz)	162	7	17	13
Caramel Hirise	1 med (16 oz)	414	13	59	56
Chai Latte 2%	1 med (16 oz)	286	5	50	47
Chai Skim	1 med (16 oz)	236	–	48	42
Cooler Caramel	1 med (12 oz)	450	10	83	77
Cooler Chocolate	1 med (12 oz)	257	3	54	44
Cooler Coffee	1 med (16 oz)	230	3	48	40
Cooler Espresso	1 med (16 oz)	193	2	40	33
Cooler Mint Oreo	1 med (12 oz)	614	19	108	89
Cooler Vanilla	1 med (16 oz)	257	4	52	45
Glacier Gum	2 pieces	5	0	2	0
Hot Apple Blast	1 med	379	8	76	41
Latte 2%	1 med (16 oz)	171	6	17	14
Latte Skim	1 med (16 oz)	121	1	17	13
Latte Skinny Bou Low Cal	1 med	120	1	17	17
Lite White Berry	1 med (16 oz)	311	5	57	51
Mint Condition	1 med (16 oz)	520	19	75	69
Mints All Flavors	3 pieces	5	0	1	0
Mocha 2%	1 med (16 oz)	347	16	41	28
Mocha Skim	1 med (16 oz)	302	12	34	33
Mocha Turtle	1 med (16 oz)	559	19	82	75
Smoothie Passion Green Tea	1 med (16 oz)	252	tr	61	58
Smoothie Raspberry	1 med (12 oz)	293	tr	70	54
Smoothie Strawberry Banana	1 med (16 oz)	253	tr	61	50
Smoothie Wild Berry	1 med (16 oz)	235	tr	56	45

FOOD	PORTION	CALS	FAT	CARB	SUGAR

CARL'S JR.

BAKED SELECTIONS

FOOD	PORTION	CALS	FAT	CARB	SUGAR
Cheese Danish	1	400	23	49	21
Cheesecake Strawberry Swirl	1 serv	290	17	30	20
Chocolate Cake	1 serv	300	12	48	37
Chocolate Chip Cookie	1	350	18	46	27
Muffin Blueberry	1	340	14	49	29
Muffin Bran Raisin	1	370	13	61	35

BEVERAGES

FOOD	PORTION	CALS	FAT	CARB	SUGAR
Shake Chocolate	1 reg (32 oz)	770	15	140	121
Shake Strawberry	1 reg (32 oz)	750	15	133	117
Shake Vanilla	1 reg (32 oz)	700	16	115	98

BREAKFAST SELECTIONS

FOOD	PORTION	CALS	FAT	CARB	SUGAR
Bacon	2 strips	45	4	0	0
Breakfast Burrito	1	560	32	36	2
Breakfast Quesadilla	1	370	17	36	3
English Muffin w/ Margarine	1	210	9	28	2
French Toast Dips w/o Syrup	1 serv	370	20	42	11
Grape Jelly	1 serv (0.5 oz)	40	0	9	7
Hash Brown Nuggets	1 serv	330	21	32	1
Sausage	1 patty	190	18	2	0
Scrambled Eggs	1 serv	180	14	1	1
Sourdough Breakfast	1 serv	410	20	33	4
Strawberry Jam	1 serv (0.5 oz)	40	0	9	7
Sunrise Sandwich w/o Meat	1	360	21	28	5
Table Syrup	1 serv (1 oz)	90	0	21	16

MAIN MENU SELECTIONS

FOOD	PORTION	CALS	FAT	CARB	SUGAR
American Cheese	1 sm	50	4	1	1
BBQ Sauce	1 serv (1.1 oz)	50	0	11	7

FOOD	PORTION	CALS	FAT	CARB	SUGAR
Breadstick	1 (0.3 oz)	35	1	7	0
Carl's Famous Star	1	590	32	50	8
Chicken Stars	6 pieces	260	16	14	1
CrissCut Fries	1 serv	410	24	43	0
Croutons	1 serv (0.5 oz)	30	1	5	0
Double Sourdough Bacon Cheeseburger	1	880	59	37	7
Double Western Bacon Cheeseburger	1	920	50	65	15
Famous Bacon Cheeseburger	1	700	41	51	9
French Fries	1 kid size	250	12	32	tr
French Fries	1 med	460	22	59	1
Hamburger	1	280	9	36	5
Honey Sauce	1 serv (1 oz)	90	0	22	20
Mustard Sauce	1 serv (1 oz)	50	0	11	8
Onion Rings	1 serv	430	22	53	5
Potato Bacon & Cheese	1	640	29	75	7
Potato Broccoli & Cheese	1 serv	530	21	76	6
Potato Plain w/o Margarine	1	290	0	68	4
Potato Sour Cream & Chives	1	430	14	70	6
Salsa	1 serv (0.9 oz)	10	0	2	1
Sandwich Bacon Swiss Crispy Chicken	1	760	38	72	8
Sandwich Carl's Catch Fish	1	530	28	55	8
Sandwich Charbroiled Sirloin Steak	1	550	24	52	6
Sandwich Chargrilled Chicken Club	1	470	23	37	6
Sandwich Chargrilled Santa Fe Chicken	1	540	31	37	7

FOOD	PORTION	CALS	FAT	CARB	SUGAR
Sandwich Chargrilled BBQ Chicken	1	290	4	41	9
Sandwich Ranch Crispy Chicken	1	660	31	71	8
Sandwich Southwest Spicy Chicken	1	620	41	48	7
Sandwich Spicy Chicken	1	480	26	47	6
Sandwich Western Bacon Crispy Chicken	1	750	28	91	15
Sourdough Bacon Cheeseburger	1	640	41	37	6
Sourdough Ranch Bacon Cheeseburger	1	720	46	43	5
Super Star	1	790	47	51	9
Sweet N'Sour Sauce	1 serv (1 oz)	50	0	12	9
Swiss Cheese	1 serv	50	4	0	0
Western Bacon Cheeseburger	1	660	30	64	15
Zucchini	1 serv	320	19	31	3
SALAD DRESSINGS					
1000 Island	1 serv (2 oz)	230	23	5	3
Blue Cheese	1 serv (2 oz)	320	35	1	1
French Fat Free	1 serv (2 oz)	60	0	16	12
House	1 serv (2 oz)	220	22	1	2
Italian Fat Free	1 serv (2 oz)	15	0	4	2
SALADS					
Salad-To-Go Charbroiled Chicken	1 serv	200	7	12	3
Salad-To-Go Garden	1	50	3	4	2

CARVEL
BEVERAGES

FOOD	PORTION	CALS	FAT	CARB	SUGAR
Carvelanche w/ Topping	1 (16 oz)	600	30	71	—
Regular Fizzlers	1 (16 oz)	340	5	75	—

FOOD	PORTION	CALS	FAT	CARB	SUGAR
Thick Shake Chocolate	1 (16 oz)	720	31	96	70
Thick Shake Reduced Fat Chocolate	1 (16 oz)	520	8	100	—
Thick Shake Reduced Fat Vanilla	1 (16 oz)	460	7	84	—
ICE CREAM					
Cake Butterscotch Dream	1 slice (4 oz)	260	10	37	—
Cake Celebration	1 slice (4 oz)	200	10	24	—
Cake Cookies & Cream	1 serv (4 oz)	240	12	29	—
Cake Fudge Drizzle	1 slice (4 oz)	240	11	32	—
Cake Game Ball	1 slice (4 oz)	330	17	41	—
Cake Holiday	1 slice (4 oz)	200	10	24	—
Cake Lil'Love	1 piece (4 oz)	200	10	24	—
Cake Sinfully Chocolate	1 slice (4 oz)	240	10	34	—
Cake Strawberries & Cream	1 slice (4 oz)	270	10	40	—
Chocolate	4 oz	190	10	22	19
Chocolate No Fat	4 oz	120	0	28	25
Flying Saucer 98% Fat Free Black Raspberry	1	170	2	40	24
Flying Saucer 98% Fat Free Chocolate	1	170	2	34	17
Flying Saucer 98% Fat Free Coffee	1	190	2	40	26
Flying Saucer 98% Fat Free Maple	1	190	2	40	26
Flying Saucer 98% Fat Free Mint	1	190	2	40	26
Flying Saucer 98% Fat Free Pistachio	1	190	2	40	26
Flying Saucer 98% Fat Free Strawberry	1	190	2	40	27

FOOD	PORTION	CALS	FAT	CARB	SUGAR
Flying Saucer 98% Fat Free Vanilla	1	190	2	40	26
Flying Saucer Chocolate	1	230	9	33	19
Flying Saucer Vanilla	1	240	10	33	19
Vanilla	4 oz	200	10	21	19
Vanilla No Fat	4 oz	120	0	25	22
Vanilla No Sugar Added	4 oz	130	3	25	7
ICES					
Italian Ice Blue Raspberry	4 oz	70	0	19	18
Italian Ice Bubble Gum	4 oz	70	0	19	18
Italian Ice Cherry	4 oz	100	0	25	21
Italian Ice Chocolate Ice Cream	4 oz	90	1	20	19
Italian Ice Cotton Candy	4 oz	70	0	19	18
Italian Ice Lemon	4 oz	70	0	19	18
Italian Ice Mango	4 oz	70	0	27	22
Italian Ice Orange	4 oz	70	0	19	18
Italian Ice Vanilla Ice Cream	4 oz	90	2	20	20
Italian Ice Watermelon	4 oz	70	0	19	18
Sherbet All Flavors	4 oz	140	1	31	24

CHICKEN OUT ROTISSERIE

MAIN MENU SELECTIONS

FOOD	PORTION	CALS	FAT	CARB	SUGAR
Apple Cornbread Stuffing	1 serv (6 oz)	215	2	42	—
Baked Potato Wedges	1 serv (6 oz)	110	tr	26	—
Biscuit	1	150	4	29	—
Chicken Breast Skinless	1 serv (6 oz)	210	4	0	0
Chicken Burger w/o Cheese	1	285	7	36	—
Chunky Cinnamon Applesauce	1 serv (6 oz)	60	0	25	—
Creamed Spinach w/ Artichokes	1 serv (6 oz)	160	6	20	—

FOOD	PORTION	CALS	FAT	CARB	SUGAR
Farm Fresh Cole Slaw	1 serv (6 oz)	55	0	10	—
French Baguette	1	80	1	28	—
Fresh Fruit Salad	1 serv (6 oz)	77	tr	56	—
Mandarin Walnut Cranberry Relish	1 serv (6 oz)	240	1	66	—
Mashed Sweet Potatoes	1 serv (6 oz)	120	tr	40	—
Oriental Green Beans	1 serv (6 oz)	34	0	8	—
Pulled White Meat	1 serv (6 oz)	180	4	0	0
Real Cheese & Macaroni	1 serv (6 oz)	311	12	39	—
Red Skin Mashed Potatoes	1 serv (6 oz)	181	6	26	—
Rice Pilaf	1 serv (6 oz)	140	1	28	—
Roasted Peas Corn & Carrots	1 serv (6 oz)	120	tr	22	—
Rotisserie Chicken Quarter Dark No Skin	1 serv	232	6	0	0
Rotisserie Chicken Quarter White No Skin	1 serv	196	4	0	0
Sandwich BBQ Pulled Chicken	1	406	8	42	—
Sandwich Grilled Chicken Breast	1	350	6	28	—
Sandwich Open Faced Pulled Chicken	1	682	18	80	—
Sandwich Pulled Chicken	1	320	6	28	—
Sandwich Signature Chicken Salad	1	370	5	31	—
Steamed Broccoli & Carrots	1 serv (6 oz)	30	0	6	—
Vegetarian Baked Beans	1 serv (6 oz)	150	1	26	—
Wrap Chinese Chicken Salad w/o Dressing	1	330	9	36	—
Wrap Fajita	1	360	10	38	—

FOOD	PORTION	CALS	FAT	CARB	SUGAR
Wrap Fresh Vegetable Salad w/o Dressing	1	170	4	32	—
Wrap Grilled Chicken Caesar	1	355	11	31	—
Wrap Pesto Chicken	1	405	11	25	—
Wrap Pulled Chicken	1	300	7	24	—
Wrap Skinless Grilled Chicken	1	330	7	24	—
SALAD DRESSINGS					
Balsamic Vinaigrette	1 oz	18	0	4	—
Caesar	1 oz	55	5	1	—
Chinese	1 oz	72	7	2	—
Low Fat Honey Mustard	1 oz	23	1	5	—
Ranch	1 oz	90	6	1	—
Southwestern	1 oz	85	7	3	—
SALADS					
Caesar w/ Grilled Chicken w/o Dressing	½ serv	235	8	7	—
Caesar w/o Dressing	½ serv	140	4	9	—
Chicken Salad Apricot	1 serv (6 oz)	300	8	1	—
Chicken Salad BBQ Pulled	1 serv (6 oz)	263	5	8	—
Chicken Salad Chinese w/o Dressing	½ serv	210	6	12	—
Chicken Salad Pesto	1 serv (6 oz)	285	8	1	—
Chicken Salad Pulled w/o Dressing	½ serv	204	4	5	—
Chicken Salad Santa Fe w/o Dressing	½ serv	240	7	14	—
Chicken Salad Signature	1 serv (6 oz)	230	5	1	—
Garden w/ Grilled Chicken w/o Dressing	½ serv	200	4	5	—
Garden w/o Dressing	½ serv	25	1	4	—

FOOD	PORTION	CALS	FAT	CARB	SUGAR
Young Spinach w/ Grilled Chicken w/o Dressing	½ serv	270	4	19	—
Young Spinach w/o Dressing	½ serv	180	2	19	—
SOUPS					
Chicken Noodle	1 serv (6 oz)	130	3	8	—
Vegetable Minestrone	1 serv (6 oz)	96	2	12	—

CHICK-FIL-A
BREAKFAST SELECTIONS

FOOD	PORTION	CALS	FAT	CARB	SUGAR
Bagel Chicken Egg & Cheese	1	500	20	49	8
Bagel Wheat	1	220	3	41	6
Biscuit Bacon	1	300	14	38	5
Biscuit Bacon & Egg	1	390	20	38	5
Biscuit Bacon Egg Cheese	1	440	24	30	5
Biscuit Buttered	1	270	12	38	5
Biscuit Chicken	1	420	19	44	6
Biscuit Chicken w/ Cheese	1	470	23	45	6
Biscuit Egg	1	350	16	38	5
Biscuit Egg Cheese	1	400	21	38	5
Biscuit Sausage	1	410	23	42	5
Biscuit Sausage Egg	1	500	29	43	6
Biscuit Sausage Egg Cheese	1	550	33	43	6
Biscuit w/ Gravy	1	330	15	44	5
Burrito Chicken	1	420	19	39	2
Burrito Sausage	1	460	24	40	2
Chick-N-Minis	1 serv	270	11	28	6
Hashbrowns	1 serv	260	17	25	0
DESSERTS					
Cheesecake	1 slice	340	21	30	25
Fudge Nut Brownie	1	330	15	45	29
Icedream Cone	1 sm	160	4	28	24

FOOD	PORTION	CALS	FAT	CARB	SUGAR
Lemon Pie	1 slice	390	13	63	36
MAIN MENU SELECTIONS					
Carrot & Raisin Salad	1 sm	170	6	28	18
Chicken Filet	1	230	11	10	2
Chicken Filet Chargrilled	1	100	2	1	2
Chick-N-Strips	4	290	13	14	3
Cole Slaw	1 sm	260	21	17	11
Cool Wrap Chargrilled Chicken	1	390	7	54	7
Cool Wrap Chicken Caesar	1	460	10	52	5
Cool Wrap Spicy Chicken	1	380	6	52	5
Fruit Cup	1 serv	60	0	16	13
Hearty Breast of Chicken Soup	1 cup	140	4	18	2
Nuggets	8	260	12	12	3
Polynesian Sauce	1 pkg	110	6	13	13
Sandwich Chargrilled Chicken	1	270	4	33	7
Sandwich Chicken	1	410	16	38	5
Sandwich Chicken Deluxe	1	420	16	39	5
Sandwich Chicken Salad On Wheat Bread	1	350	15	32	6
Waffle Potato Fries	1 sm	270	13	34	0
SALAD DRESSINGS AND SAUCES					
Barbecue Sauce	1 pkg	45	0	11	9
Blue Cheese	2 tbsp	150	16	1	1
Buffalo Sauce	1 pkg	15	2	1	0
Buttermilk Ranch	2 tbsp	160	16	1	1
Buttermilk Ranch Sauce	1 pkg	110	12	1	1
Caesar	2 tbsp	160	17	1	0
Fat Free Honey Mustard	2 tbsp	60	0	14	11
Honey Mustard	1 pkg	45	0	10	10

FOOD	PORTION	CALS	FAT	CARB	SUGAR
Honey Roasted BBQ Sauce	1 pkg	60	6	2	1
Light Italian	2 tbsp	15	1	2	2
Raspberry Vinaigrette Reduced Fat	2 tbsp	80	2	15	11
Spicy	2 tbsp	140	14	2	1
Thousand Island	2 tbsp	150	14	5	4
SALADS					
Chargrilled Chicken Garden Salad	1 serv	180	6	9	6
Chick-N-Strips Salad	1 serv	390	18	22	8
Croutons Garlic & Butter	1 pkg	50	3	6	0
Honey Roasted Sunflower Kernels	1 pkg	80	7	3	2
Side Salad	1 serv	60	3	4	2
Southwest Chargrilled Salad	1 serv	240	8	17	6
Tortilla Strips	1 pkg	70	4	9	2

CHILI'S

CHILDREN'S MENU SELECTIONS

FOOD	PORTION	CALS	FAT	CARB	SUGAR
Corn Dog	1	250	17	18	—
Grilled Chicken Platter	1 serv	140	3	3	—
Little Chicken Crispers	1 serv	590	42	19	—
Little Mouth Burger	1 serv	280	15	14	—
Little Mouth Cheeseburger	1 serv	350	21	14	—
Macaroni & Cheese	1 serv	510	18	69	—
Pepper Pal Pasta w/ Alfredo	1 serv	410	19	47	—
Pepper Pal Pasta w/ Marinara	1 serv	290	5	52	—
Pizza	1	570	24	67	—
Rib Basket	1 serv	370	24	16	—
Sandwich Grilled Cheese	1 serv	420	27	26	—
Sandwich Grilled Chicken	1 serv	140	3	10	—

FOOD	PORTION	CALS	FAT	CARB	SUGAR
DESSERTS					
Cheesecake	1 serv	760	44	75	—
Chocolate Chip Paradise Pie w/ Vanilla Ice Cream	1 serv	1600	78	215	—
Frosty Chocolate Shake w/ Chocolate Sprinkles	1 serv	850	36	123	—
Molten Chocolate Cake w/ Vanilla Ice Cream	1 serv	1270	62	172	—
MAIN MENU SELECTIONS					
Awesome Blossom	1 serv	2710	203	194	—
Baby Back Ribs & Chicken	1 serv	1460	67	163	—
Black Bean Burger	1 serv	650	12	96	—
Boneless Buffalo Wings	1 serv	1250	80	55	—
Boneless Shangai Wings	1 serv	1260	71	97	—
Bottomless Tostada Chips	1 basket	400	36	18	—
Burger Bacon	1 serv	1080	71	54	—
Burger BBQ Ranch	1 serv	1110	71	60	—
Burger Chipotle Bleu Cheese Bacon	1 serv	1090	71	57	—
Burger Ground Peppercorn	1 serv	1050	68	61	—
Burger Mushroom Swiss	1 serv	1100	71	60	—
Burger Oldtimer	1 serv	800	44	54	—
Chicken Crispers	1 serv	1870	129	132	—
Chicken Tacos	1 serv	1200	41	143	—
Cinnamon Apples	1 serv	210	8	35	—
Citrus Fire Chicken & Shrimp	1 serv	760	27	68	—
Classic Nachos	1 serv	1570	115	66	—
Country Fried Steak	1 serv	1890	107	148	—
Fried Cheese w/ Marinara Sauce	1 serv	1210	89	82	—
Garlic Toast	1 piece	200	12	18	—

FOOD	PORTION	CALS	FAT	CARB	SUGAR
Grilled Baby Back Ribs	1 serv	1370	82	112	–
Grilled Salmon w/ Garlic & Herbs	1 serv	700	33	53	–
Guiltless Grill Chicken Pita	1 serv	550	9	70	–
Guiltless Grill Chicken Platter	1 serv	580	9	89	–
Guiltless Grill Chicken Sandwich	1 serv	490	8	63	–
Guiltless Grill Salmon	1 serv	480	14	31	–
Guiltless Grill Tomato Basil Pasta	1 serv	650	14	107	–
Homestyle Fries	1 serv	520	31	53	–
Kettle Black Beans	1 serv	140	1	23	–
Loaded Mashed Potatoes	1 serv	560	37	42	–
Margarita Grilled Chicken	1 serv	690	14	85	–
Monterey Chicken	1 serv	1170	71	70	–
Pasta Cajun Chicken	1 serv	1460	75	118	–
Pasta Grilled Shrimp Alfredo	1 serv	1340	72	102	–
Pasta Tomato Basil Chicken	1 serv	860	26	111	–
Pita Chicken Caesar	1 serv	650	41	31	–
Pita Chicken Fajita	1 serv	450	17	35	–
Pita Steak Fajita	1 serv	580	33	32	–
Quesadillas Fajita Chicken	1 serv	1720	82	150	–
Quesadillas Fajita Combo	1 serv	1840	94	148	–
Quesadillas Fajita Steak	1 serv	1970	106	147	–
Ribeye Cajun	1 serv	870	76	3	–
Ribeye Flame Grilled	1 serv	960	87	1	–
Rice	1 serv	210	2	45	–
Sandwich Cajun Chicken	1 serv	820	43	66	–
Sandwich Chicken Ranch	1 serv	1150	70	82	–

FOOD	PORTION	CALS	FAT	CARB	SUGAR
Sandwich Chili's Cheesesteak	1 serv	1010	55	72	—
Sandwich Grilled Chicken	1 serv	840	47	57	—
Sandwich Smoked Turkey	1 serv	930	57	65	—
Sauteed Mushrooms Onions & Bell Peppers	1 serv	120	10	6	—
Seasonal Grilled Veggies	1 serv	90	6	7	—
Seasonal Steamed Veggie w/ Parmesan Cheese	1 serv	60	1	8	—
Sirloin Chili's Classic	1 serv	530	41	1	—
Sirloin Honey BBQ	1 serv	800	56	19	—
Skillet Queso	1 serv	670	53	12	—
Southwestern Eggrolls	1 serv	810	51	59	—
Steamed Broccoli	1 serv	80	6	6	—
Sweet Corn On The Cob	1 serv	180	2	55	—
Triple Play	1 serv	2330	177	96	—
Wings Over Buffalo	1 serv	1140	100	4	—
SALAD DRESSINGS AND SAUCES					
Dressing Asian Sesame Ginger	1 serv (2 oz)	250	22	11	—
Dressing Avocado Ranch	1 serv (2 oz)	150	15	3	—
Dressing Bleu Cheese	1 serv (2 oz)	330	35	1	—
Dressing Caesar	1 serv (2 oz)	350	37	3	—
Dressing Chipotle Ranch	1 serv (2 oz)	170	18	2	—
Dressing Citrus Balsamic Vinaigrette	1 serv (2 oz)	350	35	8	—
Dressing Creamy Cilantro	1 serv (2 oz)	300	32	2	—
Dressing Honey Lime	1 serv (2 oz)	270	22	17	—
Dressing Honey Mustard	1 serv (2 oz)	260	28	2	—
Dressing Ranch	1 serv (2 oz)	240	25	3	—
Dressing Thousand Island	1 serv (2 oz)	270	26	9	—
Dressing Low Fat Ranch	1 serv (2 oz)	110	6	12	—

FOOD	PORTION	CALS	FAT	CARB	SUGAR
Dressing No Fat Balsamic Vinaigrette	1 serv (2 oz)	50	0	9	—
Dressing No Fat Honey Mustard	1 serv (2 oz)	90	1	14	—
Sauce Peanut Dipping	1 serv (2 oz)	190	13	15	—
Sauce Picante Salsa	1 serv (2 oz)	40	0	4	—
Sauce Sesame Dipping	1 serv (2 oz)	70	0	11	—
SALADS					
Boneless Buffalo Chicken	1 serv	870	55	50	—
Chicken Caesar w/ Dressing	1 serv	1010	76	39	—
Crispy Chicken	1 serv	810	47	59	—
Dinner Caesar w/ Dressing	1 serv	430	34	20	—
Dinner House	1 serv	140	7	12	—
Grilled Caribbean	1 serv	440	10	51	—
Lettuce Wraps	1 serv	330	21	29	—
Lime Grilled Shrimp Caesar w/ Dressing	1 serv	980	77	39	—
Quesadilla Explosion	1 serv	850	45	60	—
Southwestern Cobb	1 serv	650	32	49	—
SOUPS					
Broccoli Cheese	1 cup	160	9	12	—
Chicken Enchilada	1 cup	220	14	11	—
Chicken Noodle	1 cup	50	1	7	—
Chicken Tortilla	1 cup	140	7	10	—
Chili w/ Cheese	1 cup	500	35	19	—
New England Clam Chowder	1 cup	470	33	27	—
Potato	1 cup	220	16	12	—
Southwestern Vegetable	1 cup	110	5	13	—
CHIPOTLE					
Barbacoa	1 serv (5 oz)	285	16	1	—

FOOD	PORTION	CALS	FAT	CARB	SUGAR
Black Beans	1 serv (4 oz)	130	1	22	—
Carnitas	1 serv (4 oz)	227	12	0	—
Cheese	1 serv (1 oz)	110	9	tr	0
Chicken	1 serv (4 oz)	219	11	0	—
Chips	1 serv (4 oz)	490	19	71	1
Crispy Taco Shells	4	240	9	34	0
Fajita Vegetables	1 serv (3 oz)	100	8	6	3
Flour Tortilla	1 (6 inch)	300	8	45	0
Flour Tortilla	1 (13 inch)	340	9	54	1
Guacamole	1 serv (4 oz)	170	15	8	1
Lettuce	1 serv (1 oz)	5	0	tr	0
Pinto Beans	1 serv (4 oz)	138	1	23	—
Rice	1 serv (5 oz)	240	7	40	0
Salsa Corn	1 serv (4 oz)	100	1	22	3
Salsa Tomato	1 serv (4 oz)	25	0	6	3
Sour Cream	1 serv (2 oz)	120	10	2	2
Steak	1 serv (4 oz)	230	12	2	—
Tomatillo Green	1 serv (2 oz)	15	tr	3	—
Tomatillo Red	1 serv (2 oz)	28	1	4	—

CHURCH'S CHICKEN

DESSERTS

FOOD	PORTION	CALS	FAT	CARB	SUGAR
Apple Pie	1 pie	280	12	41	13
Edward's Double Lemon Pie	1 pie	300	14	39	29
Edward's Strawberry Cream Cheese Pie	1 pie	280	15	32	22

MAIN MENU SELECTIONS

FOOD	PORTION	CALS	FAT	CARB	SUGAR
Breast	1 serv	200	12	4	0
Cajun Rice	1 reg	130	7	16	0
Chicken Fried Steak w/ White Gravy	1 serv	470	28	36	4
Cole Slaw	1 reg	92	6	8	6
Collard Greens	1 reg	25	0	5	0

FOOD	PORTION	CALS	FAT	CARB	SUGAR
Corn On The Cob	1 ear	139	3	24	2
French Fries	1 reg	210	11	29	0
Honey Butter Biscuit	1	250	16	26	3
Jalapeno Cheese Bombers	4 pieces	240	10	29	5
Krispy Tender Strips	1 piece	137	5	11	0
Leg	1 serv	140	9	2	0
Macaroni & Cheese	1 reg	210	11	23	6
Mashed Potatoes & Gravy	1 reg	90	3	14	2
Okra	1 reg	210	16	19	tr
Sweet Corn Nuggets	1 reg	250	12	30	6
Tender Crunchers	6-8 pieces	411	15	32	0
Thigh	1 serv	230	16	5	0
Whole Jalapeno Peppers	2	10	0	2	tr
Wing	1 serv	250	16	8	0
SAUCES					
BBQ	1 pkg	29	0	7	2
Creamy Jalapeno	1 pkg	102	11	1	0
Honey Mustard	1 pkg	111	11	4	1
Purple Pepper	1 pkg	21	0	12	6
Sweet & Sour	1 pkg	31	0	8	2
COLD STONE CREAMERY					
Waffle Cone Dipped	1	310	15	46	31
Waffle Cone Dipped w/ Candy	1	390	20	55	31
Waffle Cone or Bowl	1	160	4	29	14
FROZEN YOGURT					
Cheesecake	1 serv (6 oz)	170	0	49	33
Low Fat Chocolate	1 serv (6 oz)	230	2	48	29
Nonfat Coffee	1 serv (6 oz)	220	0	45	31
Nonfat Sweet Cream	1 serv (6 oz)	220	0	45	31
ICE CREAM					
Amaretto	1 serv (6 oz)	390	24	40	35
Banana	1 serv (6 oz)	370	22	40	34

FOOD	PORTION	CALS	FAT	CARB	SUGAR
Black Cherry	1 serv (6 oz)	390	22	43	38
Butter Pecan	1 serv (6 oz)	390	24	40	35
Cake A Cheesecake Named Desire	1 slice (5 oz)	410	19	57	38
Cake Butterfinger Bonanza	1 slice (5 oz)	450	22	58	43
Cake Celebration Sensation	1 slice (4.5 oz)	350	17	46	34
Cake Chocolate Chipper	1 slice (4.6 oz)	450	28	50	39
Cake Coffeehouse Crunch	1 slice (5 oz)	530	31	59	36
Cake Cookie Dough Delirium	1 slice (4.8 oz)	420	21	53	34
Cake Cookies & Creamery	1 slice (4.5 oz)	390	20	48	35
Cake Midnight Delight	1 slice (5.3 oz)	510	28	61	47
Cake MMMMMM Chip	1 slice (4.5 oz)	380	20	46	36
Cake Peanut Butter Playground	1 slice (5 oz)	490	29	54	43
Cake Raspberry Truffle Temptation	1 slice (5 oz)	480	27	57	43
Cake Snicker's Supreme	1 slice (5 oz)	510	29	57	46
Cake Strawberry Passion	1 slice (5 oz)	380	19	50	35
Cake Zebra Stripes	1 slice (4.8 oz)	400	22	46	36
Cake Batter	1 serv (6 oz)	410	23	50	36
Candy Cane	1 serv (6 oz)	420	24	48	39
Caramel Latte	1 serv (6 oz)	400	22	47	39
Carrot Cake Batter	1 serv (6 oz)	450	24	54	44
Cheesecake	1 serv (6 oz)	390	22	44	37
Chocolate	1 serv (6 oz)	390	24	39	36
Cinnamon	1 serv (6 oz)	400	24	41	35
Coconut	1 serv (6 oz)	390	23	39	34
Coffee	1 serv (6 oz)	400	24	40	34
Cookie Batter	1 serv (6 oz)	450	24	53	41
Cotton Candy	1 serv (6 oz)	390	23	41	34

FOOD	PORTION	CALS	FAT	CARB	SUGAR
Dark Chocolate Peppermint	1 serv (6 oz)	410	23	41	33
Egg Nog	1 serv (6 oz)	400	22	46	38
Expresso	1 serv (6 oz)	350	21	36	30
French Vanilla	1 serv (6 oz)	400	23	45	39
Irish Cream	1 serv (6 oz)	390	24	40	35
Macadamia Nut	1 serv (6 oz)	390	24	40	35
Mango	1 serv (6 oz)	370	22	40	34
Mint	1 serv (6 oz)	400	23	43	37
Mocha	1 serv (6 oz)	390	24	40	35
Oatmeal Batter	1 serv (6 oz)	400	23	44	34
Orange Dreamsicle	1 serv (6 oz)	380	22	41	34
Peanut Butter	1 serv (6 oz)	440	29	39	33
Pecan Praline	1 serv (6 oz)	400	22	44	37
Pistachio	1 serv (6 oz)	390	24	40	35
Pumpkin	1 serv (6 oz)	390	22	42	36
Raspberry	1 serv (6 oz)	390	22	43	37
Sinless Sans Fat Sweet Cream	1 serv (6 oz)	160	0	41	11
Strawberry	1 serv (6 oz)	380	22	41	36
Sweet Cream	1 serv (6 oz)	390	24	95	35
Vanilla Bean	1 serv (6 oz)	400	23	39	34
White Chocolate	1 serv (6 oz)	390	23	40	34
MIX-INS AND TOPPINGS					
Almond Joy	1 piece	180	9	20	16
Apple Pie Filling	¾ oz	60	0	16	14
Banana	½	60	0	14	9
Black Cherries	¾ oz	80	0	19	16
Blackberries	¾ oz	10	0	2	2
Blueberries	¾ oz	10	0	2	2
Brownies	1 piece	180	6	29	19
Butterfinger	½ bar	140	6	20	15
Caramel Topping	1 oz	110	0	24	16

FOOD	PORTION	CALS	FAT	CARB	SUGAR
Cashews	1 oz	170	14	9	2
Chocolate Chips	1 oz	130	7	15	15
Cinnamon	⅛ tsp	15	0	4	0
Coconut	1 oz	80	5	7	6
Cookie Dough	1 piece	180	8	25	9
Fat Free Butterscotch	1 oz	80	0	19	14
Fat Free Caramel	1 oz	80	0	19	14
Fat Free Fudge	1 oz	80	0	20	16
Fudge Topping	1 oz	110	3	18	12
Granola	1 oz	120	2	23	0
Gumballs	1 oz	120	0	34	24
Gummi Bears	1 oz	120	0	30	13
Heath Candy	1 bar	110	7	12	0
Honey	1 oz	90	0	25	25
Kit Kat	½ bar	100	5	13	9
Krackel Candy	½ bar	130	7	15	13
M&M's	1 oz	170	7	25	22
M&M's Peanut	1 oz	150	8	18	14
Macadamia Nuts	1 oz	180	19	3	1
Maraschino Cherry	1	5	0	1	1
Marshmallow Creme	1 oz	100	0	24	20
Marshmallows	1 oz	100	0	24	24
Nestle Crunch	½ bar	130	7	16	14
Nilla Wafers	3	70	3	11	6
Oreo Cookies	2	120	5	17	10
Peach Pie Filling	1 oz	60	0	16	14
Peanut Butter	¾ oz	150	13	5	2
Peanuts	1 oz	200	17	7	0
Pecan Pralines	1 oz	210	21	5	4
Pecans	1 oz	140	14	3	1
Pie Crust Graham Cracker	1 oz	110	3	19	6
Pie Crust Oreo	1 oz	180	8	19	10
Pistachio Nuts	1 oz	210	18	10	1

FOOD	PORTION	CALS	FAT	CARB	SUGAR
Raisins	1 oz	80	0	20	16
Raspberries	¾ oz	15	0	4	2
Red Hot Candy	1 oz	130	4	24	18
Reese's Peanut Butter Cup	1 piece	190	11	19	16
Reese's Pieces	1 oz	170	7	21	18
Roasted Almonds	1 oz	190	17	5	1
Sliced Almonds	1 oz	210	20	6	0
Snickers	½ bar	170	9	21	17
Sprinkles Chocolate	1 oz	25	0	6	6
Sprinkles Rainbow	1 oz	25	0	6	6
Strawberries	¾ oz	20	0	7	4
Toasted Coconut	1 oz	180	14	13	11
Twix	1 cup	150	7	20	14
Walnuts	1 oz	130	12	4	0
Whip Topping	1 serv	50	4	4	4
White Chocolate Chips	1 oz	160	9	18	18
Whoppers	1 oz	100	4	16	13
Yellow Sponge Cake	1 piece	70	1	15	12
York Peppermint Patties	2 pieces	120	2	24	18
SORBET					
Sinless Lemon	1 serv	180	0	48	41
Sinless Raspberry	1 serv (6 oz)	200	0	50	43
Sinless Tangerine	1 serv (6 oz)	200	0	52	44

COLOMBO FROZEN YOGURT

Strawberry Lowfat	½ cup	110	2	21	16
Strawberry Nonfat	½ cup	100	0	20	16

D'ANGELO'S SANDWICH SHOP
CHILDREN'S MENU SELECTIONS

D'Lite Turkey	1 kidz	217	3	30	2
Sub Cheeseburger	1 kidz	294	13	28	2
Sub Ham & Cheese	1 kidz	214	4	31	2
Sub Meatball	1 kidz	330	15	37	5

FOOD	PORTION	CALS	FAT	CARB	SUGAR
Sub Tuna	1 kidz	450	30	30	2
SALAD DRESSINGS AND TOPPINGS					
Bacon	1 serv	64	5	0	0
Bleu Cheese	1 serv (1 oz)	152	15	3	2
Buffalo Sauce	1 serv (1 oz)	10	0	2	0
Caesar	1 serv (1 oz)	140	15	2	2
Caesar Fat Free	1 serv (1 oz)	20	0	3	3
Creamy Italian	1 serv (1 oz)	122	13	3	2
Cucumbers	3 slices	2	0	0	0
Greek Dressing w/ Feta	1 serv (3 oz)	227	26	6	3
Honey Mustard Dressing	1 serv (1 oz)	150	142	7	6
Hot Peppers	1 serv	0	0	1	1
Mayonnaise	2 tbsp	236	26	0	0
Mayonnaise Fat Free	1 pkg	10	0	2	0
Mustard Honey Dijon	2 tbsp	60	0	18	18
Mustard Yellow	2 tbsp	20	1	2	0
Olive Oil Vinaigrette	1 serv (3 oz)	170	17	9	6
Olive Oil Blend	2 tbsp	239	27	0	0
Ranch Lite	1 serv (3 oz)	240	19	6	4
Sesame Ginger	1 serv (1 oz)	170	7	10	10
SALADS					
Antipasto Salad w/o Dressing	1 serv	275	16	15	5
Asian Chicken w/o Dressing	1 serv	224	4	23	7
Caesar w/ Dressing	1 serv	474	39	20	2
Chef w/o Dressing	1 serv	273	12	17	5
Chicken Caesar w/ Dressing	1 serv	532	38	13	2
Chicken Stir Fry w/o Dressing	1 serv	166	3	10	5
Cobb w/o Dressing	1 serv	289	17	9	5
Greek w/o Dressing	1 serv	298	23	16	6

FOOD	PORTION	CALS	FAT	CARB	SUGAR
Lobster w/o Dressing	1 serv	385	27	11	4
Roast Beef w/o Dressing	1 serv	146	3	9	4
Tossed Garden w/o Dressing	1 serv	47	1	9	4
Turkey w/o Dressing	1 serv	157	2	9	4
SANDWICHES					
D'Lite Chicken Stir Fry	1 sm	426	6	57	8
D'Lite Fresh Veggie	1	348	7	62	14
D'Lite Grilled Chicken Breast	1 sm	387	7	52	5
D'Lite Ham & Cheese	1 sm	351	6	52	5
D'Lite Roast Beef	1 sm	353	5	51	5
D'Lite Turkey	1 sm	364	4	51	5
D'Lite Turkey Cranberry	1 sm	460	4	75	22
Pokket BLT & Cheese	1 sm	421	18	44	3
Pokket Caesar Salad	1 sm	643	40	55	1
Pokket Capacola & Cheese	1 sm	426	14	52	5
Pokket Cheeseburger	1 sm	481	25	37	2
Pokket Chicken Caesar Salad	1 sm	701	39	48	2
Pokket Chicken Club	1 sm	559	28	47	2
Pokket Chicken Honey Dijon	1 sm	527	20	45	5
Pokket Chicken Salad	1 sm	705	42	39	1
Pokket Chicken Stir Fry	1 sm	425	10	45	4
Pokket Classic Veggie No Cheese	1 sm	238	2	50	6
Pokket Greek	1 sm	812	61	54	6
Pokket Grilled Chicken	1 sm	328	5	41	1
Pokket Ham & Cheese	1 sm	349	9	41	2
Pokket Ham & Salami	1 sm	412	17	39	2
Pokket Hamburger	1 sm	422	21	35	1

FOOD	PORTION	CALS	FAT	CARB	SUGAR
Pokket Italian	1 sm	574	33	42	2
Pokket Lobster	1 sm	568	32	39	0
Pokket Meatball	1 sm	600	31	56	9
Pokket Mortadella & Cheese	1 sm	505	28	42	2
Pokket Seafood Salad	1 sm	532	28	56	5
Pokket Steak	1 sm	335	13	29	0
Pokket Steak & Cheese	1 sm	407	18	31	1
Pokket Tuna	1 sm	791	58	28	38
Sub Cheeseburger	1 sm	542	27	47	5
Sub Chicken Club	1 sm	619	30	52	5
Sub Chicken Honey Dijon	1 sm	587	22	56	8
Sub Chicken Salad	1 sm	769	44	50	4
Sub Chicken Stir Fry	1 sm	487	11	57	8
Sub Classic Veggie	1 sm	465	15	64	11
Sub Grilled Chicken	1 sm	387	7	52	5
Sub Ham & Cheese	1 sm	412	11	53	5
Sub Ham & Salami	1 sm	474	19	51	5
Sub Hamburger	1 sm	482	22	45	4
Sub Italian	1 sm	637	34	54	5
Sub Lobster	1 sm	628	33	50	3
Sub Meatball	1 sm	663	33	70	13
Sub Mortadella & Cheese	1 sm	568	29	54	5
Sub Number 9	1 sm	475	19	44	6
Sub Pastrami	1 sm	526	27	51	3
Sub Pepperoni	1 sm	614	34	53	5
Sub Roast Beef	1 sm	350	5	50	4
Sub Salad	1 sm	298	3	60	10
Sub Salami & Cheese	1 sm	597	32	51	5
Sub Seafood Salad	1	595	29	67	9
Sub Steak	1 sm	383	14	37	2
Sub Steak & Cheese	1 sm	455	19	40	4
Sub Steak Tip	1 sm	486	14	63	13

FOOD	PORTION	CALS	FAT	CARB	SUGAR
Sub Stuffed Turkey	1 sm	1036	37	136	18
Sub Tuna	1 sm	853	59	49	4
Sub Turkey	1 sm	361	4	50	4
Sub Turkey Club	1 sm	360	8	37	4
Wrap Asian Chicken Salad	1	914	24	105	26
Wrap BLT & Cheese	1	500	18	58	5
Wrap Buffalo Chicken Salad	1	778	36	71	7
Wrap Caesar Salad	1	669	37	64	3
Wrap Capacola & Cheese	1	451	12	57	4
Wrap Cheese	1	631	27	63	7
Wrap Cheeseburger	1	569	26	52	4
Wrap Chef	1	832	40	82	18
Wrap Chicken Caesar Salad	1	788	39	65	4
Wrap Chicken Cobb	1	855	46	69	17
Wrap Chicken Filet & Bacon	1	643	28	57	3
Wrap Chicken Honey Dijon	1	619	20	63	8
Wrap Chicken Salad	1	780	41	55	3
Wrap Chicken Stir Fry	1	511	10	61	7
Wrap Classic Veggie	1	490	14	69	10
Wrap Greek	1	761	61	43	6
Wrap Grilled Chicken	1	420	5	56	4
Wrap Ham & Cheese	1	436	9	58	4
Wrap Ham & Salami	1	499	17	56	4
Wrap Hamburger	1	509	21	50	3
Wrap Italian	1	654	32	59	4
Wrap Lobster	1	766	44	56	2
Wrap Meatball	1	687	31	75	11
Wrap Mortadella & Cheese	1	592	28	58	4

FOOD	PORTION	CALS	FAT	CARB	SUGAR
Wrap Number 9	1	494	18	48	5
Wrap Pastrami	1	550	25	55	2
Wrap Pepperoni	1	638	33	58	4
Wrap Roast Beef	1	374	4	55	3
Wrap Salad	1	322	2	65	8
Wrap Salami & Cheese	1	605	29	56	4
Wrap Seafood Salad	1	619	28	72	7
Wrap Steak	1	402	13	41	2
Wrap Steak & Cheese	1	474	18	43	3
Wrap Steak Tip	1	374	12	40	11
Wrap Tuna	1	881	58	55	3
Wrap Turkey	1	385	3	55	3
Wrap Turkey Club	1	435	8	52	4
SOUPS					
#9 Steak & Cheese	1 sm	280	21	11	2
Chicken Noodle	1 sm	130	2	8	5
Hearty Vegetable	1 sm	40	0	7	4
Lobster Bisque	1 sm	360	29	16	3
New England Clam Chowder	1 sm	270	20	15	2
Santa Fe Chipotle Vegetable	1 sm	130	1	22	3
Shrimp & Roasted Corn	1 sm	250	16	23	6
Thanksgiving Everyday	1 sm	250	17	18	4
DENNY'S					
BEVERAGES					
Cappuccino French Vanilla	8 oz	100	2	28	24
Cappuccino Original	8 oz	100	3	17	13
Malted Milk Shake Chocolate or Vanilla	12 oz	583	26	82	71
BREAKFAST SELECTIONS					
All American Slam	1 serv	816	67	3	0
Applesauce	1 serv	60	0	15	15

FOOD	PORTION	CALS	FAT	CARB	SUGAR
Bacon	4 strips	162	18	1	1
Bagel Dry	1	235	1	46	0
Banana	1	110	0	29	21
Belgian Waffle	1	619	45	28	1
Breakfast Dagwood	1 serv	1446	90	81	5
Buttermilk Hotcakes	3	466	23	47	0
Cantaloupe	¼	32	0	8	7
Chicken Fajita Skillet	1 serv	855	49	30	5
Corned Beef Hash Slam	1 serv	668	55	11	2
Country Fish Potatoes	1 serv	394	20	23	2
Egg	1	120	10	tr	tr
English Muffin Dry	1	125	1	24	0
Fabulous French Toast	1 serv	1146	71	104	20
Farmer's Slam	1 serv	1200	80	82	5
French Slam	1 serv	1119	77	71	17
Fruit Mix	1 serv	36	0	9	9
Grand Slam Slugger	1 serv	927	55	74	24
Grapefruit	½	60	0	16	10
Grapes	1 serv	55	1	15	14
Grits	1 serv	80	0	18	0
Ham & Cheddar Omelette	1 serv	595	47	5	2
Ham & Cheese Omelette w/ Eggbeaters	1 serv	468	32	5	2
Ham Slice	1	94	3	2	0
Hashed Browns	1 serv	197	12	20	1
Hashed Browns Covered	1 serv	280	19	21	1
Hashed Browns Covered & Smothered	1 serv	493	25	54	12
Honeydew	¼	31	0	8	7
Lumberjack Slam w/ Hash Browns	1 serv	1035	58	73	7
Meat Lover's Skillet	1 serv	1031	74	27	3
Moon Over My Hammy	1 serv	841	51	42	4

FOOD	PORTION	CALS	FAT	CARB	SUGAR
Oatmeal	1 serv	100	2	18	0
Oatmeal Deluxe	1 serv	460	6	95	63
Original Grand Slam	1 serv	665	49	33	1
Ready To Eat Cereal	1 serv	100	0	23	5
Sausage	4 links	354	32	0	4
Scram Slam	1 serv	827	68	8	4
Senior Belgian Waffle Slam	1 serv	399	33	12	2
Senior Omelette	1 serv	429	20	8	6
Sirloin Steak & Eggs	1 serv	675	45	1	0
Slim Slam	1 serv	438	6	56	15
T-Bone Steak & Eggs	1 serv	991	77	1	0
Toast Dry	1 slice	92	1	17	1
Two Egg Breakfast w/ Hash Browns	1 serv	825	67	24	1
Ultimate Omelette	1 serv	611	50	11	6
Veggie Cheese Omelette	1 serv	494	39	11	6
CHILDREN'S MENU SELECTIONS					
Burgerlicious	1 serv	296	17	24	2
Burgerlicious w/ Cheese	1 serv	341	20	24	2
Dennysaur Chicken Nuggets	1 serv	190	13	9	0
Frenchtastic Slam	1 serv	452	33	22	3
Junior Fish & Chips	1 serv	698	45	55	0
Junior Grand Slam	1 serv	397	25	33	2
Junior Shrimps Ahoy!	1 serv	411	18	50	4
Oreo Blender Blaster	1 serv	580	29	72	60
Pizza Party	1 serv	400	15	47	8
Smiley-Face Hotcakes w/ Meat	1 serv	463	22	63	7
Smiley-Face Hotcakes w/o Meat	1 serv	344	9	62	6
The Big Cheese	1 serv	334	20	28	3

FOOD	PORTION	CALS	FAT	CARB	SUGAR
DESSERTS					
Apple Pie	1 serv	470	24	64	36
Banana Split	1	894	43	121	29
Carrot Cake	1 serv	799	45	99	75
Cheesecake	1 serv	580	38	51	36
Chocolate Topping	1 serv	317	25	27	27
Chocolate Peanut Butter Pie	1 serv	653	39	64	45
Double Scoop Sundae	1 serv	375	27	29	8
Float Rootbeer or Coke	12 oz	280	10	47	33
Hot Fudge Brownie A La Mode	1 serv	997	42	147	105
Milkshake Vanilla or Chocolate	12 oz	560	26	76	71
Oreo Blender Blaster	1 serv	895	46	112	93
Single Scoop Sundae	1 serv	188	14	14	4
MAIN MENU SELECTIONS					
Albacore Tuna Melt	1 serv	640	39	42	3
Applesauce	1 serv	60	0	15	15
Bacon Lettuce & Tomato	1	610	38	50	5
Baked Potato Plain	1	220	0	51	3
BBQ Chicken Sandwich	1 serv	1089	62	86	20
Bread Stuffing Plain	1 serv	100	1	19	3
Buffalo Chicken Sandwich	1 serv	708	28	80	20
Buffalo Chicken Strips	5 pieces	734	42	43	0
Buffalo Wings	12 pieces	856	54	1	0
Burger Bacon Cheddar	1	875	52	58	9
Burger BBQ	1 serv	953	52	72	12
Burger Boca	1 serv	601	27	64	10
Burger Classic	1	694	35	56	11
Burger Classic w/ Cheese	1	852	48	57	11
Burger Mushroom Swiss	1 serv	880	49	63	14
Carrots In Honey Glaze	1 serv	80	3	12	7

FOOD	PORTION	CALS	FAT	CARB	SUGAR
Chicken Strips	5 pieces	720	33	56	14
Chicken Ranch Melt	1 serv	758	45	44	4
Chicken Strips	1 serv	635	25	55	13
Club Sandwich	1	718	38	62	6
Coleslaw	1 serv	274	30	14	11
Corn In Butter Sauce	1 serv	120	4	19	4
Cottage Cheese	1 serv	72	3	2	0
Country Fried Steak	1 serv	644	48	30	7
Fish & Chips Dinner	1 serv	955	57	77	11
French Fries Unsalted	1 serv	423	20	57	0
Fried Shrimp Dinner	1 serv	219	10	18	5
Fried Shrimp & Shrimp Scampi	1 serv	346	20	15	5
Green Beans w/ Bacon	1 serv	60	4	6	2
Grilled Cheese Sandwich	1	510	30	40	2
Grilled Chicken Dinner	1 serv	130	4	0	0
Grilled Chicken Sandwich	1	469	14	53	8
Ham & Swiss On Rye	1	417	16	39	8
Herb Toast	1 serv	170	11	15	1
Hoagie Chicken Melt	1	751	44	43	2
Hoagie Philly Melt	1 serv	874	50	58	14
Mashed Potatoes Plain	1 serv	168	7	23	1
Mozzarella Sticks	8 pieces	710	41	49	0
Onion Rings	1 serv	381	23	38	2
Patty Melt	1	798	51	37	10
Pot Roast Dinner w/ Gravy	1 serv	292	11	5	0
Roast Turkey & Stuffing w/ Gravy	1 serv	388	3	38	17
Sampler	1 serv	1405	80	124	4
Seasoned Fries	1 serv	261	12	35	0
Senior Chicken Strip Dinner	1 serv	285	10	31	13

FOOD	PORTION	CALS	FAT	CARB	SUGAR
Senior Club	1 serv	540	31	34	4
Senior Country Fried Steak	1 serv	341	23	18	6
Senior Fish & Chips	1 serv	756	47	64	11
Senior French Slam	1 serv	820	65	40	8
Senior Fried Shrimp Dinner	1 serv	129	5	13	4
Senior Grilled Chicken Breast	1 serv	200	5	15	0
Senior Pot Roast	1 serv	160	6	3	0
Senior Starter	1 serv	544	42	23	1
Senior Turkey & Stuffing	1 serv	220	2	25	9
Shrimp Scampi Skillet Dinner	1 serv	289	19	3	tr
Sirloin Steak Dinner	1 serv	337	28	1	0
Sliced Tomatoes	3 slices	13	0	3	2
Smoothered Cheese Fries	1 serv	767	48	69	1
Steak & Shrimp Dinner	1 serv	645	42	31	4
T-Bone Steak Dinner	1 serv	860	65	0	0
The Super Bird Sandwich	1	620	32	48	4
Turkey Breast On Multigrain w/o Mayo	1	277	4	41	6
SALAD DRESSINGS AND TOPPINGS					
BBQ Sauce	1.5 oz	47	1	11	5
Bleu Cheese	1 oz	163	18	1	0
Blueberry Topping	1 serv	71	0	17	17
Caesar	1 oz	133	14	1	1
Cherry Topping	1 serv	57	0	14	6
Cream Cheese	1 oz	100	10	1	1
French	1 oz	106	10	3	3
Fudge Topping	1 serv	201	10	30	27
Gravy Brown	1 serv	13	0	2	1
Gravy Chicken	1 serv	14	1	2	1

FOOD	PORTION	CALS	FAT	CARB	SUGAR
Gravy Country	1 serv	17	1	2	0
Honey Mustard	1 serv	160	15	20	4
Low Calorie Italian	1 oz	15	1	3	2
Marinara Sauce	1 serv	48	2	7	5
Ranch	1 oz	129	14	1	0
Ranch Fat Free	1 serv	25	tr	6	2
Sour Cream	1.5 oz	91	9	2	0
Strawberry Topping	1 serv	77	1	17	13
Syrup	3 tbsp	143	0	36	36
Syrup Sugar Free	1 serv	23	0	9	0
Tartar Sauce	1 serv	225	23	3	3
Thousand Island	1 oz	118	11	5	5
Thousand Island	2 tbsp	170	18	2	–
Whipped Margarine	1 serv	87	10	0	0
Whipped Cream	2 tbsp	23	2	2	0
SALADS					
Garden Salad w/ Albacore Tuna	1 serv	444	29	12	6
Garden Salad w/ Fried Chicken Strips	1 serv	438	26	26	5
Garden Salad w/ Grilled Chicken Breast	1 serv	264	11	10	5
Grilled Chicken Caesar Salad w/ Dressing	1 serv	600	41	19	3
Side Caesar w/ Dressing	1 serv	362	26	20	2
Side Garden Salad w/o Dressing	1 serv	113	4	16	4
SOUPS					
Chicken Noodle	1 serv	60	2	8	0
Clam Chowder	1 serv	624	42	55	7
Cream Of Broccoli	1 serv	574	43	41	6
Vegetable Beef	1 serv	79	1	11	2

FOOD	PORTION	CALS	FAT	CARB	SUGAR

DESERT MOON CAFE
CHILDREN'S MENU SELECTIONS

FOOD	PORTION	CALS	FAT	CARB	SUGAR
Burrito Bean & Cheese	1 serv	650	26	83	2
Kids Nachos	1 serv	500	23	59	0
Kids Taco w/ Chicken	1	280	7	38	1
Kids Taco w/ Steak	1	290	8	38	1
Kidsadilla	1 serv	630	30	70	1

MAIN MENU SELECTIONS

FOOD	PORTION	CALS	FAT	CARB	SUGAR
Alamo Burger	1	810	51	35	8
Burrito Adobe Moon w/ Chicken	1	730	28	85	4
Burrito Adobe Moon w/ Steak	1	750	31	85	4
Burrito Black Bean w/ Chicken	1	770	25	98	6
Burrito Black Bean w/ Steak	1	790	27	98	6
Burrito Full Moon w/ Chicken	1	620	24	66	5
Burrito Full Moon w/ Steak	1	640	26	66	5
Burrito Get It Smothered	1	120	9	4	3
Burrito Harvest Wrap w/ Chicken	1	620	30	57	5
Burrito Harvest Wrap w/ Steak	1	300	33	57	5
Enchilada Mesa	1	710	27	74	3
Enchilada Queso	1	730	26	74	6
Enchilada Shrimp	1	830	28	110	10
Fajita Platter w/ Chicken	1 serv	1160	51	109	13
Fajita Platter w/ Shrimp	1 serv	1060	49	109	13
Fajita Platter w/ Steak	1	1190	55	109	13
Hell Canyon Chili	1 serv	260	14	20	12

FOOD	PORTION	CALS	FAT	CARB	SUGAR
Mucho Nachos	1 serv	800	47	71	9
Mucho Nachos w/ Chicken	1 serv	900	49	71	9
Mucho Nachos w/ Steak	1 serv	920	52	71	9
Pizza Texas BBQ	1	330	37	68	18
Quesadilla Baja Chicken	1	650	32	53	4
Quesadilla Coyote w/ Chicken	1	660	32	53	3
Quesadilla Coyote w/ Steak	1	680	35	53	3
Quesadilla Sonoran	1	660	39	60	6
Rice Bowl Black Bean w/ Chicken	1 serv	790	14	123	4
Rice Bowl Black Bean w/ Steak	1 serv	820	17	123	4
Rice Bowl Chili w/ Chicken	1 serv	760	17	109	6
Rice Bowl Chili w/ Steak	1 serv	790	20	109	6
Rice Bowl Shrimp Creole	1 serv	910	19	124	13
Shrimp Dippers	1 serv	430	15	50	12
Soup Black Bean	1 serv	360	7	55	7
Soup Tortilla	1 serv	330	13	45	21
Taco Acapulco Shrimp	1	230	9	30	11
Taco Classic w/ Chicken	1	190	6	17	1
Taco Classic w/ Steak	1	200	7	17	1
Taco Fajita w/ Chicken	1	200	6	19	2
Taco Fajita w/ Steak	1	210	8	19	2
SALAD DRESSINGS AND SAUCES					
BBQ Sauce	1 serv (1 oz)	50	1	12	11
Buffalo Wing Sauce	1 serv (1 oz)	45	5	1	0
Dressing Bleu Cheese	1 serv (2 oz)	300	32	2	2
Dressing Creamy Caesar	1 serv (2 oz)	320	36	0	0
Dressing Honey Dijon Fat Free	1 serv (2 oz)	80	0	17	11

FOOD	PORTION	CALS	FAT	CARB	SUGAR
Dressing Lite Ranch	1 serv (2 oz)	150	13	4	2
Dressing Lite Raspberry Vinaigrette	1 serv (2 oz)	150	11	6	4
Dressing Poblano	1 serv (1 oz)	150	16	2	0
Guacamole	1 serv (2 oz)	100	9	4	1
Pepper Cream Sauce	1 serv (2 oz)	100	9	4	1
Pico De Gallo	1 serv (2 oz)	15	0	3	2
Salsa Black Bean	1 serv (2 oz)	20	0	4	2
Salsa Fruit	1 serv (2 oz)	60	2	12	10
Salsa Mild Tomato	1 serv (2 oz)	15	0	3	3
Salsa Rattlesnake	1 serv (2 oz)	15	0	3	0
SALADS W/O TORTILLA BOWL					
Caesar	1 serv	530	47	15	3
Caesar w/ Chicken	1 serv	640	49	15	3
Caesar w/ Shrimp	1 serv	570	48	15	3
Chopped Chicken	1 serv	520	35	21	10
Taco w/ Chicken	1 serv	310	15	15	10
Taco w/ Steak	1 serv	340	17	15	10

DOMINO'S PIZZA

12 INCH MEDIUM PIZZAS

FOOD	PORTION	CALS	FAT	CARB	SUGAR
Deep Dish Cheese Only	2 slices	482	22	56	6
Hand Tossed America's Favorite Feast	1 serv	508	22	57	5
Hand Tossed Bacon Cheeseburger Feast	2 slices	549	26	55	5
Hand Tossed Barbeque Feast	2 slices	506	20	62	9
Hand Tossed Cheese Only	2 slices	375	11	55	5
Hand Tossed Deluxe Feast	2 slices	465	18	57	5
Hand Tossed ExtravaganZZa Feast	2 slices	576	27	59	5
Hand Tossed Hawaiian Feast	2 slices	450	16	58	7

FOOD	PORTION	CALS	FAT	CARB	SUGAR
Hand Tossed MeatZZa Feast	2 slices	560	26	57	5
Hand Tossed Pepperoni Feast	2 slices	534	25	56	5
Hand Tossed Vegi Feast	2 slices	439	16	57	5
Thin Crust Cheese	¼ pie	273	12	31	4
Toppings Pineapple	1 serv	12	0	3	3
DESSERTS					
Cinna Stix	1 serv	111	5	15	3
Sweet Icing	1 serv	283	5	60	51
MAIN MENU SELECTIONS					
Breadstick	1	116	4	18	1
Buffalo Chicken Kickers	1 piece	47	2	3	tr
Buffalo Wings Barbeque	1 piece	50	2	2	1
Buffalo Wings Hot	1 piece	45	2	1	tr
Cheesy Bread	1 piece	142	6	18	1
TOPPINGS					
Blue Cheese	1 serv	223	23	2	2
Hot Sauce	1 serv	14	tr	4	1
Medium Pizza Anchovies	1 serv	34	1	0	0
Medium Pizza Bacon	1 serv	102	9	tr	tr
Medium Pizza Banana Peppers	1 serv	5	tr	1	0
Medium Pizza Beef	1 serv	78	7	tr	tr
Medium Pizza Cheddar Cheese	1 serv	57	5	tr	tr
Medium Pizza Extra Cheese	1 serv	49	4	1	tr
Medium Pizza Green Olives	1 serv	19	2	tr	tr
Medium Pizza Green Peppers	1 serv	4	tr	1	0
Medium Pizza Ham	1 serv	23	1	tr	tr

FOOD	PORTION	CALS	FAT	CARB	SUGAR
Medium Pizza Italian Sausage	1 serv	77	6	2	tr
Medium Pizza Mushrooms	1 serv	6	tr	1	tr
Medium Pizza Onion	1 serv	5	tr	1	0
Medium Pizza Pepperoni	1 serv	74	7	tr	tr
Medium Pizza Ripe Olives	1 serv	21	2	1	tr
Ranch	1 serv	197	20	2	2

DONATOS PIZZA
PIZZA

FOOD	PORTION	CALS	FAT	CARB	SUGAR
Dessert Apple	¼ pie	722	20	137	66
Dessert Cherry	¼ pie	818	20	149	70
Original	¼ pie	660	33	58	6
Original Chicken Vegy Medley	¼ pie	500	19	56	6
Original Chicken Vegy Medley No Cheese	¼ pie	392	10	54	6
Original Founders	¼ pie	737	42	71	6
Original Hawaiian	¼ pie	620	30	58	16
Original Hawaiian No Cheese	¼ pie	411	13	58	10
Original Mariachi Beef	¼ pie	613	30	56	6
Original Mariachi Chicken	¼ pie	580	25	56	6
Original Serious Cheese	¼ pie	640	28	62	4
Original Serious Meat	¼ pie	817	47	68	6
Original Vegy	¼ pie	564	24	60	8
Original Vegy No Cheese	¼ pie	370	9	59	7
Original Works	¼ pie	729	41	75	6
Traditional Chicken Vegy Medley	¼ pie	647	17	90	8
Traditional Founders	¼ pie	900	40	107	11
Traditional Hawaiian	¼ pie	794	30	98	17
Traditional Mariachi Beef	¼ pie	797	31	95	11

FOOD	PORTION	CALS	FAT	CARB	SUGAR
Traditional Mariachi Chicken	¼ pie	770	26	95	11
Traditional Original	¼ pie	928	39	89	11
Traditional Serious Cheese	¼ pie	830	36	123	8
Traditional Serious Meat	¼ pie	977	46	104	11
Traditional Vegy	¼ pie	752	26	98	12
Traditional Works	¼ pie	892	39	111	11
SALAD DRESSINGS					
Italian	1 serv (1.5 oz)	230	24	1	1
Italian Lite	1 serv (1.5 oz)	20	1	2	0
SALADS					
Grilled Chicken w/o Dressing	1 serv	314	18	12	8
Italian Chef w/o Dressing	1 serv	338	23	13	8
Side w/o Dressing	1 serv	106	7	6	4
SIDE ORDERS					
Breadsticks	2	220	5	29	1
Chicken Wings Hot	5	449	29	6	–
Chicken Wings Mild	5	451	29	6	–
Three Cheese Garlic Bread	1 bun	605	28	66	3
SUBS					
Big Don Italian	1 serv	705	33	68	6
Big Don Lite Italian	1 serv	631	25	69	6
Grilled Chicken	1 serv	786	43	68	5
Ham & Cheese Italian	1 serv	609	22	70	8
Ham & Cheese Lite Italian	1 serv	534	14	70	8
Southwest Turkey	1 serv	710	33	74	12
Steak & Cheese	1 serv	929	52	107	4
Vegy Italian	1 serv	730	36	75	8
Vegy Lite Italian	1 serv	661	28	78	6

FOOD	PORTION	CALS	FAT	CARB	SUGAR
DUNKIN' DONUTS					
BAGELS AND CREAM CHEESE					
Bagel Blueberry	1	330	3	66	10
Bagel Cinnamon Raisin	1	330	3	65	11
Bagel Everything	1	370	6	67	4
Bagel Harvest	1	350	6	61	15
Bagel Onion	1	320	4	61	5
Bagel Plain	1	320	3	62	4
Bagel Poppyseed	1	370	7	65	4
Bagel Reduced Carb w/ Cheese	1	380	12	45	8
Bagel Salsa	1	310	3	60	5
Bagel Salt	1	370	3	62	4
Bagel Sesame	1	380	8	64	4
Bagel Wheat	1	330	4	62	7
Cream Cheese Chive	2 oz	170	17	4	2
Cream Cheese Garden Vegetable	2 oz	170	15	4	2
Cream Cheese Lite	2 oz	110	9	6	0
Cream Cheese Plain	2 oz	190	17	4	2
Cream Cheese Salmon	2 oz	170	17	2	0
Cream Cheese Strawberry	2 oz	190	17	9	9
BAKED SELECTIONS					
Apple Fritter	1	300	14	41	12
Biscuit	1	250	13	29	3
Bismark Chocolate Iced	1	340	15	50	31
Coffee Roll	1	270	14	33	10
Coffee Roll Chocolate Frosted	1	290	15	36	12
Coffee Roll Maple Frosted	1	290	14	36	13
Coffee Roll Vanilla Frosted	1	290	14	36	13
Cookie Chocolate Chunk	2	220	11	28	17

FOOD	PORTION	CALS	FAT	CARB	SUGAR
Cookie Chocolate Chunk w/ Walnuts	2	230	12	27	16
Cookie Oatmeal Raisin Pecan	2	220	10	29	18
Cookie White Chocolate Chunk	2	230	12	28	19
Croissant Plain	1	330	18	37	3
Danish Apple	1	330	20	32	10
Danish Cheese	1	340	22	30	8
Danish Strawberry Cheese	1	320	20	31	9
Donut Apple Crumb	1	230	10	34	12
Donut Apple Crumb Cake	1	290	15	41	22
Donut Apple N' Spice	1	200	8	29	7
Donut Bavarian Kreme	1	210	9	30	9
Donut Black Raspberry	1	210	8	32	10
Donut Blueberry	1	290	16	35	16
Donut Blueberry Crumb	1	240	10	36	15
Donut Boston Kreme	1	240	9	36	14
Donut Bow Tie	1	300	17	34	10
Donut Chocolate Coconut	1	300	19	31	12
Donut Chocolate Frosted	1	360	20	40	15
Donut Chocolate Glazed	1	290	16	33	14
Donut Chocolate Kreme Filled	1	270	13	35	16
Donut Cinnamon	1	330	20	34	14
Donut Double Chocolate	1	310	17	37	18
Donut Frosted Lemon	1	240	14	28	17
Donut Glazed	1	350	19	41	21
Donut Glazed Gingerbread	1	260	11	35	18
Donut Glazed Lemon	1	240	14	28	16
Donut Jelly Filled	1	210	8	32	14
Donut Lemon Burst	1	300	14	35	25

FOOD	PORTION	CALS	FAT	CARB	SUGAR
Donut Maple Frosted	1	210	9	30	12
Donut Marble Frosted	1	200	9	29	11
Donut Old Fashioned	1	300	19	28	9
Donut Powdered	1	330	19	36	17
Donut Strawberry	1	210	8	32	11
Donut Strawberry Frosted	1	210	9	30	12
Donut Sugar Raised	1	170	8	22	4
Donut Vanilla Kreme Filled	1	270	13	36	17
Donut Whole Wheat Glazed	1	310	19	32	14
Eclair	1	270	11	39	17
English Muffin	1	160	2	31	1
French Cruller	1	150	8	17	8
Fritter Glazed	1	260	14	31	7
Muffin Banana Walnut	1	540	25	69	31
Muffin Blueberry	1	470	17	73	38
Muffin Chocolate Chip	1	630	26	89	49
Muffin Coffee Cake	1	580	19	78	40
Muffin Corn	1	510	18	77	32
Muffin Cranberry Orange	1	440	17	66	30
Muffin Honey Bran Raisin	1	480	15	79	43
Muffin Reduced Fat Blueberry	1	400	5	78	33
Munchkins Chocolate Glazed	3	200	10	26	13
Munchkins Cinnamon	4	270	19	31	14
Munchkins Glazed	3	280	13	38	22
Munchkins Jelly Filled	5	210	9	30	15
Munchkins Lemon Filled	4	170	8	23	9
Munchkins Plain	4	270	16	27	9
Munchkins Powdered	4	270	14	31	15
Munchkins Sugar Raised	7	220	12	26	5

FOOD	PORTION	CALS	FAT	CARB	SUGAR
Stick Cinnamon	1	450	30	42	17
Stick Glazed	1	490	29	51	26
Stick Glazed Chocolate	1	470	29	49	24
Stick Jelly	1	530	29	61	32
Stick Plain	1	420	29	35	12
Stick Powdered	1	450	29	42	18
BEVERAGES					
Cappuccino	1 (10 oz)	60	5	7	7
Cappuccino w/ Soy Milk	1 (10 oz)	70	3	6	5
Cappuccino w/ Soy Milk Sugar	1 (10 oz)	120	3	20	19
Cappuccino w/ Sugar	1 (10 oz)	130	4	21	20
Coffee Blueberry	1 (10 oz)	20	0	4	0
Coffee Caramel	1 (10 oz)	20	0	4	0
Coffee Chocolate	1 (10 oz)	20	0	4	0
Coffee Cinnamon	1 (10 oz)	20	0	4	0
Coffee Coconut	1 (10 oz)	20	0	4	0
Coffee French Vanilla	1 (10 oz)	20	0	4	0
Coffee Hazelnut	1 (10 oz)	20	0	4	0
Coffee Marshmallow	1 (10 oz)	20	0	4	0
Coffee Regular	1 (10 oz)	15	0	3	0
Coffee Toasted Almond	1 (10 oz)	20	0	4	0
Coffee w/ Cream	1 (10 oz)	70	6	3	0
Coffee w/ Cream Sugar	1 (10 oz)	120	6	15	12
Coffee w/ Milk	1 (10 oz)	35	1	4	2
Coffee w/ Milk Sugar	1 (10 oz)	80	1	16	13
Coffee w/ Skim Milk	1 (10 oz)	25	0	4	1
Coffee w/ Skim Milk Sugar	1 (10 oz)	70	0	16	13
Coffee w/ Sugar	1 (10 oz)	60	0	15	12
Coolatta Lemonade	1 (16 oz)	240	0	59	56
Coolatta Strawberry Fruit	1 (16 oz)	290	0	72	65
Coolatta Tropicana Orange	1	370	0	92	87

FOOD	PORTION	CALS	FAT	CARB	SUGAR
Coolatta Vanilla Bean	1 (16 oz)	440	17	70	69
Coolatta Coffee w/ 2% Milk	1 (16 oz)	190	2	41	40
Coolatta Coffee w/ Cream	1 (16 oz)	350	22	40	35
Coolatta Coffee w/ Milk	1 (16 oz)	210	4	42	40
Coolatta Coffee w/ Skim Milk	1 (16 oz)	170	0	41	40
Dunkaccino	1 (10 oz)	230	10	35	25
Expresso	1 (2 oz)	0	0	1	1
Expresso w/ Sugar	1 (2 oz)	30	0	7	7
Hot Chocolate	1 (10 oz)	220	8	38	28
Ice Coffee w/ Milk	1 (16 oz)	35	1	4	2
Iced Coffee	1 (16 oz)	15	0	3	0
Iced Coffee w/ Cream	1 (16 oz)	70	6	4	0
Iced Coffee w/ Cream Sugar	1 (16 oz)	120	6	16	12
Iced Coffee w/ Milk Sugar	1 (16 oz)	80	1	16	13
Iced Coffee w/ Skim Milk	1 (16 oz)	25	0	4	0
Iced Coffee w/ Skim Milk Sugar	1 (16 oz)	70	0	16	12
Iced Coffee w/ Sugar	1 (16 oz)	60	0	15	12
Iced Latte	1 (16 oz)	120	7	11	10
Iced Latte Caramel Creme	1 (16 oz)	260	9	40	40
Iced Latte Caramel Swirl	1 (16 oz)	240	7	37	36
Iced Latte Caramel Swirl w/ Skim Milk	1 (16 oz)	180	0	36	35
Iced Latte Lite	1 (16 oz)	80	0	13	10
Iced Latte Mocha Almond	1 (16 oz)	290	10	46	45
Iced Latte Mocha Swirl	1 (16 oz)	240	8	38	36
Iced Latte Mocha Swirl w/ Skim Milk	1 (16 oz)	180	1	37	35
Iced Latte w/ Skim Milk	1 (16 oz)	70	0	11	10

FOOD	PORTION	CALS	FAT	CARB	SUGAR
Iced Latte w/ Skim Milk Sugar	1 (16 oz)	120	0	23	22
Iced Latte w/ Sugar	1 (16 oz)	170	7	23	21
Latte	1 (10 oz)	120	6	10	9
Latte Caramel Creme	1 (10 oz)	260	9	40	40
Latte Caramel Swirl	1 (10 oz)	230	6	36	35
Latte Caramel Swirl w/ Soy Milk	1 (10 oz)	210	4	34	32
Latte Lite	1 (10 oz)	70	0	11	9
Latte Mocha Almond	1 (10 oz)	290	10	46	45
Latte Mocha Swirl	1 (10 oz)	230	7	37	35
Latte Mocha Swirl w/ Soy Milk	1 (10 oz)	210	5	35	32
Latte w/ Soy Milk	1 (10 oz)	90	4	8	6
Latte w/ Soy Milk Sugar	1 (10 oz)	150	4	22	20
Latte w/ Sugar	1 (10 oz)	160	6	22	21
Tea Regular or Decaffeinated	1 (10 oz)	0	0	1	0
Tea w/ Milk	1 (10 oz)	25	1	2	2
Tea w/ Milk Sugar	1 (10 oz)	70	1	14	13
Tea w/ Skim Milk	1 (10 oz)	25	0	4	1
Tea w/ Skim Milk Sugar	1 (10 oz)	60	0	14	13
Tea w/ Sugar	1 (10 oz)	50	0	13	12
Turbo Ice	1 (16 oz)	120	7	14	13
Vanilla Chai	1 (10 oz)	230	8	40	32
SANDWICHES					
Bagel Bacon Egg Cheese	1	540	18	69	11
Bagel Egg Cheese	1	470	15	65	10
Bagel Ham Egg Cheese	1	510	16	65	10
Bagel Sausage Egg Cheese	1	660	35	63	8
Biscuit Egg Cheese	1	410	25	32	9
Biscuit Sausage Egg Cheese	1	610	43	32	9

FOOD	PORTION	CALS	FAT	CARB	SUGAR
Croissant Bacon Egg Cheese	1	520	33	40	9
Croissant Egg Cheese	1	550	34	41	9
Croissant Ham Egg Cheese	1	520	32	40	9
Croissant Sausage Egg Cheese	1	490	51	40	8
English Muffin Bacon Egg Cheese	1	360	16	36	8
English Muffin Egg Cheese	1	280	9	34	3
English Muffin Ham Egg Cheese	1	310	10	34	3
English Muffin Sausage Egg Cheese	1	530	32	37	8
Panini Meatball	1	480	19	56	6
Panini Southwestern Chicken	1	420	10	57	4
Panini Steak	1	450	12	56	4

EINSTEIN BROS BAGELS
BAGELS AND BREADS

FOOD	PORTION	CALS	FAT	CARB	SUGAR
Bagel Asiago Cheese	1	360	3	71	4
Bagel Cranberry Special	1	350	1	78	13
Bagel Egg	1	340	3	69	5
Bagel Honey Whole Wheat	1	320	1	71	11
Bagel Jalapeno	1	330	1	71	4
Bagel Lucky Green	1	320	1	71	4
Bagel Mango	1	360	1	80	14
Bagel Marble Rye	1	340	2	73	3
Bagel Potato	1	350	5	69	5
Bagel Power	1	410	5	81	18
Bagel Power w/ Peanut Butter	1	750	34	92	22

FOOD	PORTION	CALS	FAT	CARB	SUGAR
Bagel Pumpkin	1	330	2	72	6
Bagel Roasted Red Pepper & Pesto	1	410	7	73	5
Bagel Six Cheese	1	390	6	72	4
Bagel Spicy Nacho	1	450	9	77	5
Bagel Spinach Florentine	1	410	7	72	5
Bagel Croutons	¼ cup	25	1	4	0
Bagel Twist	1	220	4	39	3
Bread Ciabatta	1 serv	320	3	64	0
Chocolate Chip	1	370	3	76	10
Chopped Garlic	1	380	3	79	3
Chopped Onion	1	330	1	71	4
Cinnamon Raisin Swirl	1	350	1	78	14
Cinnamon Sugar	1	330	1	74	10
Dark Pumpernickel	1	320	1	68	3
Everything	1	340	2	75	5
Focaccia Cheese Pizza	1 serv	500	11	75	6
Focaccia Margherita	1 serv	400	17	76	6
Focaccia Pepperoni Pizza	1 serv	590	19	76	6
Nutty Banana	1	360	3	74	5
Plain	1	320	1	71	4
Poppy Dip'd	1	350	2	74	3
Roll Challah	1	300	5	55	7
Salt	1	330	1	73	3
Sesame Dip'd	1	380	5	75	3
Sun Dried Tomato	1	320	1	69	3
Wild Blueberry	1	350	1	77	9
DESSERTS					
Brownie Iced	1	550	24	81	56
Brownie Iced w/ Walnuts	1	600	29	82	57
Cherry Figure 8	1	400	18	51	26
Cinnamon Roll	1	810	32	118	50
Cookie Chocolate Chunk	1	640	31	87	48

FOOD	PORTION	CALS	FAT	CARB	SUGAR
Cookie Oatmeal Raisin	1	600	27	82	40
Cookie Peanut Butter	1	640	34	75	36
Muffin Banana Nut	1	640	32	81	32
Muffin Blueberry	1	540	22	80	35
Muffin Chocolate Chip	1	620	27	89	48
Pound Cake Lemon Iced	1 slice	540	25	74	50
Pound Cake Marble	1 slice	460	24	57	33
Rice Krispy Bar	1	420	8	83	29
Scone Blueberry w/ Icing	1	450	18	64	21
Scone Lemon Currant	1	430	15	69	25
Strudel Cinnamon Walnut	1 piece	550	31	63	25
Sweetie Pie	1	620	20	106	72
SALAD DRESSINGS					
Asian Sesame	2 tbsp	80	2	16	13
Caesar	2 tbsp	150	16	1	1
Chipotle Vinaigrette	2 tbsp	110	10	5	4
Horseradish Sauce	2 tbsp	170	18	1	0
Raspberry Vinaigrette	2 tbsp	160	14	8	8
Thousand Island	2 tbsp	110	9	5	4
SALADS					
Asian Chicken Salad	1 serv (14.5 oz)	550	9	88	23
Bros Bistro	1 serv (9.5 oz)	520	43	25	18
Chicken Caesar	1 serv (12.5 oz)	750	53	26	8
Chicken Chipotle Salad	1 serv	710	43	48	18
Chicken Salad On Greens	1 serv (10.5 oz)	210	9	11	6
Egg Salad	1 serv (4 oz)	200	17	5	2
Fresh Fruit Cup	1 serv (8 oz)	110	1	25	24
Mixed Greens	1 serv (3.5 oz)	228	18	13	4
Potato	½ cup	290	21	21	1
Tuna Salad On Greens	1 serv (10.5 oz)	170	5	10	6
SANDWICHES					
12 Grain Bread Deli Chicken Salad	1	440	13	55	8

FOOD	PORTION	CALS	FAT	CARB	SUGAR
12 Grain Bread Deli Egg Salad	1	490	21	57	8
12 Grain Bread Deli Ham	1	560	25	55	8
12 Grain Bread Deli Roast Beef	1	560	24	56	8
12 Grain Bread Deli Smoked Turkey	1	530	21	56	9
12 Grain Bread Deli Tuna Salad	1	440	13	56	8
12 Grain Bread Deli Turkey Pastrami	1	540	21	55	9
12 Grain Bread Ultimate Toasted Cheese w/ Tomato	1	870	50	77	7
Bagel Chicken Salad	1	500	10	78	8
Bagel Egg Bacon	1	580	19	74	6
Bagel Egg Ham	1	530	13	74	6
Bagel Egg Salad	1	560	18	79	7
Bagel Egg Sausage	1	550	14	74	6
Bagel Ham	1	450	6	74	6
Bagel Holey Cow	1	900	50	77	6
Bagel Hummus & Feta	1	540	13	89	10
Bagel New York Lox	1	660	27	79	10
Bagel Original	1	480	10	74	6
Bagel Roast Beef	1	460	4	76	6
Bagel Rueben Deli	1	660	19	83	8
Bagel Salmon & Shmear	1	650	22	82	10
Bagel Sante Fe	1	650	24	78	6
Bagel Smoked Turkey	1	420	2	75	6
Bagel Tasty Turkey	1	570	15	83	9
Bagel The Veg Out	1	490	13	77	11
Bagel Tuna Salad	1	470	6	77	7
Bagel Turkey Pastrami	1	440	2	76	7

FOOD	PORTION	CALS	FAT	CARB	SUGAR
Challah Club Mex	1	750	45	47	3
Challah Cobbie	1	630	33	45	5
Challah Deli Chicken Salad	1	480	14	62	11
Challah Deli Egg Salad	1	430	20	45	7
Challah Deli Pastrami	1	480	21	43	8
Challah Deli Roast Beef	1	500	23	44	7
Challah Deli Smoked Turkey	1	470	21	44	8
Challah Deli Tuna Salad	1	370	10	42	6
Challah Deli Turkey Ham	1	500	25	43	7
Challah EBBQ Chicken	1	380	8	52	17
Challah Roasted Chicken & Smoked Gouda	1	440	13	47	10
Chicago Bagel Dog Asiago	1	740	34	78	6
Chicago Bagel Dog Chili Cheese	1	810	38	83	9
Chicago Bagel Dog Everything	1	730	34	80	6
Chicago Bagel Dog Onion w/o Cheese	1	680	30	78	6
Country White Deli Chicken Salad	1	540	15	75	8
Country White Deli Egg Salad	1	590	23	77	8
Country White Deli Ham	1	660	27	75	8
Country White Deli Roast Beef	1	660	26	76	8
Country White Deli Smoked Turkey	1	630	23	76	9
Country White Deli Tuna Salad	1	510	11	74	7

FOOD	PORTION	CALS	FAT	CARB	SUGAR
Country White Deli Turkey Pastrami	1	640	23	75	9
Country White Ultimate Toasted Cheese w/ Tomato	1	870	51	73	7
Panini Cali Club	1	730	24	90	15
Panini Cuban Ham	1	700	31	68	2
Panini Denver Omelet Breakfast	1	740	33	70	4
Panini Italian Chicken	1	770	36	69	3
Panini Taos Turkey	1	740	25	93	15
Panini Ultimate Toasted Cheese	1	900	44	96	19
Roll Ups Albuquerque Turkey	1	790	39	81	28
Roll Ups Thai Vegetable w/ Chicken	1	670	18	99	26
Roll Ups Thai Vegetables	1	630	21	97	17
SOUPS					
Broccoli Sharp Cheddar	1 cup	230	15	13	8
Chicken & Wild Rice	1 cup	190	4	29	3
Chicken Noodle	1 cup	220	9	17	2
Clam Chowda	1 cup	160	11	11	1
Minestroni Low Fat	1 cup	180	3	32	7
Tomato Bisque	1 cup	190	10	23	9
Tortilla	1 cup	90	3	14	5
Turkey Chili	1 cup	140	5	14	4
SPREADS					
Butter	1 tbsp	100	11	0	0
Butter & Margarine Blend	1 tbsp	60	7	0	0
Cream Cheese Blueberry	1 tbsp	70	5	6	5
Cream Cheese Cappuccino	2 tbsp	70	5	4	4

FOOD	PORTION	CALS	FAT	CARB	SUGAR
Cream Cheese Garden Vegetable	2 tbsp	60	5	2	1
Cream Cheese Honey Almond Reduced Fat	2 tbsp	70	5	5	4
Cream Cheese Jalapeno Salsa	1 tbsp	60	5	3	1
Cream Cheese Maple Walnut Raisin	2 tbsp	60	5	4	3
Cream Cheese Onion & Chive	2 tbsp	70	6	3	1
Cream Cheese Plain	2 tbsp	60	7	1	1
Cream Cheese Plain Reduced Fat	2 tbsp	60	5	2	1
Cream Cheese Pumpkin	2 tbsp	100	8	6	5
Cream Cheese Smoked Salmon	2 tbsp	60	5	3	1
Cream Cheese Strawberry	2 tbsp	70	5	5	4
Cream Cheese Sun Dried Tomato & Basil	2 tbsp	60	5	2	1
Fruit Spread Apricot	1 serv	75	0	19	0
Fruit Spread Grape	1 serv (1 oz)	75	0	19	0
Fruit Spread Strawberry	1 serv (1 oz)	75	0	19	0
Honey Butter	1 tbsp	90	8	4	3
Hummus	1 serv	110	7	9	2
Mayo Ancho Lime	1 tbsp	50	5	1	0
Mustard French Dijon	1 tsp	10	0	0	0
Mustard Grain Dijon	1 tsp	5	0	0	0
Mustard Honey	1 tsp	15	0	2	0
Mustard Raspberry	2 tbsp	50	2	7	5
Mustard Yellow	1 tbsp	5	0	0	0
Peanut Butter	2 tbsp	190	15	8	3
Salsa Ancho Lime	¼ cup	20	1	3	0

FOOD	PORTION	CALS	FAT	CARB	SUGAR
EL POLLO LOCO					
DESSERTS					
Churro	1	179	11	18	0
Fosters Freeze Soft Serve	1 cup	180	5	30	26
MAIN MENU SELECTIONS					
Bowl Chicken Caesar	1 serv	535	28	46	4
Bowl Pollo	1 serv	545	10	84	1
Bowl Veggie	1 serv	570	16	91	3
Bowl Veggie w/o Cheese	1 serv	529	12	91	3
Burrito Classic Chicken	1	580	22	66	1
Burrito Twice Grilled	1 serv	835	39	60	3
Burrito BRC	1 serv	530	15	79	1
Burrito Caesar	1 serv	895	45	76	3
Burrito Chicken Lover's	1 serv	525	18	55	2
Burrito Spicy	1 serv	555	19	64	2
Burrito Ultimate Chicken	1 serv	685	23	84	2
Chicken Breast	1 piece	153	4	0	0
Chicken Leg	1 piece	86	3	0	0
Chicken Thigh	1 piece	120	7	0	0
Chicken Wing	1	83	3	0	0
Cole Slaw	1 serv	206	16	12	5
Corn Cobbette	1 serv	80	1	18	4
French Fries	1 serv	444	19	61	0
Fresh Vegetables	1 serv	70	4	6	2
Gravy	1 serv (1 oz)	107	4	15	4
Mashed Potatoes	1 serv	97	1	21	1
Nachos Chicken	1 serv	1420	91	105	6
Pinto Beans	1 serv	165	4	26	0
Popcorn Chicken	1 serv	226	12	15	0
Potato Salad	1 serv	256	14	30	6
Quesadilla Cheese	1 serv	495	25	45	2
Quesadilla Chicken	1 serv	593	29	48	2
Smokey Black Beans	1 serv	306	16	35	19

FOOD	PORTION	CALS	FAT	CARB	SUGAR
Spanish Rice	1 serv	165	1	34	0
Taco Al Carbon Chicken	1 serv	135	3	18	0
Taco Soft Chicken	1	237	12	15	1
Taquitos Chicken	2	370	17	43	2
Tortilla Chips	1 serv	426	24	48	1
Tortilla Corn	1 (4.5 inch)	40	1	8	0
Tortilla Corn	1 (6 inches)	70	1	14	0
Tortilla Flour	1 (6.5 inch)	110	4	13	0
Tortilla Flour	1 (12 inches)	325	8	51	1
Tortilla Spicy Tomato	1 (12 inches)	270	7	43	1
Tostada Salad	1 serv	700	32	76	8
SALAD DRESSINGS AND TOPPINGS					
Bleu Cheese	1 serv (1.5 oz)	230	24	2	2
Buttermilk Ranch	1 serv (1.5 oz)	220	24	2	2
Creamy Chipotle	1 (0.5 oz)	75	8	1	0
Creamy Cilantro	1 serv (0.5 oz)	80	8	0	0
Guacamole	1 serv (1 oz)	30	2	3	0
Hot Sauce Jalapeno	1 pkg (0.5 oz)	5	0	1	0
Light Italian	1 serv (1.5 oz)	20	1	2	2
Salsa Avocado	1 serv (1 oz)	20	1	1	0
Salsa House	1 serv (1 oz)	6	tr	1	1
Salsa Pico De Gallo	1 serv (1 oz)	10	tr	1	1
Salsa Spicy Chipotle	1 serv (1 oz)	7	0	1	1
Sour Cream	1 serv (1 oz)	60	5	1	1
Thousand Island	1 serv (1.5 oz)	220	21	7	7
SALADS					
Caesar	1 serv	565	45	18	5
Ceasar w/o Dressing	1 serv	250	11	16	4
Fiesta Salad	1 serv	755	58	28	6
Fiesta Salad w/o Dressing	1 serv	450	26	25	5
Garden Salad	1 serv	110	7	8	2
Macaroni & Cheese	1 serv	381	26	25	3
Tostada Salad w/o Shell	1 serv	360	14	34	3

FOOD	PORTION	CALS	FAT	CARB	SUGAR
IHOP					
Pancake Buckwheat	1 (1.7 oz)	110	4	15	—
Pancake Buttermilk	1 (1.7 oz)	110	3	17	—
Pancake Country Griddle	1 (2 oz)	120	4	19	—
Pancake Harvest Grain 'N Nut	1 (2.25 oz)	180	9	20	—
JACK IN THE BOX					
BEVERAGES					
Ice Cream Shake Caramel	1 serv (16 oz)	660	30	86	74
Ice Cream Shake Chocolate	1 serv (16 oz)	660	29	89	79
Ice Cream Shake Oreo	1 serv (16 oz)	670	33	81	62
Ice Cream Shake Strawberry	1 serv (16 oz)	640	28	84	71
Ice Cream Shake Strawberry Banana	1 serv (16 oz)	700	28	100	67
Ice Cream Shake Vanilla	1 serv (16 oz)	570	29	65	54
BREAKFAST SELECTIONS					
Breakfast Sandwich Sourdough	1	440	26	36	3
Breakfast Sandwich Ultimate	1	730	40	66	9
Breakfast Jack	1	310	14	33	4
Croissant Sausage	1	680	50	41	5
Croissant Supreme	1	570	37	41	5
French Toast Sticks	4 pieces	430	18	57	11
Hash Brown	1 serv	150	10	13	0
Sandwich Extreme Sausage	1	720	53	35	5
DESSERTS					
Cheesecake	1 serv	310	16	34	23
Double Fudge Cake	1 serv	310	11	49	37

FOOD	PORTION	CALS	FAT	CARB	SUGAR
MAIN MENU SELECTIONS					
American Cheese	1 slice	45	4	1	0
Bacon Cheddar Potato Wedges	1 serv	770	53	52	2
Cheeseburger Bacon Bacon	1	910	59	58	10
Cheeseburger Bacon Ultimate	1	1120	75	59	12
Cheeseburger Junior Bacon	1	540	36	31	6
Cheeseburger Ultimate	1	990	66	59	12
Chicken Breast Pieces	4	360	17	24	0
Chicken Breast Strips	1 serv	500	25	36	1
Chicken Fajita Pita	1	330	11	35	4
Chicken Sandwich	1	410	21	39	4
Dipping Sauce Barbeque	1 serv (1.6 oz)	45	0	11	4
Egg Rolls	1	130	6	15	1
Fish & Chips	1 serv	610	31	66	0
French Fries	1 lg	580	28	77	0
French Fries	1 med	410	20	55	0
French Fries	1 sm	330	16	44	0
Hamburger	1	310	14	30	6
Hamburger w/ Cheese	1	360	18	31	6
Jumbo Jack	1	600	31	58	12
Jumbo Jack w/ Cheese	1	690	38	61	13
Onion Rings	1 serv	500	30	51	3
Philly Cheesesteak	1	580	22	55	6
Salsa	1 serv (1 oz)	10	0	2	1
Sandwich Roasted Turkey	1	580	25	50	5
Sandwich Ultimate Club	1	640	30	51	7
Seasoned Curly Fries	1 serv	400	23	45	1
Sour Cream	1 serv (1 oz)	60	5	2	0

FOOD	PORTION	CALS	FAT	CARB	SUGAR
Sourdough Grilled Chicken Club	1	520	28	33	5
Sourdough Jack	1	700	49	36	7
Spicy Crispy Chicken	1	730	37	69	9
Stuffed Jalapeno	3 pieces	230	13	22	2
Swiss Style Cheese	1 slice	40	3	1	0
Taco	1	170	9	15	2
Taco Monster	1	260	15	21	4
Turkey Jack	1	700	32	69	18
SALAD DRESSINGS AND TOPPINGS					
Almonds Roasted Slivered	1 serv (0.7 oz)	130	11	4	1
Asian Sesame	1 serv (2.5 oz)	230	17	20	13
Bacon Ranch	1 serv (2.5 oz)	320	33	5	2
Balsamic Vinaigrette Low Fat	1 serv (2.5 oz)	40	2	6	3
Country Crock Spread	1 pkg	25	3	0	0
Creamy Southwest Dressing	1 serv (2.5 oz)	270	26	7	2
Croutons	1 serv (0.5 oz)	60	2	10	1
Dipping Sauce Buttermilk House	1 serv (0.9 oz)	130	13	3	0
Dipping Sauce Frank's Red Hot Buffalo	1 serv (1 oz)	10	0	2	0
Dipping Sauce Sweet & Sour	1 serv (1 oz)	45	0	11	6
Grape Jelly	1 serv (0.5 oz)	35	0	9	9
Herb Mayo Sauce Low Fat	1 serv (1.5 oz)	45	4	3	1
Ketchup	1 pkg (0.3 oz)	10	0	2	2
Marinara Sauce	1 serv (0.9 oz)	15	0	3	3
Mustard	1 pkg	0	0	0	0
Ranch	1 serv (2.5 oz)	390	41	4	2
Ranch Lite	1 serv (2.5 oz)	190	18	3	2
Soy Sauce	1 serv (0.3 oz)	5	0	1	0

FOOD	PORTION	CALS	FAT	CARB	SUGAR
Syrup	1 serv (1.5 oz)	130	0	32	27
Taco Sauce	1 serv (0.3 oz)	0	0	0	0
Tartar Sauce	1 serv (1.5 oz)	210	22	2	1
Thousand Island	1 serv (2 oz)	160	12	12	10
Vinegar	1 serv	0	0	0	0
Wonton Strips	1 serv (0.7 oz)	110	6	13	1
SALADS					
Asian Salad	1 serv	140	2	18	11
Chicken Club Salad	1 serv	290	16	12	5
Side Salad	1 serv	50	3	4	2
Southwest Chicken	1 serv	320	13	28	6

JERSEY MIKE'S

FOOD	PORTION	CALS	FAT	CARB	SUGAR
Ham On Wheat	1	240	4	31	—
Ham On White	1	240	5	31	—
Ham/Turkey Wheat	1	230	3	32	—
Ham/Turkey White	1	240	4	32	—
Roast Beef Wheat	1	290	5	30	—
Roast Beef White	1	280	5	30	—
Turkey On Wheat	1	230	2	30	—
Turkey On White	1	230	3	18	—
Veggie On Wheat	1	170	2	32	—
Veggie On White	1	170	2	31	—

KENTUCKY FRIED CHICKEN
DESSERTS

FOOD	PORTION	CALS	FAT	CARB	SUGAR
Cake Double Chocolate Chip	1 slice	400	29	31	27
Cherry Cheesecake Parfait	1 serv	300	11	46	37
Lil' Bucket Chocolate Creme	1 serv	270	13	37	28
Lil' Bucket Fudge Brownie	1	270	9	44	39
Lil' Bucket Lemon Creme	1 serv	400	14	65	51

FOOD	PORTION	CALS	FAT	CARB	SUGAR
Lil' Bucket Strawberry Shortcake	1 serv	200	6	34	34
Pie Apple	1 slice	270	9	45	22
Pie Lemon Meringue	1 slice	310	11	47	36
Pie Pecan	1 slice	370	15	55	20
Pie Strawberry Creme	1 slice	270	12	37	23
MAIN MENU SELECTIONS					
BBQ Beans	1 serv	230	1	46	22
Biscuit	1	190	10	23	1
Boneless Wings HBBQ Sauced	7 pieces	600	28	40	7
Chicken Pot Pie	1 serv	770	40	70	2
Cole Slaw	1 serv	190	11	22	13
Corn On The Cob	1 ear (3 inch)	70	2	13	5
Crispy Strips	3	400	24	17	0
Extra Crispy Breast	1 serv	490	28	19	0
Extra Crispy Drumstick	1	160	10	5	0
Extra Crispy Thigh	1	370	26	12	0
Extra Crispy Whole Wing	1	190	12	10	0
Green Beans	1 serv	50	2	5	2
Hot & Spicy Breast	1 serv	460	27	20	0
Hot & Spicy Drumstick	1	150	9	4	0
Hot & Spicy Thigh	1	400	28	14	0
Hot & Spicy Whole Wing	1	180	11	9	0
Hot Wings	6 pieces	450	29	23	1
Mac & Cheese	1 serv	130	8	15	1
Mashed Potatoes w/o Gravy	1 serv	110	4	16	0
Mashed Potatoes w/ Gravy	1 serv	120	5	18	tr
Original Recipe Breast	1 serv	380	19	11	0
Original Recipe Breast w/o Skin or Breading	1 serv	140	3	0	0

FOOD	PORTION	CALS	FAT	CARB	SUGAR
Original Recipe Drumstick	1	140	8	4	0
Original Recipe Thigh	1	360	25	12	0
Original Recipe Whole Wing	1	150	9	5	0
Popcorn Chicken	1 reg serv	450	30	25	0
Potato Salad	1 serv	180	9	22	5
Potato Wedges	1 sm	240	12	30	0
Sandwich HBBQ	1	300	8	41	16
Sandwich Original Recipe w/ Sauce	1	450	27	22	0
Sandwich Tender Roast w/ Sauce	1	390	19	24	0
Sandwich Tender Roast w/o Sauce	1	260	5	23	0
Sandwich Twister	1	670	38	55	7
Sandwich Zinger w/ Sauce	1	680	41	42	3
Sandwich Zinger w/o Sauce	1	540	26	41	2
Sandwiches Original Recipe w/o Sauce	1	320	13	21	0
Wings HBBQ Sauced	6 pieces	540	33	36	15

KOO-KOO-ROO

FOOD	PORTION	CALS	FAT	CARB	SUGAR
Original Breast	1 piece	187	6	tr	—
Original Chicken Dark	3 pieces	320	16	5	—
Rotisserie Chicken Breast & Wing	1 serv	355	16	1	—
Rotisserie Chicken Leg & Thigh	1 serv	300	18	1	—
Rotisserie Half Chicken	1 serv	655	34	2	—
Sandwich BBQ Chicken	1	562	12	71	—
Sandwich Chicken Caesar	1	781	36	63	—

FOOD	PORTION	CALS	FAT	CARB	SUGAR
Sandwich Original Chicken	1	661	29	63	−
Traditional Turkey Dinner	1 serv	692	29	67	−
Turkey Pot Pie	1 serv	883	44	83	−
Turkey Sandwich Hand Carved	1	599	32	31	−
Wrap Caesar Chicken	1	757	39	59	−
Wrap Chipotle Chicken	1	924	43	89	−

KRISPY KREME

FOOD	PORTION	CALS	FAT	CARB	SUGAR
Apple Fritter	1	380	21	46	23
Caramel Kreme Crunch	1	350	19	43	25
Chocolate Iced Glazed w/ Sprinkles	1	260	12	38	24
Chocolate Malted Kreme	1	390	21	49	30
Chocolate Iced	1	250	12	33	21
Chocolate Iced Cake	1	270	14	36	20
Chocolate Iced Creme Filled	1	350	21	39	23
Chocolate Iced Cruller	1	290	15	37	25
Chocolate Iced Custard Filled	1	300	17	35	17
Chocolated Iced w/ Sprinkles	1	290	14	40	23
Cinnamon Apple Filled	1	290	16	32	14
Cinnamon Bun	1	260	16	28	13
Cinnamon Sugar Cake	1	280	14	37	18
Cinnamon Twist	1	230	9	33	19
Coffee & Kreme	1	360	20	43	27
Dulce De Leche	1	290	18	30	12
Glazed Blueberry	1	340	18	42	27
Glazed Blueberry Filled	1	290	16	35	18
Glazed Cinnamon	1	210	12	24	12
Glazed Creme Filled	1	340	20	39	23

FOOD	PORTION	CALS	FAT	CARB	SUGAR
Glazed Cruller	1	240	14	26	14
Glazed Custard Filled	1	290	16	34	17
Glazed Devil's Food	1	340	18	42	27
Glazed Lemon Filled	1	290	16	34	18
Glazed Raspberry Filled	1	300	16	39	21
Glazed Sour Cream	1	340	18	42	27
Glazed Strawberry Filled	1	290	16	35	17
Glazed Twist	1	210	9	28	16
Honey & Oat	1	340	18	42	27
Key Lime Pie	1	330	18	40	23
Maple Iced	1	240	12	32	20
Maple Iced Cake	1	270	13	35	19
New York Cheesecake	1	330	19	36	17
Original Glazed	1	200	12	22	10
Powdered Blueberry Filled	1	290	16	32	14
Powdered Strawberry Filled	1	260	16	26	9
Powdered Cake	1	280	14	37	19
Powdered Creme Filled	1	340	21	36	19
Powdered Raspberry	1	300	16	36	17
Pumpkin Spice Cake	1	340	18	42	27
Sugar Coated	1	200	12	21	10
Traditional Cake	1	230	13	25	9
Vanilla Iced Cake w/ Sprinkles	1	270	13	35	19
Vanilla Iced Creme Filled	1	340	20	38	23
Vanilla Iced Custard Filled	1	290	16	33	16
Vanilla Iced Glazed	1	240	12	32	20
Vanilla Iced Raspberry Filled	1	350	16	50	31
Vanilla Iced Raspberry Glazed	1	350	16	50	31

FOOD	PORTION	CALS	FAT	CARB	SUGAR
KRYSTAL					
BREAKFAST SELECTIONS					
Biscuit	1	270	13	33	2
Biscuit And Gravy	1	280	14	34	2
Biscuit Bacon Egg & Cheese	1	390	23	33	2
Biscuit Chik	1	360	15	40	2
Biscuit Sausage	1	480	33	33	2
Country Breakfast	1 serv	660	42	46	3
Kryspers	1 serv	190	13	17	0
Krystal Sunriser	1	240	14	14	1
Scrambler	1 serv	440	26	33	tr
DESSERTS					
Fried Apple Turnover	1	220	10	31	7
Lemon Icebox Pie	1 serv	260	9	41	37
MAIN MENU SELECTIONS					
Chik'n Bites	1 sm	310	19	16	0
Chik'n Bites Salad	1 serv	290	20	12	1
Fries	1 med	470	20	53	0
Fries Chili Cheese	1 serv	540	28	59	1
Krystal	1	160	7	17	1
Krystal Bacon Cheese	1	190	10	16	2
Krystal Cheese	1	180	9	17	1
Krystal Chik	1	240	11	24	1
Krystal Chili	1 serv	200	7	22	2
Krystal Double	1	260	13	24	2
Krystal Double Cheese	1	310	16	26	2
Pup	1	170	9	15	—
Pup Chili Cheese	1	210	12	17	2
Pup Corn	1	260	19	19	5
LITTLE CAESARS					
MAIN MENU SELECTIONS					
Baby Pan! Pan!	1 piece	360	16	34	3

FOOD	PORTION	CALS	FAT	CARB	SUGAR
Crazy Bread	1 piece	90	3	15	tr
Crazy Bread Cinnamon	2 pieces	100	2	19	5
Crazy Sauce	1 serv (4 oz)	45	0	9	5
Deli Sandwich Ham & Cheese	1	640	29	66	5
Deli Sandwich Italian	1	800	45	66	6
Deli Sandwich Veggie	1	600	28	67	5
Italian Cheese Bread	1 piece	130	6	13	tr
PIZZA					
14 Inch Round Meatsa	1/10 pie	280	13	26	2
14 Inch Round Supreme	1/10 pie	270	10	31	4
14 Inch Round Veggie	1/10 pie	240	8	32	5
14 Inch Thin Crust Cheese	1/10 pie	160	7	14	1
16 Inch Round Cheese	1/12 pie	220	7	27	2
18 Inch Round Cheese	1/14 pie	230	7	30	2
Deep Dish Large	1/8 pie	320	12	37	3
Deep Dish Medium	1/8 pie	230	9	27	2
SALAD DRESSINGS					
Caesar	1 serv (1.5 oz)	230	25	1	0
Greek	1 serv (1.5 oz)	270	29	0	0
Italian	1 serv (1.5 oz)	220	23	2	2
Italian Fat Free	1 serv (1.5 oz)	25	0	5	3
Ranch	1 serv (1.5 oz)	230	24	2	1
SALADS					
Antipasto	1 serv	140	8	6	4
Caesar	1 serv	90	3	12	2
Greek	1 serv	128	7	11	8
Tossed Salad	1 serv	100	3	15	4
TOPPINGS PER SLICE					
Bacon	1 serv	41	4	tr	tr
Beef	1 serv	20	2	tr	tr
Black Olives	1 serv	12	2	tr	—
Extra Cheese	1 serv	26	2	tr	tr

FOOD	PORTION	CALS	FAT	CARB	SUGAR
Green Peppers	1 serv	2	tr	tr	tr
Ham	1 serv	5	tr	tr	tr
Italian Sausage	1 serv	22	2	tr	tr
Mushrooms	1 serv	2	tr	tr	tr
Onion	1 serv	3	tr	1	tr
Pepperoni	1 serv	26	2	tr	—
Pineapple	1 serv	7	—	2	2
Tomato	1 serv	2	tr	tr	tr

LONG JOHN SILVER'S
DESSERTS

FOOD	PORTION	CALS	FAT	CARB	SUGAR
Pie Chocolate Cream	1 pie	310	44	24	19
Pie Pecan	1 pie	370	15	55	20
Pie Pineapple Cream	1 pie	290	13	39	26

MAIN MENU SELECTIONS

FOOD	PORTION	CALS	FAT	CARB	SUGAR
Baked Cod	1 piece	120	5	0	0
Battered Chicken	1 piece	140	8	9	0
Battered Fish	1 piece	230	13	16	0
Battered Shrimp	1 piece	45	3	3	0
Breaded Clams	1 serv	240	13	22	5
Cheesesticks	3 pieces	140	8	12	0
Clam Chowder	1 bowl	220	10	23	8
Corn Cobbette	1 piece	90	3	14	6
Crumblies	1 serv	170	12	14	0
Crunchy Shrimp	21 pieces	330	18	31	1
Fries	1 reg	230	10	34	0
Hushpuppy	1 piece	60	3	9	1
Rice	1 serv	180	4	34	1
Sandwich Chicken	1	360	15	41	4
Sandwich Fish	1	440	20	48	2
Sandwich Ultimate Fish	1	500	28	48	4
Slaw	1 serv	200	15	15	10

FOOD	PORTION	CALS	FAT	CARB	SUGAR
MAGGIE MOO'S					
Ice Cream Fat Free	½ cup	80	0	18	13
Ice Cream Low Carb Sugar Added	½ cup	100	6	11	4
Ice Cream Udderly Cream	½ cup	180	11	18	16
Sorbet	½ cup	90	0	22	20
MANHATTAN BAGEL					
Blueberry	1	260	tr	54	4
Cheddar Cheese	1	270	4	48	3
Chocolate Chip	1	290	3	56	3
Cinnamon Raisin	1	280	tr	57	9
Cranberry Orange	1	270	1	55	5
Egg	1	270	2	53	3
Everything	1	290	3	54	3
Garlic	1	270	tr	55	3
Jalapeno Cheddar	1	260	2	53	2
Marble	1	260	tr	52	3
Oat Bran	1	260	1	53	3
Oat Bran Raisin Walnut	1	270	3	54	5
Onion	1	270	tr	55	3
Plain	1	260	tr	52	3
Poppy	1	300	4	54	3
Pumpernickel	1	250	1	52	3
Rye	1	260	1	52	3
Salt	1	260	tr	53	3
Sesame	1	310	5	55	3
Spinach	1	270	tr	54	3
Sun-Dried Tomato	1	260	1	53	3
Whole Wheat	1	260	tr	52	3
MARBLE SLAB CREAMERY					
Cone Honey Wheat	1	130	3	24	12
Cone Sugar	1	130	3	23	12

FOOD	PORTION	CALS	FAT	CARB	SUGAR
Cone Vanilla Cinnamon	1	130	3	24	12
Frozen Yogurt Nonfat	½ cup	100	1	22	17
Frozen Yogurt Nonfat No Sugar Added	½ cup	90	1	17	6
Ice Cream Reduced Fat	1 serv (6.75 oz)	390	20	47	45
Ice Cream Superpremium	1 serv (6.75 oz)	450	28	44	43
Sorbet	½ cup	90	0	22	19

MAUI WOWI

Smoothie Rip Sticks All Flavors	1	88	0	22	17

MCDONALD'S
BAKED SELECTIONS

Cinnamon Roll Warm	1	420	18	57	26

BEVERAGES

Triple Shake Chocolate	1 (16 oz)	580	14	102	84
Triple Shake Strawberry	1 (16 oz)	560	13	97	84
Triple Shake Vanilla	1 (16 oz)	550	13	96	72

BREAKFAST SELECTIONS

Big Breakfast	1 serv	730	46	53	2
Biscuit	1	240	11	31	2
Biscuit Bacon Egg Cheese	1	440	24	36	3
Biscuit Sausage	1	410	26	34	2
Biscuit Sausage w/ Egg	1	500	32	36	2
Deluxe Breakfast	1 serv	1220	60	136	43
English Muffin Buttered	1	150	2	27	2
Hash Browns	1 serv	140	8	15	0
Hotcakes Margarine & Syrup	1 serv	600	17	102	45
Hotcakes & Sausage	1 serv	770	33	104	45
Hotcakes Plain	1 serv	340	8	57	12
McGriddles Sausage	1	420	22	44	15

FOOD	PORTION	CALS	FAT	CARB	SUGAR
McGriddles Sausage Egg Cheese	1	560	32	48	16
McMuffin Egg	1	290	11	30	3
McMuffin Sausage	1	370	21	31	2
McMuffin Egg	1	450	26	31	3
Sausage	1 patty	170	15	2	0
Sausage Burrito	1	300	16	26	3
Scrambled Eggs	2	180	11	5	0
DESSERTS					
Apple Dippers	1 pkg	35	0	8	6
Apple Pie Baked	1	250	11	34	13
Caramel Dip Low Fat	1 pkg	70	1	15	9
Cinnamon Roll Deluxe Warm	1	590	24	36	86
Cookie Chocolate Chip	1 pkg	270	11	39	19
Cookie Chocolate Chip	1 (1.1 oz)	160	7	22	14
Cookie Oatmeal	1 (1.1 oz)	140	5	22	12
Cookie Sugar	1 (1.1 oz)	150	6	22	11
Fruit 'n Yogurt Parfait	1 serv	160	2	31	21
Ice Cream Cone Reduced Fat Vanilla	1	150	5	24	18
McDonaldland Cookies	1 pkg	250	8	42	14
McFlurry M&M	1 (12 oz)	620	20	96	85
McFlurry Oreo	1 (12 oz)	560	16	88	71
Peanuts For Sundae	1 serv	4540	4	2	0
Sundae Hot Caramel	1	340	7	62	43
Sundae Hot Fudge	1	340	9	55	48
Sundae Strawberry	1	280	6	51	45
MAIN MENU SELECTIONS					
Big Mac	1	560	30	47	8
Big N' Tasty	1	470	23	41	9
Big N' Tasty w/ Cheese	1	520	26	43	9
Cheeseburger	1	310	12	35	7

FOOD	PORTION	CALS	FAT	CARB	SUGAR
Cheeseburger Double	1	460	23	37	8
Chicken McNuggets	4 pieces	170	10	10	0
Chicken Selects	3 pieces	380	20	28	0
Crispy Chicken Classic	1	500	16	63	11
Crispy Chicken Club	1	680	29	64	11
Crispy Chicken Ranch BLT	1	580	20	64	12
Filet-O-Fish	1	400	18	42	8
French Fries	1 sm (2.6 oz)	230	11	30	0
Grilled Chicken Classic	1	420	9	52	11
Grilled Chicken Club	1	590	22	54	12
Grilled Chicken Ranch BLT	1	490	13	54	13
Hamburger	1	260	9	33	7
McChicken	1	370	16	41	5
McChicken Hot 'n Spicy	1	380	17	42	5
Quarter Pounder	1	420	18	40	8
Quarter Pounder Double w/ Cheese	1	730	40	46	9
Quarter Pounder w/ Cheese	1	510	25	43	9
SALAD DRESSINGS AND SAUCES					
Honey	1 pkg (0.5 oz)	50	0	12	11
Newman's Own Cobb	1 pkg (2 oz)	120	9	9	5
Newman's Own Creamy Caesar	1 pkg (2 oz)	190	18	4	2
Newman's Own Low Fat Balsamic Vinaigrette	1 pkg (1.5 oz)	40	3	4	3
Newman's Own Low Fat Family Recipe Italian	1 pkg (1.6 oz)	50	3	7	2
Newman's Own Ranch	1 pkg (2 oz)	170	15	9	4
Sauce Barbecue	1 pkg (1 oz)	45	0	11	10
Sauce Chipotle Barbecue	1 pkg	70	0	16	14
Sauce Creamy Ranch	1 pkg (1.5 oz)	200	21	3	1
Sauce Hot Mustard	1 pkg (1 oz)	50	2	9	6

FOOD	PORTION	CALS	FAT	CARB	SUGAR
Sauce Spicy Buffalo	1 pkg (1.5 oz)	60	6	1	0
Sauce Sweet 'N Sour	1 pkg (1 oz)	50	0	11	10
Sauce Tangy Honey Mustard	1 pkg (1.5 oz)	70	2	13	9
SALADS					
Bacon Ranch w/ Crispy Chicken	1 serv	340	16	23	4
Bacon Ranch w/ Grilled Chicken	1 serv	260	9	12	3
Bacon Ranch w/o Chicken	1 serv	140	7	10	4
Caesar w/ Crispy Chicken	1 serv	300	13	22	4
Caesar w/ Grilled Chicken	1 serv	220	6	12	5
Caesar w/o Chicken	1 serv	90	4	9	4
California Cobb w/ Crispy Chicken	1 serv	360	18	22	5
California Cobb w/ Grilled Chicken	1 serv	280	11	12	4
California Cobb w/o Chicken	1 serv	160	9	9	5
Croutons Butter Garlic	1 pkg	60	1	10	1
Fruit & Walnut	1 serv	310	13	44	32
Side Salad	1 serv	20	0	4	2
MIAMI SUBS					
Burger Deluxe	1	784	59	31	3
Cheeseburger Deluxe	1	859	65	32	3
Cheeseburger Deluxe Bacon	1	919	70	32	3
Cheesesteak Classic	1 (6 inch)	420	11	48	5
Cheesesteak Original	1 (6 inch)	409	11	45	5
Cheesesteak Works	1 (6 inch)	532	23	51	7
Chicken Philly Classic	1 (6 inch)	551	27	47	4
Mozzarella Sticks	1 serv	757	57	34	9
Onion Rings	1 serv	869	68	56	7

FOOD	PORTION	CALS	FAT	CARB	SUGAR
Pita Chicken	1	392	13	34	6
Pita Gyros	1	662	39	47	6
Platter Chicken Breast	1 serv	743	41	57	3
Platter Gyros	1 serv	1420	93	81	3
Salad Caesar w/ Dressing	1 serv	459	34	26	4
Salad Chicken Caesar w/ Dressing	1 serv	609	39	28	4
Salad Chicken Club	1 serv	490	25	23	6
Salad Garden	1 serv	310	18	21	6
Salad Greek	1 serv	284	15	24	6
Salad Greek Side w/ Dressing	1 serv	78	5	4	2
Spicy Fries	1 reg	532	39	39	0
Subs 6 Inch Ham And Cheese	1	452	18	49	6
Subs 6 Inch Italian Deli	1	516	25	49	6
Subs 6 Inch Meatball	1	491	22	49	4
Subs 6 Inch Tuna	1	468	18	44	3
Subs 6 Inch Turkey	1	484	18	51	6
Wings w/ Fries Celery & Blue Cheese	1 serv	1020	67	50	1

MR. PITA

FOOD	PORTION	CALS	FAT	CARB	SUGAR
Cranberry Turkey	1 reg	424	1	77	17
Grilled Raspberry Chicken	1 reg	342	3	56	5
Grilled Chicken & Broccoli	1 reg	373	4	57	4
Grilled Chicken Caesar	1 reg	353	4	50	3
Grilled Hawaiian Chicken	1 reg	375	4	57	5
Ultra Combo	1 reg	354	3	56	4
Ultra Grilled Chicken	1 reg	367	4	56	5
Ultra Supreme	1 reg	350	3	56	5
Ultra Turkey	1 reg	343	1	56	4

FOOD	PORTION	CALS	FAT	CARB	SUGAR
MRS. FIELDS					
Brownie Double Fudge	1 (2.7 oz)	360	19	59	49
Brownie Frosted Fudge	1 (3.7 oz)	440	21	62	41
Brownie Pecan Fudge	1 (2.7 oz)	340	21	40	30
Brownie Pecan Pie	1 (2.7 oz)	340	20	40	30
Brownie Walnut Fudge	1 (2.7 oz)	380	23	45	23
Bundt Cake Banana Walnut	1 piece (2.9 oz)	350	21	35	18
Bundt Cake Banana Walnut w/ Chocolate Chips	1 piece (2.9 oz)	370	22	39	25
Bundt Cake Blueberry	1 piece (2.9 oz)	270	12	36	19
Bundt Cake Raspberry	1 piece (2.9 oz)	270	12	36	19
Bundt Cake White w/ Chocolate Chips	1 piece (2.9 oz)	350	17	45	27
Cookie Butter Toffee	1 (2.3 oz)	290	13	40	24
Cookie Cinnamon Sugar	1 (2.3 oz)	300	12	41	23
Cookie Coconut Macadamia	1 (2.3 oz)	280	13	39	23
Cookie Debra's Special	1 (2.3 oz)	280	12	39	25
Cookie Milk Chocolate	1 (2.3 oz)	280	13	38	18
Cookie Milk Chocolate & Walnuts	1 (2.3 oz)	320	17	37	26
Cookie Milk Chocolate Macadamia	1 (2.3 oz)	320	18	36	25
Cookie Oatmeal Chocolate Chip	1 (2.3 oz)	280	13	40	17
Cookie Oatmeal Raisin & Walnuts	1 (2.3 oz)	280	12	39	25
Cookie Peanut Butter	1 (2.3 oz)	310	16	34	18
Cookie Peanut Butter w/ Milk Chocolate Chips	1 (2.3 oz)	300	17	35	16

FOOD	PORTION	CALS	FAT	CARB	SUGAR
Cookie Semi-Sweet Chocolate	1 (2.3 oz)	280	14	40	26
Cookie Semi-Sweet Chocolate & Walnuts	1 (2.3 oz)	310	16	38	25
Cookie White Chunk Macadamia	1 (2.3 oz)	310	17	37	25
Jumbo Cookie Snickerdoodle	1 (5 oz)	640	29	90	49
Nibbler Cookies	2 (0.9 oz)	110	5	15	9
Nibbler Cookies Chewy Chocolate Fudge	2 (0.9 oz)	110	5	15	10
Nibbler Cookies Cinnamon Sugar	2 (0.9 oz)	120	5	17	11
Nibbler Cookies Debra's Special	2 (0.9 oz)	100	5	13	8
Nibbler Cookies M&M	2 (0.9 oz)	110	5	16	10
Nibbler Cookies Milk Chocolate	2 (0.9 oz)	110	5	15	10
Nibbler Cookies Milk Chocolate w/ Walnuts	2 (0.9 oz)	120	6	14	9
Nibbler Cookies Peanut Butter	2 (0.9 oz)	110	6	13	7
Nibbler Cookies Semi-Sweet Chocolate	2 (0.9 oz)	110	5	15	10
Nibbler Cookies Triple Chocolate	2 (0.9 oz)	110	6	15	11
Nibbler Cookies White Chunk Macadamia	2 (0.9 oz)	120	7	13	5

MY FAVORITE MUFFIN
BAGELS

FOOD	PORTION	CALS	FAT	CARB	SUGAR
Blueberry	1	320	2	66	8
Cinnamon Raisin	1	310	1	66	13
Honey Grain	1	310	3	61	5

FOOD	PORTION	CALS	FAT	CARB	SUGAR
Plain	1	310	1	64	9
Russian Black Bread	1	320	1	67	8
Sour Dough	1	310	1	64	9
Whole Wheat	1	310	2	66	7
MUFFINS					
Banana Nut	⅓ jumbo	195	11	21	12
Blueberry	⅓ jumbo	168	8	22	12
Blueberry Cheesecake	⅓ jumbo	199	12	20	9
Boston Cream Pie	⅓ jumbo	176	7	26	17
Cheery Cheesecake	⅓ jumbo	170	10	19	10
Chocolate Cheesecake	⅓ jumbo	202	12	22	11
Chocolate Chip	⅓ jumbo	211	11	27	16
Cinnamon Crumb Cake	⅓ jumbo	212	13	21	11
Cinnamon Swirl Cheesecake	⅓ jumbo	214	11	28	15
Deep Dish Apple Pie	⅓ jumbo	177	8	25	14
Double Chocolate	⅓ jumbo	201	9	28	17
Fat Free Blueberry	⅓ jumbo	108	0	26	12
Fat Free Cherry Pie	⅓ jumbo	109	0	26	14
Fat Free Chocolate Eclair	⅓ jumbo	120	0	28	17
Fat Free Chocolate Marble	⅓ jumbo	125	0	29	15
Fat Free Cinnamon Bun	⅓ jumbo	168	0	42	11
Fat Free Raspberry Amaretto	⅓ jumbo	127	0	31	18
Golden Corn Bread	⅓ jumbo	197	9	26	12
Lemon Poppyseed	⅓ jumbo	201	10	25	14
Pumpkin Spice	⅓ jumbo	181	8	26	10
NATHAN'S					
¼ Pound Burger	1	537	30	42	11
¼ Pound Burger w/ Cheese	1	850	61	45	11
Bacon Cheeseburger	1	707	44	43	11
Cheesesteak Chicken	1 serv	565	19	62	11

FOOD	PORTION	CALS	FAT	CARB	SUGAR
Cheesesteak Original	1	741	43	50	7
Cheesesteak Supreme	1 serv	786	43	61	11
Chicken Tender Pita	1	610	38	45	8
Chicken Tenders	3 pieces	512	37	24	8
Cole Slaw	1 serv	213	9	34	30
Corn Muffin	1	163	6	25	10
Famous Hot Dog	1	309	20	23	0
Fish N Chips	1 serv	1538	101	132	39
French Fries	1 reg	547	38	46	0
Hot Dog Nuggets	6 pieces	351	28	20	5
Hush Puppy	2 pieces	277	10	42	7
Onion Rings	1 sm	559	44	36	5
Platter Chicken Breast	1 serv	943	54	89	32
Platter Chicken Tender	1 serv	1301	83	109	32
Sandwich Chicken Tender	1	725	47	56	9
Sandwich Fish	1	469	20	42	14
Sandwich Grilled Chicken	1	524	29	42	9
Seafood Sampler	1 serv	3379	270	227	49
Shrimp N Chips	1 serv	2051	124	225	51
Super Burger	1	864	62	42	13

OLD SPAGHETTI FACTORY
CHILDREN'S MENU SELECTIONS

Grilled Cheese Sandwich	1 serv	360	22	28	–
Macaroni & Cheese	1 serv	350	9	57	–
Spaghetti w/ Tomato Sauce	1 serv	300	4	56	–
Spaghetti w/ Tomato Sauce & Meatballs	1 serv	440	13	59	–

DESSERTS

Caramel Turtle Pie	1 serv	660	29	93	–
Mud Pie	1 serv	680	32	90	–
New York Cheese Cake w/ Strawberry Topping	1 serv	690	40	72	–

FOOD	PORTION	CALS	FAT	CARB	SUGAR
MAIN MENU SELECTIONS					
Baked Chicken	1 dinner serv	880	47	55	—
Caesar Salad	1 sm	330	30	8	—
Caesar Salad Dinner Chicken	1 serv	1280	85	42	—
Chicken Marsala	1 dinner serv	960	44	55	—
Fettuccine Alfredo	1 dinner serv	1130	83	71	—
Fettuccine Chicken	1 dinner serv	960	56	74	—
Lasagne	1 dinner serv	630	33	36	—
Parmigiana Chicken	1 dinner serv	840	34	84	—
Parmigiana Eggplant	1 dinner serv	670	32	75	—
Pot Pourri	1 dinner serv	710	30	84	—
Ravioli Spinach & Cheese	1 dinner serv	480	15	59	—
Salmon Tuscany	1 dinner serv	680	43	21	—
Sandwich Meatball	1	860	41	74	—
Sandwich Sausage	1	730	40	53	—
Sandwich Tuscan Chicken	1	1060	60	53	—
Seafood Cheddar Melt	1 serv	790	42	65	—
Spaghetti w/ Clam Sauce	1 dinner serv	690	28	84	—
Spaghetti w/ Clam Sauce & Mizithra	1 dinner serv	960	54	81	—
Spaghetti w/ Meat & Clam Sauces	1 dinner serv	980	17	84	—
Spaghetti w/ Meat Sauce	1 dinner serv	470	5	83	—
Spaghetti w/ Meat Sauce & Mizithra	1 dinner serv	850	42	80	—
Spaghetti w/ Meat Sauce & Sausage	1 dinner serv	830	35	85	—
Spaghetti w/ Meatballs	1 dinner serv	840	33	86	—
Spaghetti w/ Mizithra	1 dinner serv	1010	64	74	—
Spaghetti w/ Mushroom & Clam Sauces	1 dinner serv	830	18	83	—

FOOD	PORTION	CALS	FAT	CARB	SUGAR
Spaghetti w/ Mushroom & Meat Sauces	1 dinner serv	460	6	83	—
Spaghetti w/ Mushroom Sauce	1 dinner serv	460	7	83	—
Spaghetti w/ Mushroom Sauce & Mizithra	1 dinner serv	850	43	80	—
Spaghetti w/ Tomato & Mizithra	1 dinner serv	840	42	81	—
Spaghetti w/ Tomato & Meat Sauces	1 dinner serv	460	5	84	—
Spaghetti w/ Tomato Sauce	1 dinner serv	440	5	84	—
Spaghetti w/ Tomato Sauce & Clam Sauce	1 dinner serv	560	17	84	—
Starter Garlic Cheese Bread	1 serv	1220	85	105	—
Starter Meatballs	1 serv	910	61	23	—
Starter Sausage	1 serv	690	56	7	—
Starter Tortellini	1 serv	930	56	82	—
Tortellini Mortadella & Chicken	1 dinner serv	930	56	82	—
SOUPS					
Chicken Mulligatawny	1 serv	250	14	20	—
Chicken Orzo	1 serv	90	3	9	—
Clam Chowder	1 serv	380	29	25	2
Cream Of Broccoli	1 serv	220	12	19	—
Mediterranean White Bean	1 serv	150	6	19	—
Minestrone	1 serv	120	5	15	—

ON THE BORDER
CHILDREN'S MENU SELECTIONS

FOOD	PORTION	CALS	FAT	CARB	SUGAR
Border Chicken Strips	1 serv	570	36	36	—
Corn Dog	1	320	21	11	—

FOOD	PORTION	CALS	FAT	CARB	SUGAR
Crispy Taco Mexican Dinner Beef	1 serv	740	31	77	—
Crispy Taco Mexican Dinner Chicken	1 serv	740	28	85	—
Hamburger	1	390	23	23	—
Nachos Bean & Cheese	1 serv	980	57	71	—
Nachos Cheese	1 serv	670	47	28	—
Quesadillas Chicken	1 serv	720	48	36	—
Sandwich Grilled Chicken	1	630	21	63	—
Soft Taco Mexican Dinner Beef	1 serv	840	35	91	—
Soft Taco Mexican Dinner Chicken	1 serv	750	27	89	—
Sundae w/ Chocolate Syrup	1 serv	300	13	40	—
Sundae w/ Strawberry Puree	1 serv	340	13	52	—
DESSERTS					
Border Brownie Sundae	1	440	25	51	—
Chocolate Turtle Empanadas	1 serv	1280	81	131	—
Dulce De Leche Cheesecake	1 serv	1160	72	122	—
Kahlua Ice Cream Pie	1 serv	850	44	100	—
Sizzling Apple Crisp	1 serv	960	36	157	—
Sopapillas	1 serv	1230	56	136	—
Vanilla Ice Cream	1 scoop	180	10	19	—
MAIN MENU SELECTIONS					
Bacon Wrapped Shrimp	1 serv	730	62	6	—
Baja Chicken	1 serv	610	43	50	—
Bandera Sirloin	1 serv	640	43	13	—
Beans Black	1 serv	180	7	19	—
Beans Refried	1 serv	290	11	36	—

FOOD	PORTION	CALS	FAT	CARB	SUGAR
Black Bean & Corn Relish	1 serv	80	4	6	—
Border Chimichanga Fajita Chicken w/ Onions & Mushrooms	1 serv	1230	93	51	—
Border Chimichanga Ground Beef	1 serv	1310	98	49	—
Border Chimichanga Spicy Chicken	1 serv	1160	85	46	—
Border Sampler	1 serv	1940	120	110	—
Bordurrito Big Beef w/ Side Salad	1 serv	1600	103	119	—
Bordurrito Big Chicken w/ Side Salad	1 serv	1420	57	121	—
Burrito Beef	1 serv	1080	57	71	—
Burrito Chicken	1 serv	880	56	55	—
Burrito Three Sauce Fajita Chicken	1 serv	870	45	59	—
Burrito Three Sauce Fajita Steak	1 serv	1050	61	57	—
Carne Asada & Shrimp	1 serv	1040	74	22	—
Cheese Chile Relleno	1	880	61	60	—
Cheesy Pepper Jack Mashed Potatoes	1 serv	380	27	26	—
Chicken Flautas Appetizer	1 serv	970	66	50	—
Chile Con Queso	1 bowl	390	29	14	—
Chile Con Queso	1 cup	250	18	8	—
Corona Extra Dinner	1 serv	2040	128	136	—
Crispy Taco Beef	1	330	20	19	—
Crispy Taco Chicken	1	240	12	16	—
Crispy Taco Veggie	1	250	16	20	—
Dos XX Fish Tacos	1 serv	1590	113	100	—
Empanadas Beef	1	440	31	26	—
Empanadas Chicken	1	390	26	25	—

FOOD	PORTION	CALS	FAT	CARB	SUGAR
Empanadas Chicken	1 serv	1090	74	68	—
Empanadas Ground Beef	1 serv	1150	81	68	—
Enchilada Beef	1	340	17	27	—
Enchilada Cheese & Onion	1	410	24	27	—
Enchilada Chicken	1	350	23	21	—
Fajitas 7 Pepper Steak	1 serv	910	62	30	—
Fajitas Blackened Chicken w/ Portobello Mushrooms	1 serv	640	29	27	—
Fajitas Carnitas	1 serv	830	62	19	—
Fajitas Chicken Con Queso	1 skillet	1130	82	7	—
Fajitas Grilled Vegetables w/ Portobello Mushrooms	1 serv	390	28	30	—
Fajitas Jalapeno BBQ Chicken	1 serv	760	32	53	—
Fajitas Mesquite Grilled Chicken	1 serv	440	18	20	—
Fajitas Mesquite Grilled Steak	1 serv	620	41	18	—
Fajitas Monterey Ranch Chicken	1 serv	840	21	21	—
Fajitas Shrimp	1 serv	750	63	18	—
Fajitas Ultimate	1 serv	1230	102	20	—
Firecracker Stuffed Jalapenos	1 serv	980	56	70	—
French Fries	1 serv	390	25	40	—
Grande Fajita Nachos Beef	1 serv	1970	127	109	—
Grande Fajita Nachos Chicken	1 serv	1890	113	109	—
Grande Fajita Nachos Combo	1 serv	1940	121	109	—
Guacamole	1 serv	130	10	9	—
Guacamole Live	1 serv	570	50	33	—
Margarita Chicken	1 serv	290	11	21	—

FOOD	PORTION	CALS	FAT	CARB	SUGAR
Mexican Rice	1 serv	220	6	33	—
Mexican Shrimp Scampi	1 serv	740	64	8	—
Pico Chicken & Shrimp	1 serv	730	51	9	—
Quesadillas Combo Fajita	1 serv	1450	96	59	—
Quesadillas Double Stacked Club	1 serv	1860	123	88	—
Quesadillas Fajita Chicken	1 serv	1430	91	59	—
Quesadillas Fajita Steak	1 serv	1530	107	59	—
Quesadillas Spinach & Mushroom	1 serv	1420	105	66	—
Ranchiladas	1 serv	1360	86	53	—
Red Chili Ribeye	1 serv	900	72	12	—
Salmon Mexican	1 serv	650	50	4	—
Sandwich Chicken Blackened w/ French Fries	1 serv	1510	93	101	—
Sandwich Chicken Grilled w/ French Fries	1 serv	1430	92	101	—
Sauteed Shrimp	4	170	10	1	—
Shaken Margarita Shrimp Cocktail	1 serv	280	13	22	—
Shaken Margarita Shrimp Cocktail w/ Tortilla Chips	1 serv	780	40	57	—
Soft Taco Beef	1	340	19	23	—
Soft Taco Chicken	1	250	11	20	—
Soft Taco Veggie	1	210	9	24	—
Superior Dinner	1 serv	1350	85	80	—
Tamale	1	310	17	26	—
Tortilla Corn	3	230	4	43	—
Tortilla Flour	3	300	9	45	—
Tortilla Soup	1 bowl	350	22	24	—
Tres Enchilada Dinner Beef	1 serv	1010	52	80	—
Tres Enchilada Dinner Cheese	1 serv	1210	73	80	—

FOOD	PORTION	CALS	FAT	CARB	SUGAR
Tres Enchilada Dinner Chicken	1 serv	1040	68	64	—
Ultimate Loaded Queso	1 serv	900	59	46	—
Vegetables Grilled	1 serv	50	1	8	—
Vegetables Sauteed	1 serv	70	4	9	—
SALAD DRESSINGS AND SAUCES					
Chili Con Carne Sauce	1 serv (2 oz)	70	3	6	—
Chipotle Mayonnaise	1 serv (1 oz)	190	21	1	—
Dressing Chipotle Honey Mustard	1 serv (2 oz)	310	29	11	—
Dressing Fat Free Balsamic Vinaigrette	1 serv (2 oz)	50	0	10	—
Dressing Lo Fat Ranch	1 serv (2 oz)	110	6	11	—
Dressing Ranch	1 serv (2 oz)	220	23	2	—
Dressing Smoked Jalapeno Vinaigrette	1 serv (2 oz)	230	22	8	—
Dressing Sweet Pepper Vinaigrette	1 serv (2 oz)	270	25	10	—
Parrila Butter	1 serv (1 oz)	120	13	1	—
Pico De Gallo	1 scoop	20	1	2	—
Ranchero Sauce	1 serv (2 oz)	18	1	3	—
Salsa	1 serv (2 oz)	25	1	3	—
Sour Cream	1 serv (2 oz)	140	14	2	—
SALADS					
Chopped Chicken w/ Dressing	1 serv	1330	89	54	—
Fiesta Blackened Chicken w/ Dressing	1 serv	1150	75	54	—
Fiesta Chicken w/ Dressing	1 serv	1140	74	52	—
Grande Taco Beef	1 serv	1450	102	78	—
Grande Taco Chicken	1 serv	1280	89	74	—
House	1 serv	170	10	15	—

FOOD	PORTION	CALS	FAT	CARB	SUGAR
Sizzling Fajita Chicken	1 serv	760	48	23	—
Sizzling Fajita Steak	1 serv	910	65	24	—

PANDA EXPRESS
MAIN MENU SELECTIONS

FOOD	PORTION	CALS	FAT	CARB	SUGAR
BBQ Pork	1 serv	350	19	13	5
Beef & Broccoli	1 serv	150	8	9	2
Beef w/ String Beans	1 serv	170	9	11	0
Black Pepper Chicken	1 serv	180	10	10	2
Chicken w/ Mushrooms	1 serv	130	7	7	2
Chicken w/ Potato	1 serv	220	11	17	1
Chicken w/ String Beans	1 serv	170	8	12	2
Egg Roll Chicken	1 (3 oz)	190	8	21	tr
Fried Shrimp	6 pieces	260	12	26	0
Mandarin Chicken	1 serv	250	9	8	2
Mixed Vegetables	1 serv	70	3	8	1
Orange Chicken	1 serv	480	21	50	5
Spicy Chicken w/ Peanuts	1 serv	200	7	17	2
Spring Roll Veggie	1 (1.7 oz)	80	3	14	0
Steamed Rice	1 serv	330	1	74	0
String Beans w/ Fried Tofu	1 serv	180	11	11	3
Sweet & Sour Chicken	1 serv	310	14	28	0
Sweet & Sour Pork	1 serv	410	30	17	0
Vegetable Chow Mein	1 serv	330	11	48	6
Vegetable Fried Rice	1 serv	390	12	61	0
SAUCES					
Hot	2 tsp	10	1	2	1
Hot Mustard	1 serv	18	0	1	0
Mandarin	1 serv	70	0	16	14
Soy	1 tbsp	16	0	2	2
Sweet & Sour	1 serv	60	0	15	13

FOOD	PORTION	CALS	FAT	CARB	SUGAR

PANERA BREAD
BAGELS AND SPREADS

FOOD	PORTION	CALS	FAT	CARB	SUGAR
Bagel Asiago Cheese	1	330	5	58	5
Bagel Blueberry	1	320	2	67	11
Bagel Cinnamon Crunch	1	490	9	91	35
Bagel Dutch Apple & Raisin	1	340	3	70	21
Bagel Everything	1	290	2	58	4
Bagel French Toast	1	340	5	65	16
Bagel Mochachip Swirl	1	340	4	68	13
Bagel Nine Grain	1	290	1	58	4
Bagel Peanut Butter Crunch	1	400	6	77	27
Bagel Plain	1	280	1	57	4
Bagel Sesame	1	310	3	60	4
Cream Cheese Hazelnut Reduced Fat	1 serv (2 oz)	150	11	6	6
Cream Cheese Honey Walnut Reduced Fat	1 serv (2 oz)	150	11	9	6
Cream Cheese Mocha Reduced Fat	1 serv (2 oz)	160	11	10	8
Cream Cheese Plain	1 serv (2 oz)	190	18	2	1
Cream Cheese Plain Reduced Fat	1 serv (2 oz)	130	12	2	1
Cream Cheese Raspberry Reduced Fat	1 serv (2 oz)	120	10	3	2
Cream Cheese Smoked Salmon Reduced Fat	1 serv (2 oz)	120	10	2	1
Cream Cheese Sun Dried Tomato Reduced Fat	1 serv (2 oz)	140	11	4	2
Cream Cheese Veggie Reduced Fat	1 serv (2 oz)	130	11	4	2
Hummus Roasted Garlic	1 serv (2 oz)	100	5	11	7

FOOD	PORTION	CALS	FAT	CARB	SUGAR
BREADS					
Artisan Country	1 slice	120	0	25	1
Artisan French	1 slice (2 oz)	110	0	23	1
Artisan Kalamata Olive	1 slice (2 oz)	140	2	26	1
Artisan Multigrain	1 slice (2 oz)	120	1	24	1
Artisan Raisin Pecan	1 slice (2 oz)	140	3	25	5
Artisan Sesame Semolina	1 slice (2 oz)	120	0	24	1
Artisan Stone Milled Rye	1 slice (2 oz)	110	0	22	1
Artisan Three Cheese	1 slice (2 oz)	120	2	21	1
Artisan Three Seed	1 slice	130	2	23	1
Ciabatta	1 (6 oz)	430	10	70	2
Cinnamon Raisin	1 slice (2 oz)	160	3	31	12
Focaccia Asiago Cheese	1 slice (2 oz)	150	6	19	1
Focaccia Basil Pesto	1 slice (2 oz)	150	6	19	1
Focaccia Rosemary & Onion	1 slice (2 oz)	140	5	19	1
French	1 slice (2 oz)	130	1	24	1
French Roll	1 (2.25 oz)	140	1	28	1
Holiday	1 slice (2 oz)	150	1	33	23
Honey Wheat	1 slice (2 oz)	140	3	25	3
Nine Grain	1 slice (2 oz)	150	3	26	3
Rye	1 slice (2 oz)	140	3	25	3
Sourdough	1 slice (2 oz)	120	0	25	1
Sourdough Roll	1 (2.5 oz)	160	0	32	1
Sourdough Soup Bowl	1 serv (8 oz)	500	2	102	2
Sunflower	1 slice (2 oz)	160	5	24	4
Tomato Basil	1 slice (2 oz)	130	1	27	1
DESSERTS					
Bear Claw	1	380	21	37	14
Brownie Caramel Pecan	1	470	24	60	47
Brownie Chocolate Raspberry	1	370	18	47	37
Brownie Very Chocolate	1	460	22	62	47

FOOD	PORTION	CALS	FAT	CARB	SUGAR
Cinnamon Roll	1	560	26	64	21
Cobblestone	1	560	9	100	42
Coffee Cake Cherry Cheese	1	190	10	21	11
Cookie Chocolate Chipper	1	420	22	51	21
Cookie Chocolate Duet w/ Walnuts	1	410	25	47	24
Cookie Nutty Chocolate Chipper	1	440	26	46	20
Cookie Nutty Oatmeal Raisin	1	350	14	51	22
Cookie Shortbread	1	340	21	36	11
Croissant Apple	1	260	11	34	17
Croissant Cheese	1	300	16	34	11
Croissant Chocolate	1	440	23	56	27
Croissant French	1	265	15	28	3
Croissant Raspberry Cheese	1	280	13	37	14
Danish Apple	1	510	30	50	17
Danish Cheese	1	590	35	55	25
Danish Cherry	1	520	26	60	31
Danish Georgia Peach	1	580	30	67	28
Danish German Chocolate	1	770	46	83	37
Macaroon Chocolate Hazelnut	1	270	15	30	18
Mini Bundt Cake Carrot Walnut	1	430	21	51	31
Mini Bundt Cake Lemon Poppyseed	1	460	20	62	33
Mini Bundt Cake Pineapple Upside Down	1	450	20	64	36
Muffie Banana Nut	1	260	12	34	15
Muffie Chocolate Chip	1	240	10	36	18

FOOD	PORTION	CALS	FAT	CARB	SUGAR
Muffie Pumpkin	1	270	6	43	26
Muffin Banana Nut	1	470	20	57	31
Muffin Blueberry	1	450	15	73	33
Muffin Chocolate Chip	1	540	22	83	42
Muffin Pumpkin	1	510	12	80	48
Muffin Low Fat Tripleberry	1	300	3	63	28
Pecan Roll	1	520	31	60	26
Scone Cinnamon Chip	1	560	27	70	23
Scone Orange	1	530	25	67	22
Strudel Apple Raisin	1	390	22	40	18
Strudel Cherry	1	400	24	38	20
SALADS					
Asian Sesame Chicken	1 serv	370	19	45	19
Caesar	1 serv	350	26	15	1
Caesar Grilled Chicken	1 serv	470	27	22	1
Classic Cafe	1 serv	380	36	15	10
Fandango	1 serv	400	28	21	15
Greek	1 serv	520	48	17	4
SANDWICHES					
Asiago Roast Beef	1	730	35	54	4
Bacon Turkey Bravo	1	770	28	84	6
Chicken Salad On Artisan Sesame Semolina	1	730	26	80	12
Chicken Salad On Nine Grain	1	640	29	56	15
Garden Veggie	1	570	23	74	6
Italian Combo	1	1050	54	80	5
Panini Coronado Carnitas	1	810	35	77	4
Panini Frontega Chicken	1	860	42	71	5
Panini Portobello & Mozzarella	1	650	29	73	7
Panini Turkey Artichoke	1	810	38	76	10

FOOD	PORTION	CALS	FAT	CARB	SUGAR
Peanut Butter & Jelly On French	1	450	15	63	23
Sierra Turkey	1	950	55	71	4
Smoked Ham On Artisan Stone Milled Rye	1	930	31	106	6
Smoked Ham On Rye	1	650	34	47	7
Smoked Turkey Breast On Artisan Country	1	590	16	73	4
Smoked Turkey On Sourdough	1	440	15	44	4
Tuna Salad On Artisan Multigrain	1	830	41	78	7
Tuna Salad On Honey Wheat	1	720	43	50	10
Turkey Fresco	1	580	17	74	5
Tuscan Chicken	1	950	56	76	8
SOUPS					
Baked Potato	1 serv	260	16	23	2
Boston Clam Chowder	1 serv	210	11	19	2
Broccoli Cheddar	1 serv	230	16	13	4
Cream Of Chicken & Wild Rice	1 serv	200	12	19	2
Forest Mushroom	1 serv	140	7	15	3
French Onion	1 serv	220	10	23	6
Low Fat Chicken Noodle	1 serv	100	2	15	1
Low Fat Vegetarian Garden Vegetable	1 serv	90	1	17	4
Low Fat Vegetarian Black Bean	1 serv	100	1	29	2
Vegetarian Santa Fe Roasted Corn	1 serv	130	4	22	4

FOOD	PORTION	CALS	FAT	CARB	SUGAR
PAPA JOHN'S					
OTHER MENU SELECTIONS					
Bread Sticks	1 serv	140	2	26	3
Cheese Sticks	1 serv	180	8	20	2
Chickenstrips	1	83	4	5	tr
Cinnapie	1 serv	114	6	14	6
PIZZA 14 INCH					
Original All The Meats	⅛ pie	405	20	39	5
Original BBQ Chicken & Bacon	⅛ pie	369	14	44	6
Original Cheese	⅛ pie	290	10	39	5
Original Chicken Alfredo	⅛ pie	310	12	37	4
Original Garden Fresh	⅛ pie	287	9	40	6
Original Hawaiian BBQ Chicken	⅛ pie	376	14	46	6
Original Pepperoni	⅛ pie	343	15	39	5
Original Sausage	⅛ pie	336	14	38	5
Original Spinach Alfredo	⅛ pie	303	12	37	4
Original The Works	⅛ pie	370	16	40	6
Thin Crust All The Meat	⅛ pie	371	24	24	3
Thin Crust BBQ Chicken & Bacon	⅛ pie	336	18	30	4
Thin Crust Cheese	⅛ pie	238	13	23	3
Thin Crust Chicken Alfredo	⅛ pie	276	15	22	1
Thin Crust Garden Fresh	⅛ pie	228	11	24	2
Thin Crust Hawaiian BBQ Chicken	⅛ pie	324	17	31	5
Thin Crust Pepperoni	⅛ pie	294	18	23	3
Thin Crust Sausage	⅛ pie	303	18	24	3
Thin Crust Spinach Alfredo	⅛ pie	251	15	22	1
Thin Crust The Works	⅛ pie	315	18	25	3

FOOD	PORTION	CALS	FAT	CARB	SUGAR
SALAD DRESSINGS AND SAUCES					
BBQ Sauce	1 serv	48	0	10	9
Buffalo Sauce	1 serv	25	1	3	1
Cheese Sauce	1 serv	60	5	0	0
Garlic Sauce	1 serv	235	26	0	0
Honey Mustard Dressing	1 serv	170	19	6	6
Pizza Sauce	1 serv	25	2	3	1
Ranch Dressing	1 serv	140	14	2	1
PAPA MURPHY'S					
PIZZA					
Deeper Dish Traditional	⅛ pie	440	24	34	1
Delite Large Cheese	⅒ pie	130	6	11	0
Delite Large Hawaiian	⅒ pie	140	7	14	2
Delite Large Meat	⅒ pie	190	12	11	0
Delite Large Pepperoni	⅒ pie	160	9	11	0
Delite Large Veggie	⅒ pie	150	8	11	1
Family Size Cheese	⅟₁₂ pie	270	10	29	1
Gourmet Family Size Chicken Garlic	⅟₁₂ pie	320	15	30	1
Gourmet Family Size Classic Italian	⅟₁₂ pie	360	19	30	1
Gourmet Family Size Veggie	⅟₁₂ pie	300	14	31	1
Papa's Family Size All Meat	⅟₁₂ pie	370	19	31	1
Papa's Family Size Cheese	⅟₁₂ pie	270	10	29	1
Papa's Family Size Cowboy	⅟₁₂ pie	370	19	31	1
Papa's Family Size Favorite	⅟₁₂ pie	380	20	32	2
Papa's Family Size Hawaiian	⅟₁₂ pie	290	11	34	4

FOOD	PORTION	CALS	FAT	CARB	SUGAR
Papa's Family Size Murphy's Combo	1/12 pie	480	20	32	2
Papa's Family Size Pepperoni	1/12 pie	310	15	29	1
Papa's Family Size Perfect	1/12 pie	300	13	32	4
Papa's Family Size Rancher	1/12 pie	330	15	31	2
Papa's Family Size Specialty	1/12 pie	340	17	31	1
Papa's Family Size Veggie Combo	1/12 pie	300	13	32	2
Stuffed Big Murphy	1/8 pie	380	17	39	1
Stuffed Chicago Style	1/8 pie	370	16	39	2
SALADS					
Club	1 serv	190	21	11	2
Garden	1 serv	160	11	9	3
Italian	1 serv	220	17	7	2

PICCADILLY CAFETERIA

DESSERTS

FOOD	PORTION	CALS	FAT	CARB	SUGAR
Gelatin Sugar Free	1 serv	0	0	0	0
Sugar Free Blueberry Pie	1 serv	314	17	42	—
Sugar Free Cherry Pie	1 serv	334	17	45	—
Sugar Free Chocolate Almond Pie	1 serv	611	44	49	—

MAIN MENU SELECTIONS

FOOD	PORTION	CALS	FAT	CARB	SUGAR
Bass Blackened	1 serv	408	32	2	—
Bass Cajun Baked	1 serv	260	15	4	—
Bass Stuffed	1 serv	447	30	8	—
Beef Chopped Steak	1 serv	382	31	4	—
Beef Chopped Steak Fried	1 serv	225	12	2	—
Beef Roast Leg	1 sm serv	353	22	2	—
Broccoli Florets	1 serv	90	7	5	—
Broccoli w/ Cheese Sauce	1 serv	55	1	9	—

FOOD	PORTION	CALS	FAT	CARB	SUGAR
Brussels Sprouts	1 serv	92	6	8	—
Cabbage Steamed Bacon Seasoned	1 serv	108	8	6	—
Cabbage Steamed Buttered	1 serv	68	5	6	—
Catfish Filet Blackened	1 serv	523	43	2	—
Catfish Filet Cajun Baked	1 serv	401	28	5	—
Catfish Filet Stuffed	1 serv	561	41	8	—
Cauliflower Buttered	1 serv	73	4	5	—
Chicken Baked Cajun Boneless Breast	1 serv	428	27	9	—
Chicken Baked Quarters	1 serv	828	59	5	—
Chicken Barbecued Quarters	1 serv	472	52	9	—
Chicken Breast Italian Boneless Breast	1 serv	371	41	7	—
Chicken Breast Mesquite Smoke	1 serv	212	8	1	—
Chicken Breast Mesquite w/ BBQ Sauce	1 serv	240	9	6	—
Chicken Breast Southwestern	1 serv	315	35	8	—
Chicken Grilled Breast	1 serv	345	21	2	—
Chicken Half Rotisserie Herb	1 serv	833	21	4	—
Chicken Rotisserie Herb Dark Meat	1 serv	823	63	3	—
Chicken Rotisserie Herb White Meat	1 serv	602	32	3	—
Corn	1 serv	125	6	18	—
Cottage Cheese	1 serv	117	5	3	—
Filet Mignon	1 (6 oz)	184	20	1	—
Green Beans	1 serv	136	11	8	—

FOOD	PORTION	CALS	FAT	CARB	SUGAR
Greens Collard Mustard Turnip	1 serv	135	10	3	–
Greens Turnip w/ Diced Turnips	1 serv	150	12	4	–
Grouper Filet Baked	1 piece (6 oz)	305	9	8	–
New York Strip	1 (10 oz)	871	71	1	–
Okra Creole	1 serv	77	4	8	–
Okra Fried	1 serv	240	13	26	–
Peas & Sugar Snapped Mixed	1 serv	102	5	10	–
Pork Loin Marinated Boneless	1 serv	365	24	1	–
Pork Loin Roast Bone In	1 serv	373	13	10	–
Ribeye	1 (10 oz)	1038	91	2	–
Roast Beef	1 serv	481	30	3	–
Roll Parker House	1	147	5	22	–
Roll Whole Wheat	1	231	8	37	–
Shrimp Fried	1 serv	499	22	45	–
Tilapia Baked	1 serv	210	11	10	–
Tilapia Cajun Baked	1 serv	263	19	6	–
Trout Almondine Baked	1 lg serv	457	18	10	–
Trout Cajun Baked	1 lg serv	517	27	6	–
Trout Filet Baked	1 lg serv	464	19	10	–
Turkey Breast Carved	1 serv	302	11	2	–
Vegetables Mixed	1 serv	95	6	8	–
SALAD DRESSINGS AND TOPPINGS					
Au Jus	1 serv	6	0	1	–
Blue Cheese	2 tbsp	160	18	1	–
Cheese Sauce	2 oz	35	1	5	–
French	2 tbsp	130	13	5	–
Italian	2 tbsp	140	14	3	–
Ranch	2 tbsp	150	17	1	–
Ranch Fat Free	2 tbsp	36	0	7	–

FOOD	PORTION	CALS	FAT	CARB	SUGAR
SALADS					
Asparagus & Tomato	1 serv	86	5	10	—
Caesar	1 serv	141	11	7	—
Cauliflower	1 serv	118	8	9	—
Chef	1 sm serv	146	9	4	—
Cole Slaw Kosher Style	1 serv	140	13	7	—
Coleslaw Italian	1 serv	163	16	5	—
Combination	1 serv	63	3	4	—
Cucumber & Celery	1 serv	74	4	9	—
Cucumber & Tomato	1 serv	41	0	10	—
Cucumber Mix	1 serv	61	4	7	—
Cucumbers & Sour Cream	1 serv	90	7	6	—
Louisianne Bowl	1 serv	42	2	2	—
Mexican	1 serv	58	3	8	—
Piccadilly Bowl	1 serv	27	0	6	—
Piccadilly Fruit	1 serv	76	0	20	—
Shrimp Remoulade	1 serv	521	29	33	—
Spring Bowl	1 reg serv	24	0	5	—
Tomato Cucumber & Onion	1 serv	44	0	10	—
Vegetable Combo w/ Cherry Tomatoes	1 serv	66	4	9	—
SOUPS					
Gumbo Chicken & Sausage No Rice	1 serv	224	15	10	—
Gumbo Chicken No Rice	1 serv	89	2	9	—

PIZZA HUT
APPETIZERS

FOOD	PORTION	CALS	FAT	CARB	SUGAR
Breadstick	1	150	6	20	4
Breadstick Cheese	1	200	10	21	4
Hot Wings	2 pieces	110	6	1	0
Mild Wings	2 pieces	110	7	tr	0

FOOD	PORTION	CALS	FAT	CARB	SUGAR
DESSERTS					
Apple Pizza	1 slice	260	4	53	14
Cherry Pizza	1 slice	240	4	47	24
Cinnamon Sticks	2	170	5	27	10
PIZZA					
Fit 'N Delicious Diced Chicken Mushroom Jalapeno	1 med slice	170	5	22	5
Fit 'N Delicious Diced Chicken Red Onion Green Pepper	1 med slice	170	5	23	6
Fit 'N Delicious Diced Red Tomato Mushroom Jalapeno	1 med slice	150	4	22	5
Fit 'N Delicious Green Pepper Red Onion Diced Red Tomato	1 med slice	150	4	24	6
Fit 'N Delicious Ham Pineapple Diced Red Tomato	1 med slice	160	4	24	7
Fit 'N Delicious Ham Red Onion Mushroom	1 med slice	160	5	22	6
Hand Tossed Cheese	1 med slice	240	8	30	5
Hand Tossed Chicken Supreme	1 med slice	230	6	30	6
Hand Tossed Ham	1 med slice	220	6	29	5
Hand Tossed Meat Lover's	1 med slice	300	13	29	6
Hand Tossed Pepperoni	1 med slice	250	9	29	6
Hand Tossed Pepperoni Lover's	1 med slice	300	13	30	6
Hand Tossed Super Supreme	1 med slice	300	13	31	6
Hand Tossed Supreme	1 med slice	270	11	30	6

FOOD	PORTION	CALS	FAT	CARB	SUGAR
Hand Tossed Veggie Lover's	1 med slice	220	6	31	6
Pan Cheese	1 med slice	280	13	29	6
Pan Chicken Supreme	1 med slice	280	12	30	7
Pan Ham	1 med slice	260	11	29	6
Pan Meat Lover's	1 med slice	340	19	29	6
Pan Pepperoni	1 med slice	290	15	29	6
Pan Pepperoni Lover's	1 med slice	340	19	29	6
Pan Super Supreme	1 med slice	340	18	30	7
Pan Supreme	1 med slice	320	16	30	7
Pan Veggie Lover's	1 med slice	260	12	30	7
Personal Pan Cheese	1 pie	630	27	71	14
Personal Pan Chicken Supreme	1 pie	620	23	73	15
Personal Pan Meat Lover's	1 pie	800	41	71	15
Personal Pan Pepperoni	1 pie	660	30	70	14
Personal Pan Pepperoni Lover's	1 pie	800	42	71	15
Personal Pan Super Supreme	1 pie	790	40	74	16
Personal Pan Supreme	1 pie	750	36	73	15
Personal Pan Veggie Lover's	1 pie	580	23	73	15
Stuffed Crust Cheese	1 lg slice	360	13	43	8
Stuffed Crust Chicken Supreme	1 lg slice	380	13	44	10
Stuffed Crust Ham	1 lg slice	340	11	43	8
Stuffed Crust Meat Lover's	1 lg slice	450	21	43	9
Stuffed Crust Pepperoni	1 lg slice	370	15	42	8
Stuffed Crust Pepperoni Lover's	1 lg slice	420	19	43	8
Stuffed Crust Super Supreme	1 lg slice	440	20	45	10

FOOD	PORTION	CALS	FAT	CARB	SUGAR
Stuffed Crust Supreme	1 lg slice	400	16	44	9
Stuffed Crust Veggie Lover's	1 lg slice	360	14	45	10
Thin 'N Crispy Cheese	1 med slice	200	8	21	4
Thin 'N Crispy Chicken Supreme	1 med slice	200	7	22	5
Thin 'N Crispy Ham	1 med slice	180	6	21	5
Thin 'N Crispy Meat Lover's	1 med slice	270	14	21	5
Thin 'N Crispy Pepperoni	1 med slice	210	10	21	5
Thin 'N Crispy Pepperoni Lover's	1 med slice	260	14	21	5
Thin 'N Crispy Super Supreme	1 med slice	260	13	23	6
Thin 'N Crispy Supreme	1 med slice	240	11	22	5
Thin 'N Crispy Veggie Lover's	1 med slice	180	7	23	5
XL Full House Cheese	1 slice	280	12	30	3
XL Full House Chicken Supreme	1 slice	270	10	31	4
XL Full House Ham	1 slice	260	10	30	3
XL Full House Meat Lover's	1 slice	380	21	30	4
XL Full House Pepperoni	1 slice	290	13	30	3
XL Full House Pepperoni Lover's	1 slice	310	15	30	3
XL Full House Super Supreme	1 slice	330	16	32	4
XL Full House Supreme	1 slice	310	15	31	4
XL Full House Veggie Lover's	1 slice	280	11	32	4
SALAD DRESSINGS AND SAUCES					
Dipping Cup White Icing	1 serv	170	0	46	39

FOOD	PORTION	CALS	FAT	CARB	SUGAR
Dipping Sauce Breadstick	1 serv	45	0	9	6
Dipping Sauce Wing Blue Cheese	1 serv	230	24	2	2
Dipping Sauce Wing Ranch	1 serv	210	22	4	2
Dressing Caesar	2 tbsp	150	16	1	tr
Dressing French	2 tbsp	140	11	11	9
Dressing Italian	2 tbsp	140	15	2	2
Dressing Lite Italian	2 tbsp	60	5	5	0
Dressing Lite Ranch	1 tbsp	70	7	0	tr
Dressing Ranch	2 tbsp	100	10	1	1
Dressing Thousand Island	2 tbsp	110	9	6	6

P.J. CHANG'S CHINA BISTRO

FOOD	PORTION	CALS	FAT	CARB	SUGAR
Cantonese Scallops	1 serv	305	8	15	–
Chicken w/ Black Bean Sauce	1 serv	426	11	19	–
Pin Rice Noodles	1 serv	270	2	55	–
Vegetable Chow Fun	1 serv	677	18	112	–

QUIZNO'S

FOOD	PORTION	CALS	FAT	CARB	SUGAR
Cookie Oatmeal Chocolate Chip	1	360	17	48	23
Cookie w/ Reese's Pieces	1	360	17	48	22
Sub Honey Burbon Chicken	1 sm	329	6	45	–
Sub Sierra Turkey w/ Raspberry Chipotle Sauce	1 sm	350	6	53	–
Sub Turkey Lite	1 sm	334	6	52	–

RANCH 1

MAIN MENU SELECTIONS

FOOD	PORTION	CALS	FAT	CARB	SUGAR
Baked Potato w/ Broccoli	1 serv	510	1	117	8
Baked Potato w/ Cheese	1 serv	790	25	118	9
Baked Potato w/ Chicken	1 serv	610	4	114	7

FOOD	PORTION	CALS	FAT	CARB	SUGAR
Chicken Tenders	1 serv	370	15	7	0
Fajita Grilled Chicken	1	330	16	25	4
Fruit Cup	1 serv	90	1	21	18
Hot Pasta Grilled Chicken	1 serv	590	10	86	7
Platter Grilled Chicken & Vegetables	1 serv	790	7	129	12
Ranch Fries	1 lg	420	17	62	2
Ranch Fries	1 reg	350	14	51	1
Sandwich American Rancher	1	390	10	51	4
Sandwich Grilled Chicken Philly	1	450	14	53	4
Sandwich Ranch Classic	1	370	5	53	4
Sandwich Spicy Grilled Chicken	1	420	11	58	7
Sandwich Club	1	470	16	53	4
SALADS					
Gourmet Greens	1 serv	220	7	31	7
Gourmet Greens w/ Chicken	1 serv	350	11	31	7
Zesty Caesar	1 serv	180	3	31	4
Zesty Chicken Caesar	1 serv	290	6	31	4

RAX
MAIN MENU SELECTIONS

FOOD	PORTION	CALS	FAT	CARB	SUGAR
Baked Potato	1	207	0	60	—
Baked Potato w/ Butter	1	306	11	60	—
Baked Potato w/ Cheese	1 serv	270	tr	70	—
Baked Potato w/ Cheese Bacon	1 serv	336	19	70	—
Baked Potato w/ Cheese Broccoli	1 serv	281	tr	71	—
Baked Potato w/ Sour Topping	1 serv	257	4	62	—

FOOD	PORTION	CALS	FAT	CARB	SUGAR
BBC Sandwich	1	716	51	37	–
BBQ Beef Sandwich	1	399	20	43	–
Cheddar Melt	1	346	23	26	–
Deluxe Sandwich	1	521	34	34	–
Grilled Chicken Sandwich	1	526	33	32	–
Jr. Deluxe Sandwich	1	367	25	25	–
Mushroom Melt	1	599	37	35	–
Philly Melt	1	537	32	35	–
Regular Rax	1	388	22	31	–
Turkey Bacon Club	1	680	47	37	–
Turkey Sandwich	1	484	32	32	–
SALAD DRESSINGS					
1000 Island	1 serv	130	13	5	–
Blue Cheese	1 serv	145	16	1	–
Buttermilk Ranch	1 serv	175	20	1	–
Catalina Fat Free	1 serv	32	0	6	–
Creamy Caesar	1 serv	140	15	1	–
Honey French	1 serv	140	5	9	–
Italian Fat Free	1 serv	12	0	2	–
Ranch Fat Free	1 serv	30	0	6	–
Vinaigrette	1 serv	30	2	4	–
SALADS					
Garden	1 serv	220	9	12	–
Grilled Chicken	1 serv	160	5	6	–
Side Salad	1 serv (19 oz)	40	4	2	–
SOUPS					
Chicken Noodle	1 serv	113	1	20	–
Chili	1 serv	158	9	11	–
Cream Of Broccoli	1 serv	95	4	14	–

RED LOBSTER
BEVERAGES

FOOD	PORTION	CALS	FAT	CARB	SUGAR
Michelob Ultra	1 glass	95	0	2	–

FOOD	PORTION	CALS	FAT	CARB	SUGAR
Sutter Home Cabernet Sauvignon	1 glass	138	0	5	—
Sutter Home Chardonnay	1 glass	147	0	5	—
MAIN MENU SELECTIONS					
Baked Potato Plain	1	170	2	36	—
Baked Potato w/ Pico De Gallo Topping	1 serv	185	2	37	—
Cheddar Bay Biscuit	1	160	9	17	—
Fresh Buttered Vegetables	1 serv	143	12	9	—
Garden Salad	1 serv	52	2	9	—
Light House Broiled Flounder	1 serv	240	5	0	0
Light House Grilled Chicken	1 serv	527	14	38	—
Light House Jumbo Shrimp Cocktail Dinner	1 serv	243	3	2	—
Light House King Crab Legs	1 serv	490	9	0	0
Light House Live Maine Lobster	1 serv	145	1	2	—
Light House Maine Lobster Tail	1 serv	104	5	2	—
Light House Rainbow Trout	1 lunch serv	273	14	2	—
Light House Rock Lobster Tail	1 serv	256	3	2	—
Light House Salmon	1 lunch serv	258	12	0	0
Light House Salmon	1 serv	578	31	0	0
Light House Snow Crab Legs	1 serv	262	5	0	0
Light House Tilapia	1 lunch serv	186	6	0	0
Light House Tilapia	1 serv	346	10	0	0
Seasoned Fresh Broccoli	1 serv	60	0	12	—

FOOD	PORTION	CALS	FAT	CARB	SUGAR
Shrimp Cocktail	1 jumbo	146	2	2	—
Wild Rice Pilaf	1 serv	208	5	36	—
SALAD DRESSINGS AND TOPPINGS					
Large Cocktail Sauce	1 serv	68	0	17	—
Lemon Wedge	1 serv	8	0	2	—
Melted Butter	1 serv	183	21	0	—
Red Wine Vinaigrette	1 serv	49	3	5	—
Topping Petite Shrimp	1 serv	30	1	1	—

RUBIO'S
MAIN MENU SELECTIONS

FOOD	PORTION	CALS	FAT	CARB	SUGAR
Black Beans	1 serv	220	3	37	0
Burritos Baja Carne Asada	1	710	33	63	6
Burritos Baja Carnitas	1	660	30	64	8
Burritos Baja Chicken	1	640	28	61	5
Burritos Carne Asada Especial w/ Black Beans	1	970	37	117	6
Burritos Carne Asada Especial w/ Pinto	1	950	38	118	6
Burritos Chicken Especial w/ Black Beans	1	920	32	116	5
Burritos Chicken Especial w/ Pinto	1	900	32	116	5
Burritos Fish	1	780	41	76	4
Burritos HealthMex Chicken	1	520	11	75	6
Burritos HealthMex Veggie	1	470	8	81	12
Burritos Lobster	1	660	26	82	5
Burritos Mahi	1	630	30	58	4
Burritos Shrimp	1	650	25	77	4
Carne Asada	1 serv	1430	87	114	3
Chips	1 serv	430	22	56	0

FOOD	PORTION	CALS	FAT	CARB	SUGAR
Grilled Grande Bowl Asada Black Beans	1 serv	770	37	70	3
Grilled Grande Bowl Asada Pinto	1 serv	760	37	70	4
Grilled Grande Bowl Chicken Black Beans	1 serv	710	31	69	3
Grilled Grande Bowl Chicken Pinto	1 serv	700	32	69	3
Guacamole	1 sm	170	16	8	1
Nachos Grande	1 serv	1270	79	112	3
Nachos Grande w/ Chicken	1 serv	1380	82	112	2
Pinto Beans	1 serv	190	3	44	1
Quesadillas Carne Asada	1	1010	61	62	4
Quesadillas Cheese	1	860	53	60	3
Quesadillas Grilled Chicken	1	860	56	61	3
Quesadillas Lobster	1	820	54	62	3
Quesadillas Shrimp	1	810	54	61	3
Roasted Chipotle	1 serv (1.5 oz)	10	0	2	1
Salsa Picante	1 serv (1.5 oz)	30	2	3	0
Salsa Regular	1 serv (1.5 oz)	15	0	2	2
Salsa Verde	1 serv (1.5 oz)	5	0	1	0
Tacos Carne Asada	1	220	8	23	1
Tacos Fish	1	310	18	28	1
Tacos Fish Especial	1	370	21	38	2
Tacos Grilled Chicken	1	300	16	23	1
Tacos Grilled Fish	1	310	16	24	1
Tacos HealthMex w/ Chicken	1	170	3	23	2
Taquitos	3	310	11	37	1

FOOD	PORTION	CALS	FAT	CARB	SUGAR
SALADS AND SALAD DRESSINGS					
Grilled Chicken Chopped Salad	1 serv	540	33	33	4
HealthMex Chicken	1 serv	220	4	27	16
Low Carb Chicken	1 serv	480	34	11	3
Serrano Grape Dressing	1 serv (1.3 oz)	10	0	2	1
RUBY TUESDAY'S					
Cajun Chicken Salad w/ Ranch Dressing	1 serv	636	46	16	—
Peppercorn Mushroom Sirloin	1 serv	947	57	19	—
SKIPPERS					
CHILDREN'S MENU SELECTIONS					
Kids Catch Chicken Tenderloin + Chips & Kids Side	1 serv	560	11	79	24
Kids Catch Fish Bites + Chips & Kids Side	1 serv	490	15	84	26
Kids Catch Sandwich Grilled Cheese + Chips & Kids Side	1 serv	620	19	97	27
Kids Catch Shrimp + Chips & Kids Side	1 serv	520	11	91	25
MAIN MENU SELECTIONS					
Baked Potato Plain	1	210	0	48	3
Basket Chicken & Fish + Chips & Slaw	1 serv	620	27	59	5
Basket Chicken & Shrimp + Chips & Slaw	1 serv	760	25	84	5
Basket Chicken + Chips & Slaw	1 piece	730	25	60	4

FOOD	PORTION	CALS	FAT	CARB	SUGAR
Basket Clam Strips + Chips & Slaw	1 serv	890	34	113	4
Basket Clams & Fish + Chips & Slaw	1 serv	740	32	91	5
Basket Original Recipe Shrimp + Chips & Slaw	1 serv	800	25	107	6
Basket Popcorn Shrimp + Chips & Slaw	1 serv	750	25	96	5
Basket Prawn & Fish + Chips & Slaw	1 serv	730	41	61	5
Basket Prawn Seafood + Chips & Slaw	1 serv	720	40	52	4
Basket Shrimp & Fish + Chips & Slaw	1 serv	650	27	83	6
Basket Shrimp Trio + Chips & Slaw	1 serv	1040	38	123	7
Clam Chowder	1 cup	120	8	14	1
Clam Strips	1 serv	270	6	39	0
Fish Bites + Chips & Slaw	6 pieces	490	17	94	0
French Fries	1 reg	180	6	27	0
Grilled Veggies	1 serv	35	0	8	3
Halibut + Chips & Slaw	1 serv	580	30	51	4
Homestyle Chicken Tenderloin	1 piece	190	2	13	0
Hush Puppies	3 pieces	240	9	47	0
Original Fish Fillet	1 piece	80	4	12	1
Original Fish + Chips & Slaw	2 pieces	510	29	59	6
Original Shrimp	9 pieces	220	2	36	1
Sandwich Fish + Chips & Slaw	1 serv	800	34	105	14
Sandwich Fried Chicken + Chips & Slaw	1	1260	49	117	12

FOOD	PORTION	CALS	FAT	CARB	SUGAR
Sandwich Grilled Chicken + Chips & Slaw	1	1070	50	92	12
Skipper's Platter + Chips & Slaw	1 serv	930	33	122	6
SALADS					
Caesar	1 sm	150	13	8	4
Caesar w/ Chicken	1 sm	340	17	8	4
Caesar w/ Salmon	1 sm	350	19	8	4
Green Salad w/o Dressing	1 sm	25	0	5	3
SMOOTHIE KING					
Activator Chocolate	1 (20 oz)	429	1	90	—
Activator Strawberry	1 (20 oz)	559	1	123	—
Activator Vanilla	1 (20 oz)	429	1	90	—
Banana Boat	1 (20 oz)	520	14	93	—
Coconut Surprise	1 (20 oz)	457	6	99	—
Coffee Smoothies Amaretto	1 (20 oz)	118	tr	23	—
Coffee Smoothies French Roast	1 (20 oz)	164	tr	35	—
Coffee Smoothies French Vanilla	1 (20 oz)	118	tr	23	—
Coffee Smoothies Hazelnut	1 (20 oz)	118	tr	23	—
Coffee Smoothies Irish Creme	1 (20 oz)	118	tr	23	—
Coffee Smoothies Mocha	1 (20 oz)	206	1	42	—
HeaterZ Banana Nut	1	400	22	67	—
HeaterZ Blueberry Muffin	1	370	26	15	—
HeaterZ Chocolate Peanut Butter Cup	1	380	13	48	—
HeaterZ Cinnamon Oatmeal Raisin	1	420	3	36	—
HeaterZ Coconut	1	440	13	3	—
HeaterZ Coffee Amaretto	1 (12 oz)	177	2	34	—

FOOD	PORTION	CALS	FAT	CARB	SUGAR
HeaterZ Coffee French Roast	1 (12 oz)	172	2	33	—
HeaterZ Coffee French Vanilla	1 (12 oz)	177	2	34	—
HeaterZ Coffee Hazelnut	1 (12 oz)	177	2	34	—
HeaterZ Coffee Irish Creme	1 (12 oz)	177	2	34	—
HeaterZ Coffee Mocha	1 (12 oz)	266	2	55	—
High Protein Almond Mocha	1 (20 oz)	402	13	45	—
High Protein Banana	1 (20 oz)	412	14	44	—
High Protein Chocolate	1 (20 oz)	401	13	45	—
High Protein Lemon	1 (20 oz)	390	13	41	—
High Protein Pineapple	1 (20 oz)	380	13	41	—
Hot Coffee Amaretto	1 (12 oz)	168	tr	35	—
Hot Coffee French Roast	1 (12 oz)	164	tr	35	—
Hot Coffee French Vanilla	1 (12 oz)	168	tr	35	—
Hot Coffee Hazelnut	1 (12 oz)	168	tr	35	—
Hot Coffee Irish Creme	1 (12 oz)	168	tr	35	—
Hot Coffee Mocha	1 (12 oz)	209	1	44	—
Iced Coffee Amaretto	1 (20 oz)	168	tr	35	—
Iced Coffee French Roast	1 (20 oz)	164	tr	35	—
Iced Coffee French Vanilla	1 (20 oz)	168	tr	35	—
Iced Coffee Hazelnut	1 (20 oz)	168	tr	35	—
Iced Coffee Irish Creme	1 (20 oz)	168	tr	35	—
Iced Coffee Mocha	1 (20 oz)	209	1	44	—
Kid Cup Berry Interesting	1	150	0	37	—
Kid Cup Choc-A-Laka	1	210	2	44	—
Kid Cup Gimmi-Grape	1	170	0	42	—
Kid Cup Smarti Tarti	1	150	0	36	—
Low Carb All Flavors	1 (20 oz)	225	6	4	—
Low Fat Angel Food	1 (20 oz)	330	1	79	—
Low Fat Blackberry Dream	1 (20 oz)	343	tr	86	—

FOOD	PORTION	CALS	FAT	CARB	SUGAR
Low Fat Caribbean Way	1 (20 oz)	392	tr	96	—
Low Fat Celestial Cherry High	1 (20 oz)	285	tr	69	—
Low Fat Cherry Picker	1 (20 oz)	360	1	98	—
Low Fat Cranberry Cooler	1 (20 oz)	538	tr	132	—
Low Fat Cranberry Supreme	1 (20 oz)	577	1	139	—
Low Fat Grape Expectations	1 (20 oz)	399	tr	96	—
Low Fat Grape Expectations II	1 (20 oz)	529	tr	129	—
Low Fat Healthy Apple	1 (20 oz)	380	2	81	—
Low Fat Immune Builder	1 (20 oz)	333	1	80	—
Low Fat Instant Vigor	1 (20 oz)	359	1	87	—
Low Fat Island Treat	1 (20 oz)	334	1	81	—
Low Fat Lemon Twist Banana	1 (20 oz)	339	tr	82	—
Low Fat Lemon Twist Strawberry	1 (20 oz)	399	tr	97	—
Low Fat Light & Fluffy	1 (20 oz)	389	tr	98	—
Low Fat Mangofest	1 (20 oz)	320	0	78	—
Low Fat Muscle Punch	1 (20 oz)	339	1	80	—
Low Fat Muscle Punch Plus	1 (20 oz)	340	1	80	—
Low Fat Orange Ka-BAM	1 (20 oz)	320	0	104	—
Low Fat Peach Slice	1 (20 oz)	341	tr	80	—
Low Fat Peach Slice Plus	1 (20 oz)	471	tr	113	—
Low Fat Pep Upper	1 (20 oz)	334	1	80	—
Low Fat Pineapple Pleasure	1 (20 oz)	331	tr	76	—
Low Fat Pineapple Surf	1 (20 oz)	440	1	104	—
Low Fat Raspberry Sunrise	1 (20 oz)	335	1	85	—

FOOD	PORTION	CALS	FAT	CARB	SUGAR
Low Fat Strawberry Kiwi Breeze	1 (20 oz)	300	0	70	—
Low Fat Strawberry X-Treme	1 (20 oz)	370	0	91	—
Low Fat Youth Fountain	1 (20 oz)	267	tr	65	—
Malts	1 (20 oz)	887	41	119	—
Mo'cuccino	1 (20 oz)	420	12	71	—
Peanut Power	1 (20 oz)	502	21	72	—
Peanut Power Plus Grape	1 (20 oz)	703	21	119	—
Peanut Power Plus Strawberry	1 (20 oz)	632	21	104	—
Pina Colada Island	1 (20 oz)	550	11	102	—
Power Punch	1 (20 oz)	430	1	102	—
Power Punch Plus	1 (20 oz)	499	2	113	—
Shakes	1 (20 oz)	875	41	117	—
Slim-N-Trim Chocolate	1 (20 oz)	270	2	55	—
Slim-N-Trim Orange Vanilla	1 (20 oz)	199	1	43	—
Slim-N-Trim Strawberry	1 (20 oz)	357	1	79	—
Slim-N-Trim Vanilla	1 (20 oz)	227	1	51	—
Super Punch	1 (20 oz)	425	tr	95	—
Super Punch Plus	1 (20 oz)	516	tr	118	—
The Hulk Chocolate	1 (20 oz)	846	29	129	—
The Hulk Strawberry	1 (20 oz)	953	29	156	—
The Hulk Vanilla	1 (20 oz)	846	29	129	—
Yogurt D-Lite	1 (20 oz)	335	4	58	—

SONIC DRIVE-IN
ADD-ONS

FOOD	PORTION	CALS	FAT	CARB	SUGAR
Bacon	1 serv (0.5 oz)	80	7	0	0
Cheddar Cheese Shredded	1 serv (1 oz)	104	9	1	0
Cheese	1 serv (0.7 oz)	70	6	1	0
Chili	1 serv (1 oz)	52	4	1	0

FOOD	PORTION	CALS	FAT	CARB	SUGAR
Cone Coat Chocolate	1 serv (1 oz)	143	8	16	15
Green Chilies	1 serv (1 oz)	10	0	3	0
Hickory Barbecue Sauce	1 serv (1 oz)	41	0	10	1
Honey Mustard Dressing	1 serv (1.1 oz)	110	9	9	7
Jalapenos Nachos Sliced	1 serv (1 oz)	5	0	1	0
Malt	1 serv (1 oz)	104	1	22	—
Maraschino Cherry	1 serv (8 g)	10	0	3	3
Marinara Sauce	1 serv (1 oz)	15	0	3	2
Ranch Dressing	1 serv (1 oz)	147	16	2	1
Slaw	1 serv (0.9 oz)	45	3	4	3
Sweet Pickle Relish	1 serv (1.1 oz)	40	0	11	10
Syrup Blue Coconut	1 serv (1 oz)	65	0	16	15
Syrup Cherry	1 serv (1 oz)	64	0	16	16
Syrup Chocolate	1 serv (1 oz)	74	0	16	16
Syrup Grape	1 serv (1 oz)	63	0	16	15
Syrup Vanilla	1 serv (1 oz)	61	0	15	—
Syrup Watermelon	1 serv (1 oz)	71	0	18	12
Thousand Island Dressing	1 serv (1 oz)	150	15	3	3
Topping Pineapple	1 serv (1.5 oz)	108	0	28	28
Topping Strawberry	1 serv (1 oz)	101	4	16	15
Topping Strawberry	1 serv (1.2 oz)	38	0	10	9
BEVERAGES					
Float or Flurry Blue Coconut Slush	1 reg	424	12	57	52
Slush Blue Coconut	1 lg	521	0	134	132
Slush Watermelon	1 lg	526	0	136	130
BREAKFAST SELECTIONS					
Breakfast Burrito	1	731	47	47	2
Fruit Taquitos	1 serv	302	7	51	12
Sunrise	1 lg	368	0	100	94
Sunrise	1 reg	224	0	60	56
Toaster Bacon Egg & Cheese	1	500	20	40	3

FOOD	PORTION	CALS	FAT	CARB	SUGAR
Toaster Ham Egg & Cheese	1	436	19	41	4
Toaster Sausage Egg & Cheese	1	570	36	44	3
DESSERTS					
Banana Split	1 serv	467	11	75	72
Chocolate Covered Shake Banana	1 reg	625	25	66	60
Chocolate Covered Shake Cherry	1 reg	587	24	59	51
Chocolate Covered Shake Peanut Butter	1 reg	678	34	57	50
Chocolate Covered Shake Strawberry	1 reg	608	24	64	56
Cream Pie Shake Banana	1 reg	775	27	92	82
Cream Pie Shake Coconut	1 reg	721	26	79	71
Dish Of Vanilla	1 serv	265	11	24	19
Float or Flurry Cherry Slush	1 reg	421	12	57	52
Float or Flurry Coca-Cola	1 reg	379	12	47	41
Float or Flurry Dr Pepper	1 reg	377	12	47	41
Float or Flurry Grape Slush	1 reg	423	12	57	52
Float or Flurry Orange Slush	1 reg	422	12	56	52
Float or Flurry Rootbeer	1 reg	386	12	50	44
Float or Flurry Watermelon Slush	1 reg	427	12	56	53
Ice Cream Cone	1	285	11	24	23
Shake Banana	1 reg	508	18	52	46
Shake Chocolate	1 reg	564	18	64	58
Shake Pineapple	1 reg	615	18	83	74
Shake Strawberry	1 reg	510	18	54	46
Shake Vanilla	1 reg	454	18	41	32

FOOD	PORTION	CALS	FAT	CARB	SUGAR
Sonic Blast Butterfinger	1 reg	636	26	59	56
Sonic Blast M&M	1 reg	641	27	64	58
Sonic Blast Oreo	1 reg	638	27	57	56
Sonic Blast Reese's	1 reg	658	30	56	52
Sundae Chocolate	1 serv	362	11	45	41
Sundae Hot Fudge	1 serv	392	15	44	40
Sundae Pineapple	1 serv	399	11	58	53
Sundae Strawberry	1 serv	322	11	37	32
MAIN MENU SELECTIONS					
Ched'R'Peppers	1 serv	256	12	29	5
Cheese Fries	1 lg	322	19	31	2
Cheese Fries	1 reg	265	17	23	2
Cheese Tater Tots	1 reg	329	22	28	1
Cheese Tots	1 lg	435	27	41	2
Chicken Strip Dinner	1 serv	749	32	86	5
Chicken Strip Snack	1 serv	272	13	22	—
Chicken Strips	2	184	9	15	—
Chili Cheese Fries	1 lg	357	22	32	2
Chili Cheese Fries	1 reg	299	19	24	2
Chili Cheese Tater Tots	1 reg	363	25	28	2
Chili Cheese Tots	1 lg	547	36	43	3
Corn Dog	1	262	17	23	5
Extra Long Coney Cheese	1	666	42	47	9
Extra Long Coney Plain	1	483	27	44	9
French Fries	1 lg	252	13	30	2
French Fries	1 reg	195	11	22	1
Fritos Chili Pie	1 serv	611	44	36	3
Hot Dog Plain	1	262	16	22	5
Jr. Burger	1	353	21	27	7
Mozzarella Sticks	1 serv	382	19	35	5
No.1 Hamburger	1	577	36	43	7
No.1 Sonic Cheeseburger	1	647	42	44	7
No.2 Hamburger	1	481	25	43	7

FOOD	PORTION	CALS	FAT	CARB	SUGAR
No.2 Sonic Cheeseburger	1	551	31	44	7
Onion Rings	1 lg	507	35	102	35
Onion Rings	1 reg	331	23	66	23
Regular Coney Cheese	1	366	24	24	5
Regular Coney Plain	1	262	16	22	5
Sandwich Breaded Chicken	1	582	23	66	6
Sandwich Country Fried Steak	1	748	47	56	7
Sandwich Grilled Chicken	1	343	13	31	6
Super Sonic No.1	1	929	66	45	7
Super Sonic No.2	1	839	56	46	7
SuperSonic Onion Rings	1 serv	706	10	141	39
SuperSonic Tots	1 serv	485	28	53	3
SuperSonic Fries	1 serv	358	18	44	2
Tater Tots	1 lg	365	21	40	2
Tater Tots	1 reg	259	16	27	1
Toaster Sandwich Bacon Cheddar Burger	1	675	38	60	6
Toaster Sandwich BLT	1	581	41	42	4
Toaster Sandwich Chicken Club	1	675	29	75	10
Toaster Sandwich Country Fried Steak	1	708	45	55	4
Toaster Sandwich Grilled Cheese	1	282	12	39	2
Wrap Chicken Strip	1	574	29	55	2
Wrap Grilled Chicken	1	539	27	40	2
Wrap w/o Ranch Chicken Strip	1	428	13	53	1
Wrap w/o Ranch Grilled Chicken	1	393	12	38	1

FOOD	PORTION	CALS	FAT	CARB	SUGAR

SOUPLANTATION

BREADS AND MUFFINS

FOOD	PORTION	CALS	FAT	CARB	SUGAR
Bread Indian Grain Low Fat	1 slice	200	2	35	5
Bread Low Fat Sourdough	1 slice	150	1	27	0
Cornbread Buttermilk Low Fat	1 piece	140	2	27	4
Focaccia Big Hearth Pizza	1	140	6	16	2
Focaccia Bruschetta	1 piece	130	6	15	1
Focaccia Pepperoni	1 piece	160	7	19	1
Focaccia Roasted Potato	1 piece	150	6	17	1
Focaccia Sauteed Vegetables	1 piece	150	7	18	3
Focaccia Tomatillo	1 piece	140	6	16	2
Focaccia Low Fat Garlic Parmesan	1 piece	100	3	15	1
Muffin Apple Cinnamon Bran 96% Fat Free	1	80	1	17	13
Muffin Apple Raisin	1	150	7	22	9
Muffin Banana Nut	1	150	7	22	9
Muffin Big Blue Blueberry	1	310	12	46	20
Muffin Black Forest	1	230	9	36	19
Muffin Cappuccino Chip	1	160	4	28	15
Muffin Caribbean Key Lime	1	170	6	28	15
Muffin Cherry Nut	1	150	7	22	9
Muffin Chocolate Brownie	1	170	8	22	10
Muffin Chocolate Chip	1	170	8	22	10
Muffin Country Blackberry	1	170	6	27	13
Muffin French Quarter Praline	1	290	15	38	21
Muffin Georgia Peach Poppyseed	1	150	6	20	10

FOOD	PORTION	CALS	FAT	CARB	SUGAR
Muffin Lemon	1	140	4	24	13
Muffin Low Fat Chile Corn	1	140	3	27	5
Muffin Macadamia Nut Spice	1	220	9	33	18
Muffin Maple Walnut	1	230	10	33	21
Muffin Nutty Peanut Butter	1	170	8	21	9
Muffin Pumpkin Raisin	1 piece	150	6	25	14
Muffin Strawberry Buttermilk	1	140	6	21	8
Muffin Sweet Orange & Cranberry	1	200	7	33	20
Muffin Taffy Apple	1	160	6	25	18
Muffin Tropical Papaya Coconut	1	180	7	28	18
Muffin Zucchini Nut	1	150	7	22	9
Muffin 96% Fat Free Cranberry Orange Bran	1	80	1	17	15
Muffin 96% Fat Free Fruit Medley Bran	1	80	1	17	15
DESSERTS					
Cobbler Apple	½ cup	350	10	64	10
Cobbler Blissful Blueberry	½ cup	380	10	70	45
Cobbler Cherry	½ cup	340	10	61	10
Cobbler Cranberry Apple	½ cup	370	10	58	42
Cobbler Peach	½ cup	360	10	65	40
Cookie Chocolate Chip	1 sm	70	3	10	6
Fat Free Apple Medley	½ cup	70	0	18	12
Fat Free Banana Royale	½ cup	80	0	20	12
Fat Free Frozen Yogurt Chocolate	½ cup	95	0	21	15
Jello Fat Free All Flavors	½ cup	80	0	20	19

FOOD	PORTION	CALS	FAT	CARB	SUGAR
Jello Fat Free Sugar Free All Flavors	½ cup	10	0	0	0
Pudding Banana	½ cup	160	4	27	26
Pudding Low Fat Butterscotch	½ cup	140	3	24	24
Pudding Low Fat Chocolate	½ cup	140	3	23	23
Pudding Low Fat Rice	½ cup	110	2	20	12
Pudding Vanilla	½ cup	140	4	24	24
Soft Serve Reduced Fat Vanilla	½ cup	140	4	22	19
Tapioca Low Fat	½ cup	140	3	24	24
MAIN MENU SELECTIONS					
Alfredo Broccoli w/ Basil	1 cup	380	17	45	5
Alfredo Fettuccine	1 cup	390	18	41	4
Alfredo Four Cheese	1 cup	390	13	50	3
Alfredo Roasted Garlic & Asiago	1 cup	330	11	45	5
Alfredo Roasted Mushroom w/ Rosemary	1 cup	380	14	44	4
Alfredo Southwestern	1 cup	350	16	42	3
Beef Stroganoff	1 cup	340	21	28	4
Carbonara Pasta	1 cup	280	8	43	3
Chili Arizona	1 cup	220	8	25	3
Chili Cheatin' Heart	1 cup	300	19	23	6
Chili Deep Kettle House Low Fat	1 cup	230	3	26	4
Chili Longhorn Beef	1 cup	190	6	25	5
Chili Rock N' Mole	1 cup	240	13	22	6
Chili Santa Fe Black Bean Low Fat	1 cup	190	3	26	2
Chili Texas Red	1 cup	240	8	30	4

FOOD	PORTION	CALS	FAT	CARB	SUGAR
Chili Three Bean Turkey Low Fat	1 cup	140	3	19	4
Chili Vegetarian	1 cup	150	3	25	6
Creamy Herb Chicken	1 cup	310	17	32	7
Creamy Pepper Jack	1 cup	290	15	35	6
Garden Vegetable w/ Italian Sausage	1 cup	300	10	42	2
Garden Vegetable w/ Meatballs	1 cup	270	7	42	2
Greek Mediterranean	1 cup	290	8	45	4
Italian Vegetable Beef	1 cup	270	6	43	3
Italian Sausage w/ Red Pepper Puree	1 cup	250	10	35	7
Lemon Cream & Asparagus	1 cup	230	9	34	4
Linguini w/ Clam Sauce	1 cup	380	10	56	3
Low Fat Oriental Green Bean & Noodle	1 cup	240	3	45	4
Macaroni & Cheese	1 cup	260	6	40	2
Nutty Mushroom	1 cup	390	20	42	4
Pasta Florentine	1 cup	360	10	54	4
Penne Arrabbiatta	1 cup	340	10	43	3
Pesto Cilantro Lime	1 cup	370	21	36	3
Roasted Eggplant Marinara	1 cup	340	10	43	3
Smoked Salmon & Dill	1 cup	360	16	41	2
Tuscany Sausage w/ Capers & Olives	1 cup	240	10	29	3
Vegetable Ragu	1 cup	250	5	41	4
Vegetarian Marinara w/ Basil	1 cup	260	4	44	3
Walnut Pesto	1 cup	310	9	42	4

FOOD	PORTION	CALS	FAT	CARB	SUGAR
SALAD DRESSINGS					
Bacon	2 tbsp	120	11	5	5
Balsamic Vinaigrette	1 tbsp	180	19	1	1
Basil Vinaigrette	2 tbsp	160	17	1	0
Blue Cheese	1 tbsp	140	14	3	2
Creamy Italian	2 tbsp	120	13	1	1
Honey Mustard	2 tbsp	150	13	8	6
Honey Mustard Fat Free	2 tbsp	45	0	10	9
Italian Fat Free	2 tbsp	20	0	5	4
Kahlena French	2 tbsp	120	9	10	9
Parmesan Pepper Cream	2 tbsp	160	17	2	1
Ranch	2 tbsp	130	13	1	1
Ranch Fat Free	2 tbsp	50	0	2	1
Reduced Calorie Cucumber	2 tbsp	80	7	4	3
Roasted Garlic	2 tbsp	140	14	2	1
Thousand Island	2 tbsp	110	11	3	2
SALADS					
Ambrosia w/ Coconut	½ cup	170	6	30	20
Antipasto w/ Peppered Salami	1 cup	140	10	6	2
Artichoke Rice	½ cup	160	8	21	2
Aunt Doris' Red Pepper Slaw Fat Free	½ cup	70	0	18	13
Baja Bean & Cilantro Low Fat	½ cup	180	3	29	2
Bartlett Pear & Walnut	1 cup	180	12	13	10
BBQ Julienne Chopped	1 cup	190	10	20	5
BBQ Smokehouse w/ Bacon & Peanuts	1 cup	190	10	19	4
Caesar Asiago	1 cup	190	14	10	4
California Cobb	1 cup	180	8	4	1

FOOD	PORTION	CALS	FAT	CARB	SUGAR
Cape Cod Spinach w/ Walnuts	1 cup	170	14	6	5
Carrot Ginger w/ Herb Vinaigrette	½ cup	150	12	9	6
Carrot Raisin Low Fat	½ cup	90	3	17	15
Chicken Tortilla	1 cup	180	10	16	4
Chinese Krab	½ cup	160	8	19	4
Citrus Noodle w/ Snow Peas	½ cup	140	6	19	5
Country French w/ Bacon	1 cup	210	18	7	1
Ensalada Azteca	1 cup	130	9	7	3
Field Corn & Very Wild Rice	½ cup	170	9	19	3
Greek	1 cup	120	9	4	2
Greek Couscous w/ Feta	½ cup	170	9	19	3
Italian Garden Vegetable	½ cup	110	8	9	2
Italian Sub Salad w/ Turkey & Salami	1 cup	260	17	18	5
Italian White Bean	½ cup	140	5	19	2
Joan's Blue BLT	1 cup	250	16	20	4
Joan's Broccoli Madness	½ cup	180	14	11	9
Lemon Rice w/ Cashews	½ cup	160	7	23	3
Mandarin Noodles w/ Broccoli Low Fat	½ cup	120	3	19	5
Mandarin Shells w/ Almonds	½ cup	120	3	19	4
Mandarin Spinach w/ Carmelized Walnuts	1 cup	170	11	14	11
Marinated Summer Vegetables Fat Free	½ cup	80	0	19	14
Mediterranean	1 cup	150	11	9	2
Monterey Blue w/ Peanuts	1 cup	200	12	20	5
Moroccan Marinated Vegetables Low Fat	½ cup	90	3	9	2

FOOD	PORTION	CALS	FAT	CARB	SUGAR
Old Fashioned Macaroni Salad w/ Ham	½ cup	180	11	15	3
Oriental Ginger Slaw w/ Krab Low Fat	½ cup	70	3	8	3
Penne w/ Chicken In Citrus Vinaigrette Low Fat	½ cup	130	3	20	5
Pesto Orzo w/ Pinenuts	1 cup	220	17	14	5
Pesto Pasta	½ cup	160	7	18	2
Pineapple Coconut Slaw	½ cup	150	10	14	10
Poppyseed Coleslaw	½ cup	120	9	9	5
Potato BBQ	½ cup	160	8	20	3
Potato Dijon w/ Garlic Dill Vinaigrette	½ cup	150	12	9	6
Potato German	½ cup	120	3	18	3
Potato Jalapeno	½ cup	140	5	20	3
Potato Picnic	½ cup	150	7	19	3
Potato Southern Dill Low Fat	½ cup	120	3	20	2
Ragin' Cajun	1 cup	200	14	12	7
Ranch House BLT Salad w/ Turkey	1 cup	180	11	10	2
Red Potato & Tomato	½ cup	120	10	8	1
Roasted Vegetables w/ Feta & Olives	1 cup	140	11	5	2
Roasted Potato Salad w/ Chipotle Chili Vinaigrette	½ cup	140	6	18	3
Roma Tomatoes Mozzarella & Basil	1 cup	120	9	7	2
San Francisco Herb Rice	½ cup	170	5	25	1
Shrimp & Seafood	½ cup	200	11	20	3
Smoked Turkey & Spinach w/ Almonds	1 cup	190	10	20	15

FOOD	PORTION	CALS	FAT	CARB	SUGAR
Sonoma Spinach w/ Honey Dijon Vinaigrette	1 cup	210	14	16	8
Southern Black Eyed Pea	½ cup	130	6	18	4
Southwestern Rice & Beans	½ cup	90	3	15	2
Spiced Pecans & Roasted Vegetables	1 cup	180	11	15	7
Spicy Southwestern Pasta Low Fat	½ cup	130	3	21	3
Spinach Gorgonzola w/ Spiced Pecans	1 cup	210	19	5	3
Strawberry Fields w/ Carmelized Walnuts	1 cup	130	8	15	12
Summer Barley w/ Black Beans Low Fat	½ cup	110	3	19	1
Summer Lemon w/ Spiced Pecans	1 cup	220	15	18	13
Thai Noodle w/ Peanut Sauce	½ cup	170	8	17	4
Three Bean Marinade	½ cup	170	6	27	11
Tomato Cucumber Marinade	½ cup	80	5	8	2
Traditional Spinach w/ Bacon	1 cup	160	11	7	3
Tuna Tarragon	½ cup	240	14	21	3
Turkey Chutney Pasta	½ cup	230	9	21	6
Watercress & Orange	1 cup	90	4	12	6
Wild Rice & Chicken	½ cup	300	22	20	4
Won Ton Chicken Happiness	1 cup	150	8	12	4
Zesty Tortellini	½ cup	190	15	18	3
SOUPS					
Albino Bean Chicken	1 cup	190	6	18	3

FOOD	PORTION	CALS	FAT	CARB	SUGAR
Albondigas Locas	1 cup	210	10	19	4
Autumn Root Vegetable w/ Wild Rice	1 cup	80	0	18	3
Baked Potato & Cheese w/ Bacon	1 cup	290	18	22	6
Be Wild With Mushroom	1 cup	220	16	14	5
Big Chunk Chicken Noodle Low Fat	1 cup	160	3	17	3
Black Bean Sausage Fling	1 cup	350	23	21	3
Black Bean & Chorizo	1 cup	230	9	27	6
Bombay Lentil Low Fat	1 cup	160	3	25	5
Broc On	1 cup	220	18	13	4
Broccoli Cheese	1 cup	280	20	15	7
Butternut Squash	1 cup	140	6	15	4
Cheese Stuffed Cappelletti	1 cup	130	4	20	8
Chesapeake Corn Chowder	1 cup	280	16	30	8
Chicken Got Smoked	1 cup	350	21	28	6
Chicken Tortilla w/ Jalapeno Chiles & Tomatoes Low Fat	1 cup	100	3	5	2
Chunky Potato Cheese w/ Thyme	1 cup	210	10	19	3
Classical French Onion	1 cup	130	5	16	12
Classical Minestrone Low Fat	1 cup	120	2	20	4
Classical Shrimp Bisque	1 cup	240	16	15	5
Country Corn & Red Potato Chowder	1 cup	160	6	24	6
Cream Of Broccoli	1 cup	210	15	14	3
Cream Of Chicken	1 cup	260	18	17	7
Cream Of Mushroom	1 cup	290	21	15	3
Cream Of Rosemary Potato	1 cup	270	19	22	4

FOOD	PORTION	CALS	FAT	CARB	SUGAR
Creamy Vegetable Chowder	1 cup	200	10	23	6
Devotion To The Ocean	1 cup	220	12	14	7
El Paso Lime & Chicken	1 cup	160	4	24	5
Field Of Creams Cauliflower w/ Cheese	1 cup	260	20	15	3
Field Of Creams Celery	1 cup	210	15	15	2
Field Of Creams Spinach	1 cup	280	22	18	3
Field Of Creams Tomato Basil	1 cup	220	15	20	4
Fire Roasted Green Chili & Corn Chowder	1 cup	230	14	21	7
Garden Fresh Vegetable Low Fat	1 cup	110	1	22	4
Garlic Kickin Roasted Chicken	1 cup	140	6	10	4
Hungarian Vegetable Low Fat	1 cup	120	2	20	5
Irish Potato Leek	1 cup	250	15	23	7
Living On The Veg	1 cup	90	1	15	3
Manhattan Clam Chowder	1 cup	130	4	16	4
Mulligatawny	1 cup	210	12	18	5
Navy Bean w/ Ham	1 cup	340	10	30	3
Neighbor Joe's Gumbo	1 cup	280	8	36	5
Posole	1 cup	150	6	8	1
Ratatouille Provencale Fat Free	1 cup	110	0	25	3
Roasted Mushroom w/ Sage	1 cup	320	25	20	7
Spicy Sausage & Pasta	1 cup	310	12	36	8
Split Pea w/ Ham	1 cup	350	10	32	3
Tomato Chipotle Bisque	1 cup	240	16	21	7

FOOD	PORTION	CALS	FAT	CARB	SUGAR
Tomato Parmesan & Vegetables Low Fat	1 cup	120	3	18	3
Toot Your Horn For Crab & Corn	1 cup	290	20	18	8
Vegetarian Lentils & Brown Rice Low Fat	1 cup	130	1	25	2
Yankee Clipper Clam Chowder w/ Bacon	1 cup	330	20	21	3

SOUTHERN TSUNAMI SUSHI BAR
SALADS

FOOD	PORTION	CALS	FAT	CARB	SUGAR
Calamari	1 serv (4 oz)	148	3	22	8
Edamame	1 serv (4 oz)	124	7	9	7
Harusame	1 serv (5 oz)	148	2	33	8
Seabreeze	1 serv (4 oz)	113	3	23	23

SUSHI

FOOD	PORTION	CALS	FAT	CARB	SUGAR
California Roll	1 (0.8 oz)	31	1	6	1
Cream Cheese Roll w/ Salmon	1 piece (0.8 oz)	43	2	5	1
Crunchy Shrimp Roll	1 piece (0.9 oz)	42	2	5	1
Dragon Roll	1 piece (0.8 oz)	42	2	6	1
Freshwater Eel Roll	1 piece (0.8 oz)	41	1	5	1
Green Horseradish	1 tsp	7	0	1	0
Inari	1 piece (1.9 oz)	105	2	18	2
Nigiri Cuttlefish	1 piece (1 oz)	42	1	9	1
Nigiri Egg Cake	1 piece (1.4 oz)	73	1	13	5
Nigiri Fish Roe	1 piece (1.4 oz)	61	1	9	1
Nigiri Fresh Salmon	1 piece (1.3 oz)	68	1	9	1
Nigiri Fresh Water Eel	1 piece (1.6 oz)	108	5	11	2
Nigiri Octopus	1 piece (1.1 oz)	57	1	9	1
Nigiri Sea Eel	1 piece (1.6 oz)	90	3	11	2
Nigiri Shrimp	1 piece (1.1 oz)	44	1	8	1
Nigiri Smoked Salmon	1 piece (1.3 oz)	68	1	9	1
Nigiri Tilapia	1 piece (1.2 oz)	49	1	8	1

FOOD	PORTION	CALS	FAT	CARB	SUGAR
Nigiri Tuna	1 piece (1.3 oz)	60	0	8	1
Nigiri Yellowtail	1 piece (1.2 oz)	54	1	8	1
Ocean Crab Roll	1 piece (0.8 oz)	33	1	5	1
Orange Roll	1 piece (0.8 oz)	32	1	6	1
Pickled Ginger	1 tbsp	9	0	2	1
Rainbow Roll	1 piece (1 oz)	41	1	6	1
Sea Eel Roll	1 piece (0.8 oz)	36	1	6	1
Soy Sauce	1 pkg	16	0	2	0
Spicy Roll Salmon	1 piece (0.8 oz)	40	1	5	1
Spicy Roll Shrimp	1 piece (0.8 oz)	31	1	5	1
Spicy Roll Tuna	1 piece (0.8 oz)	37	1	5	1
Tempura Roll	1 piece (0.9 oz)	44	1	7	2
Tofu Roll	1 piece (0.8 oz)	27	tr	5	1
Tsunami Roll Crab & Fish Roe	1 piece (0.8 oz)	39	1	6	1

STARBUCKS
BAKED SELECTIONS

FOOD	PORTION	CALS	FAT	CARB	SUGAR
Baby Bundt Cake Chocolate	1	330	15	45	29
Bagel	1	430	1	92	5
Bagel Cinnamon Raisin	1	440	1	96	14
Bagel Sesame	1	440	3	92	5
Bar Caramel Apple	1	310	16	38	21
Bar Carrot Cake	1	420	25	46	35
Bar Lemon	1	310	14	44	32
Bar Oreo Dream	1	420	30	33	22
Bar Toffee Crunch	1	430	21	56	37
Biscotti Chocolate Hazelnut	1	110	5	15	8
Biscotti Vanilla Almond	1	110	5	15	8
Brownie Caramel	1	580	36	60	44
Brownie Enrobed Espresso	1	430	25	48	32

FOOD	PORTION	CALS	FAT	CARB	SUGAR
Brownie Espresso	1	370	21	43	30
Brownie Milk Chocolate Peanut Butter	1	460	29	45	34
Bundt Cake Lemon Yogurt	1 serv	350	13	56	34
Caramel Pecan Sticky Roll	1	730	40	75	39
Cinnamon Roll	1	620	29	80	41
Cinnamon Twist	1	320	17	37	13
Coffee Cake	1 serv	570	28	75	45
Coffee Cake Apple Walnut	1 serv	320	17	41	28
Coffee Cake Blueberry Walnut	1 serv	340	18	43	30
Coffee Cake Cinnamon Walnut	1 serv	360	18	46	31
Coffee Cake Crumble Berry	1 serv	520	26	69	40
Coffee Cake Hazelnut	1 serv	630	35	74	43
Coffee Cake Sour Cream	1 serv	420	25	43	29
Cookie Black And White	1	430	17	68	53
Cookie Double Chocolate Chunk	1 serv	430	21	58	37
Cookie Oatmeal Raisin	1	390	15	65	34
Cookie White Chocolate Macadamia Nut	1	470	27	54	34
Crisp Cinnamon Twist	1	60	2	9	4
Croissant Almond	1	330	18	39	16
Croissant Butter w/ Apricot Glaze	1	320	17	37	13
Croissant Chocolate	1	350	19	43	21
Croissant Raspberry & Cream Cheese	1	260	12	34	11
Crumb Cake	1 serv	670	32	89	44
Crumb Cake Key Lime	1 serv	550	27	71	44

FOOD	PORTION	CALS	FAT	CARB	SUGAR
Danish Apple w/ Mocha Swirls	1	370	19	44	18
Danish Cheese w/ Mocha Swirls	1	460	28	44	18
Danish Raspberry w/ Mocha Swirls	1	370	19	45	17
Graham Dark Chocolate	1	140	8	17	12
Graham Milk Chocolate	1	140	8	17	12
Madeline	1	80	4	11	6
Muffin Blueberry	1	380	19	49	28
Muffin Chocolate Cream Cheese	1	450	24	53	31
Muffin Cranberry Orange	1	410	20	53	31
Muffin Morning Sunrise	1	330	12	54	32
Pound Cake Banana	1 serv	360	18	47	24
Pound Cake Cranberry Walnut	1 serv	390	21	45	26
Pound Cake Iced Carrot	1 serv	540	13	101	64
Pound Cake Iced Lemon	1 serv	500	23	69	46
Pound Cake Marble	1 serv	400	21	49	29
Pound Cake Orange Poppy	1 serv	490	27	55	32
Pound Cake Pumpkin	1 serv	310	12	47	27
Pound Cake Zucchini	1 serv	370	19	47	27
Pullman Banana	1 serv	400	17	57	31
Pullman Chocolate	1	380	17	54	33
Pullman Cranberry Walnut	1	360	15	53	28
Pullman Lemon Glazed	1	370	15	55	31
Pullman Marble Chocolate Chip	1	440	20	61	37
Pullman Orange Poppy Cheese	1	450	22	55	34

FOOD	PORTION	CALS	FAT	CARB	SUGAR
Pullman Pumpkin	1	370	17	51	22
Scone Blueberry	1	460	18	68	24
Scone Butterscotch Pecan	1	520	27	64	22
Scone Maple Oat w/ Icing	1	490	22	69	28
Scone Apricot Currant	1	450	17	67	17
Scone Raspberry	1	440	18	65	20
Shortbread	1	100	6	12	4
BEVERAGES					
Apple Juice	1 grande	230	0	57	52
Blended Coffee Of The Week	1 grande	10	0	2	0
Cafe Americano	1 grande	150	0	3	0
Cafe Au Lait Nonfat Milk	1 grande	90	0	13	11
Cafe Au Lait Soy Milk	1 grande	110	3	15	12
Cafe Latte Whole Milk	1 grande	260	14	21	19
Cafe Misto Cafe Au Lait Whole Milk	1 grande	140	8	11	11
Cafe Mocha Whip Whole Milk	1 grande	400	22	42	33
Caffe Latte Nonfat Milk	1 grande	160	0	24	20
Caffe Latte Soy Milk	1 grande	210	6	28	21
Caffe Mocha No Whip Whole Milk	1 grande	300	12	41	31
Caffe Mocha No Whip Nonfat Milk	1 grande	230	2	43	32
Caffe Mocha No Whip Soy Milk	1 grande	260	6	46	33
Caffe Mocha Whip Nonfat Milk	1 grande	330	12	44	34
Caffe Mocha Whip Soy Milk	1 grande	360	16	48	35
Cappuccino Nonfat Milk	1 grande	100	0	14	11
Cappucino Soy Milk	1 grande	120	3	17	12

FOOD	PORTION	CALS	FAT	CARB	SUGAR
Caramel Apple Cider No Whip	1 grande	300	0	72	64
Caramel Apple Cider Whip	1 grande	410	10	76	68
Caramel Macchiato Nonfat Milk	1 grande	230	2	40	35
Caramel Macchiato Soy Milk	1 grande	300	8	49	36
Caramel Macchiato Whole Milk	1 grande	320	14	37	34
Caramel Mocha No Whip Nonfat Milk	1 grande	300	3	63	51
Caramel Mocha No Whip Soy Milk	1 grande	340	6	66	52
Caramel Mocha No Whip Whole Milk	1 grande	370	11	61	50
Caramel Mocha Whip Nonfat Milk	1 grande	410	12	65	52
Caramel Mocha Whip Soy Milk	1 grande	440	16	68	54
Caramel Mocha Whip Whole Milk	1 grande	470	21	63	52
Chocolate Nonfat Milk	1 grande	240	2	45	36
Chocolate Whole Milk	1 grande	340	15	42	35
Cinnamon Spice Mocha No Whip Nonfat Milk	1 grande	250	1	47	40
Cinnamon Spice Mocha No Whip Whole Milk	1 grande	330	12	45	45
Cinnamon Spice Mocha Whip Nonfat Milk	1 grande	350	11	49	41
Cinnamon Spice Mocha Whip Whole Milk	1 grande	430	22	47	41

FOOD	PORTION	CALS	FAT	CARB	SUGAR
Cinnamon Spice No Whip Soy Milk	1 grande	290	6	51	41
Cinnamon Spice Whip Soy Milk	1 grande	390	15	53	42
Espresso Decaf Coffee Of The Week	1 grande	10	0	2	0
Frappuccino Blended Coffee	1 grande	230	3	46	38
Frappuccino Blended Coffee Mocha Coconut No Whip Whole Milk	1 grande	400	10	75	60
Frappuccino Caramel Blended Coffee No Whip	1 grande	280	4	57	48
Frappuccino Caramel Blended Coffee Whip	1 grande	430	16	61	52
Frappuccino Chocolate Blended Creme Whip	1 grande	530	19	75	65
Frappuccino Chocolate Blended Creme No Whip	1 grande	400	7	73	63
Frappuccino Chocolate Brownie Blended Coffee No Whip	1 grande	370	9	69	56
Frappuccino Chocolate Brownie Blended Coffee Whip	1 grande	510	22	72	59
Frappuccino Chocolate Malt Blended Creme No Whip	1 grande	470	10	87	69
Frappuccino Chocolate Malt Blended Creme Whip	1 grande	610	22	90	72
Frappuccino Mocha Blended Coffee No Whip	1 grande	290	4	58	48

FOOD	PORTION	CALS	FAT	CARB	SUGAR
Frappuccino Mocha Blended Coffee Whip	1 grande	420	16	61	51
Frappuccino Mocha Coconut Blended Coffee Whip	1 grande	550	22	80	64
Frappuccino Mocha Malt Blended Coffee No Whip	1 grande	430	7	91	65
Frappuccino Mocha Malt Blended Coffee Whip	1 grande	570	20	95	68
Frappuccino Tazo Chai Creme Blended Tea No Whip	1 grande	370	5	69	64
Frappuccino Tazo Chai Creme Blended Tea Whip	1 grande	500	17	72	66
Frappuccino Tazoberry Blended Tea	1 grande	190	0	49	46
Frappuccino Tazoberry Creme Blended Tea No Whip	1 grande	330	2	74	60
Frappuccino Tazoberry Creme Blended Tea Whip	1 grande	460	14	76	71
Frappuccino Vanilla Blended Creme No Whip	1 grande	350	5	64	60
Frappuccino Vanilla Blended Creme Whip	1 grande	480	17	66	62
Frappuccino White Chocolate Mocha Blended Coffee No Whip	1 grande	320	5	62	54
Frappuccino White Chocolate Mocha Blended Coffee Whip	1 grande	450	17	65	56

FOOD	PORTION	CALS	FAT	CARB	SUGAR
Hot Chocolate No Whip Whole Milk	1 grande	340	15	42	35
Hot Chocolate No Whip Nonfat Milk	1 grande	240	2	45	36
Hot Chocolate Whip Nonfat Milk	1 grande	340	12	47	37
Hot Chocolate Whip Whole Milk	1 grande	440	24	44	37
Iced Caffe Americano	1 grande	20	0	3	0
Iced Caffe Latte Nonfat Milk	1 grande	100	0	14	11
Iced Caffe Latte Soy Milk	1 grande	120	5	17	12
Iced Caffe Latte Whole Milk	1 grande	160	8	13	11
Iced Caffe Mocha No Whip Nonfat Milk	1 grande	180	2	36	26
Iced Caffe Mocha No Whip Soy Milk	1 grande	200	5	38	26
Iced Caffe Mocha No Whip Whole Milk	1 grande	220	8	35	25
Iced Caffe Mocha Whip Nonfat Milk	1 grande	310	14	38	28
Iced Caffe Mocha Whip Soy Milk	1 grande	330	17	40	28
Iced Caffe Mocha Whip Whole Milk	1 grande	350	20	37	27
Iced Caramel Macchiato Nonfat Milk	1 grande	100	1	36	32
Iced Caramel Macchiato Soy Milk	1 grande	230	5	39	33
Iced Caramel Macchiato Whole Milk	1 grande	270	10	34	31
Iced Shaken Coffee	1 grande	80	0	20	19
Iced Tazo Chai Nonfat Milk	1 grande	230	0	50	45

FOOD	PORTION	CALS	FAT	CARB	SUGAR
Iced Tazo Chai Whole Milk	1 grande	270	7	48	45
Iced White Chocolate Mocha No Whip Soy Milk	1 grande	340	8	59	53
Iced White Chocolate Mocha No Whip Whole Milk	1 grande	360	11	56	52
Iced White Chocolate Mocha Whip Nonfat Milk	1 grande	450	18	59	55
Iced White Chocolate Mocha Whip Soy Milk	1 grande	470	20	61	55
Iced White Chocolate Mocha Whip Whole Milk	1 grande	490	24	58	54
Iced White Chocolate No Whip Nonfat Milk	1 grande	320	6	57	53
Milk Nonfat	1 grande	160	0	23	22
Steamed Apple Cider	1 grande	230	0	57	52
Steamed Nonfat Milk	1 grande	160	0	23	22
Steamed Whole Milk	1 grande	270	15	21	21
Tazo Chai Whole Milk	1 grande	290	7	50	46
Tazo Chai Nonfat Milk	1 grande	230	0	51	47
Tazo Iced Tea	1 grande	80	0	20	19
Tazo Tea Lemonade	1 grande	120	0	31	29
Vanilla Creme No Whip Nonfat Milk	1 grande	240	0	43	40
Vanille Creme No Whip Whole Milk	1 grande	340	14	40	39
Vanilla Creme Whip Nonfat Milk	1 grande	340	9	44	42
Vanilla Creme Whip Whole Milk	1 grande	440	24	42	41
White Chocolate Mocha No Whip Nonfat Milk	1 grande	340	5	58	54

FOOD	PORTION	CALS	FAT	CARB	SUGAR
White Chocolate Mocha No Whip Whole Milk	1 grande	410	15	56	53
White Chocolate Mocha Whip Nonfat Milk	1 grande	440	14	60	56
White Chocolate Mocha Whip Whole Milk	1 grande	510	24	58	55
White Chocolate No Whip Soy Milk	1 grande	370	14	62	55
White Chocolate Whip Soy Milk	1 grande	440	15	65	58
White Hot Chocolate No Whip Nonfat Milk	1 grande	390	6	66	63
White Hot Chocolate No Whip Whole Milk	1 grande	480	18	63	62
White Hot Chocolate Whip Nonfat Milk	1 grande	490	15	68	65
White Hot Chocolate Whip Whole Milk	1 grande	580	28	65	64
Whole Milk	1 grande	270	15	21	21
TOPPINGS					
Caramel	1 tbsp	15	1	2	2
Chocolate	1 tsp	5	0	1	1
Flavored Sugar Free Syrup	1 pump	0	0	0	0
Flavored Syrup	1 pump	20	0	5	5
Mocha Syrup	1 pump	25	1	6	4
Sprinkles	1 serv	0	0	tr	tr

STEAK ESCAPE
CHILDREN'S MENU SELECTIONS

FOOD	PORTION	CALS	FAT	CARB	SUGAR
Kids Fries	1 serv	249	13	34	—
Kids Tenders	2 pieces	240	11	21	—
Sandwich Chicken	1	205	7	32	—
Sandwich Ham	1	183	1	32	—
Sandwich Steak	1	210	3	31	—

FOOD	PORTION	CALS	FAT	CARB	SUGAR
Sandwich Turkey	1	183	1	32	—
MAIN MENU SELECTIONS					
12 Inch Sandwich Grand Cobbler	1	680	4	116	—
12 Inch Sandwich Grand Escape	1	776	12	108	—
12 Inch Sandwich Grandest Chicken	1	770	10	110	—
12 Inch Sandwich Great Escape	1	776	12	108	—
12 Inch Sandwich Hambrosia	1	684	4	119	—
12 Inch Sandwich Ragin' Cajun	1	756	10	108	—
12 Inch Sandwich Turkey Club	1	675	4	111	—
12 Inch Sandwich Vegetarian	1	524	2	109	—
12 Inch Sandwich Wild West BBQ	1	841	12	126	—
7 Inch Sandwich Grand Cobbler	1	380	2	67	—
7 Inch Sandwich Grand Escape	1	435	6	64	—
7 Inch Sandwich Grandest Chicken	1	425	5	64	—
7 Inch Sandwich Great Escape	1	428	6	63	—
7 Inch Sandwich Hambrosia	1	382	2	69	—
7 Inch Sandwich Ragin' Cajun	1	418	5	63	—

FOOD	PORTION	CALS	FAT	CARB	SUGAR
7 Inch Sandwich Turkey Club	1	390	2	65	–
7 Inch Sandwich Vegetarian	1	302	1	64	–
7 Inch Sandwich Wild West BBQ	1	469	6	72	–
Fries	1 serv (12 oz)	498	26	67	–
Fries	1 serv (32 oz)	996	52	134	–
Fries Loaded Bacon & Cheddar	1 serv	905	44	88	–
Fries Loaded Ranch & Bacon	1 serv	1044	71	84	–
Smashed Potatoes Loaded Bacon & Cheddar	1 serv	636	26	91	–
Smashed Potatoes Loaded Ranch & Bacon	1 serv	692	34	87	–
Smashed Potatoes Plain	1 serv	246	0	53	–
Smashed Potatoes w/ Chicken	1 serv	318	4	56	–
Smashed Potatoes w/ Ham	1 serv	336	2	59	–
Smashed Potatoes w/ Steak	1 serv	391	5	56	–
Smashed Potatoes w/ Turkey	1 serv	336	2	59	–
SALAD DRESSINGS AND TOPPINGS					
American Cheese	1 slice	101	9	3	–
Bacon	1 serv (1 oz)	80	7	0	0
BBQ Sauce	1 serv (1 oz)	40	0	9	–
Black Olives	1 serv (1 oz)	32	3	2	–
Brown Mustard	1 serv (1 oz)	0	0	0	0
Cheddar Cheese	1 slice	116	9	1	–
Dressing Italian	1 serv (0.5 oz)	51	5	1	–

FOOD	PORTION	CALS	FAT	CARB	SUGAR
Dressing Ranch	1 serv (0.5 oz)	83	9	0	0
Lettuce	1 serv (1 oz)	2	0	0	0
Margarine	1 serv (1 oz)	203	23	0	0
Mayonnaise	1 serv (1 oz)	101	11	0	0
Peppers Jalapeno	1 serv (1.5 oz)	11	0	2	—
Peppers Mild	1 serv (1.5 oz)	11	0	4	—
Provolone Cheese	1 slice	80	6	0	0
Sour Cream	1 serv (1 oz)	61	6	1	—
Swiss Cheese	1 slice	100	8	1	—
Tomatoes	1 serv (2 oz)	24	0	2	—
SALADS					
Grilled Salad w/ Chicken	1 serv	175	5	11	—
Grilled Salad w/ Ham	1 serv	130	2	8	—
Grilled Salad w/ Steak	1 serv	185	6	11	—
Grilled Salad w/ Turkey	1 serv	130	2	8	—
Side	1 serv	40	5	8	—
TACO BELL					
Bean Burrito	1	370	10	55	4
Border Bowl Zesty Chicken	1 serv	730	42	65	5
Border Bowl Zesty Chicken w/o Dressing	1 serv	500	19	60	4
Burrito 7 Layer	1	530	21	66	6
Burrito Chili Cheese	1	390	18	40	3
Burrito Fiesta Chicken	1	370	12	48	4
Burrito Fiesta Steak	1	370	13	48	4
Burrito Grilled Chicken	1	680	26	76	6
Burrito Spicy Chicken	1	430	19	50	4
Burrito Supreme Beef	1	440	18	52	5
Burrito Supreme Chicken	1	410	14	50	5
Burrito Supreme Steak	1	420	16	50	5
Burrito ½ Lb Bean Especial	1	600	21	62	6

FOOD	PORTION	CALS	FAT	CARB	SUGAR
Burrito ½ Lb Beef & Potato	1	530	24	65	4
Burrito ½ Lb Combo Beef	1	470	19	52	4
Chalupa Baja Beef	1	430	27	32	4
Chalupa Baja Chicken	1	400	24	30	4
Chalupa Baja Steak	1	400	25	30	4
Chalupa Nacho Cheese Beef	1	380	22	33	4
Chalupa Nacho Cheese Chicken	1	350	18	31	4
Chalupa Nacho Cheese Steak	1	350	19	31	4
Chalupa Supreme Beef	1	390	24	31	4
Chalupa Supreme Chicken	1	370	20	30	4
Chalupa Supreme Steak	1	370	22	29	4
Cheesy Fiesta Potatoes	1 serv	280	18	27	2
Cinnamon Twists	1 serv	160	5	28	13
Empanada Caramel Apple	1	290	15	37	14
Enchirito Beef	1	380	18	35	3
Enchirito Chicken	1	350	14	33	3
Enchirito Steak	1	360	16	33	3
Express Taco Salad	1 serv	630	33	58	8
Express Taco Salad w/o Chips	1 serv	410	21	32	8
Fiesta Taco Salad	1 serv	870	47	80	10
Fiesta Taco Salad w/o Shell	1 serv	500	37	42	9
Gordita Baja Beef	1	350	19	31	7
Gordita Baja Chicken	1	320	15	29	7
Gordita Baja Steak	1	320	16	29	7
Gordita Nacho Cheese Beef	1	300	13	32	7

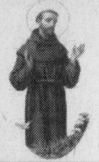
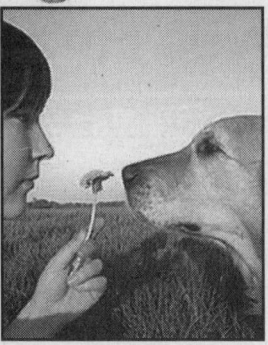
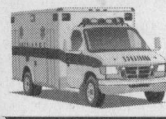

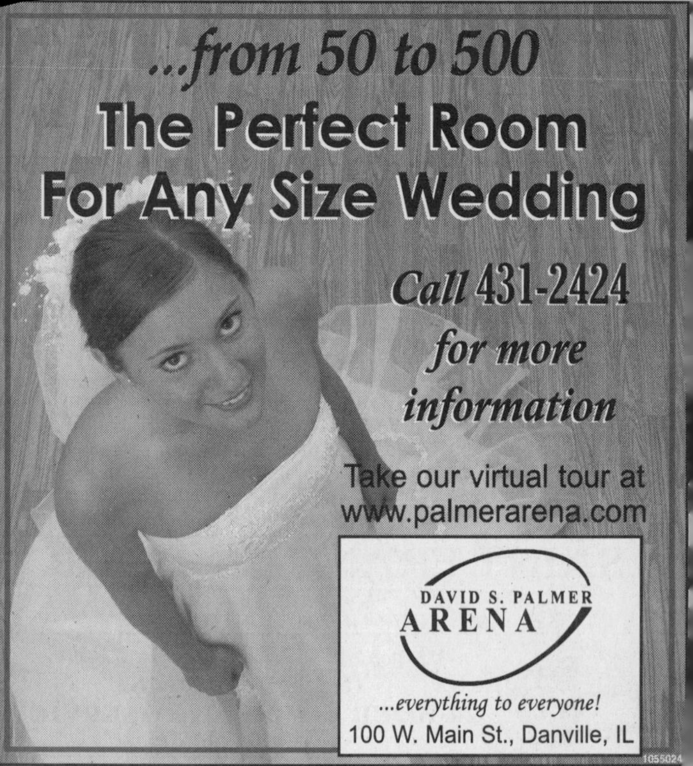
...from 50 to 500
The Perfect Room
For Any Size Wedding
Call 431-2424
for more
information
Take our virtual tour at
www.palmerarena.com
DAVID S. PALMER
ARENA
...everything to everyone!
100 W. Main St., Danville, IL
1055024

FOOD	PORTION	CALS	FAT	CARB	SUGAR
Gordita Nacho Cheese Chicken	1	270	10	30	7
Gordita Nacho Cheese Steak	1	270	11	30	7
Gordita Supreme Beef	1	310	16	30	7
Gordita Supreme Chicken	1	290	12	28	7
Gordita Supreme Steak	1	280	13	26	7
Mexican Pizza	1 serv	550	31	47	3
Mexican Rice	1 serv	210	10	23	tr
MexiMelt	1 serv	290	16	23	2
Nacho Supreme	1 serv	450	26	42	3
Nachos	1 serv	320	19	33	3
Nachos Bellgrande	1 serv	780	43	80	5
Pintos 'n Cheese	1 serv	180	7	20	1
Quesadilla Cheese	1 serv	490	28	39	4
Quesadilla Chicken	1	540	30	40	4
Quesadilla Steak	1	540	31	40	4
Soft Taco Beef	1	210	10	21	2
Soft Taco Grande	1	450	21	44	4
Soft Taco Grilled Steak	1	280	17	21	3
Soft Taco Ranchero Chicken	1	270	14	21	3
Soft Taco Supreme Beef	1	260	14	23	3
Southwest Steak Bowl	1 serv	700	32	73	4
Taco	1	170	10	13	tr
Taco Double Decker	1	340	14	39	2
Taco Spicy Chicken	1	180	7	21	2
Taco Supreme	1	220	14	14	2
Taco Supreme Double Decker	1	380	18	41	4
Tostada	1	250	10	29	2

TACO CABANA

FOOD	PORTION	CALS	FAT	CARB	SUGAR
Black Beans	1 serv (4 oz)	111	tr	21	–

FOOD	PORTION	CALS	FAT	CARB	SUGAR
Borracho Beans	1 serv (4 oz)	108	3	17	—
Breakfast Taco Bacon & Egg	1	246	12	22	—
Breakfast Taco Barbacoa	1	307	15	2	—
Breakfast Taco Chorizo & Egg	1	248	12	22	—
Breakfast Taco Potato & Egg	1	234	10	27	—
Burrito Bean & Cheese	1	710	27	85	—
Burrito Beef	1	653	24	76	—
Burrito Black Bean	1	559	11	95	—
Burrito Chicken	1	665	26	74	—
Calabacita	1 serv (4 oz)	78	5	6	—
Chips	1 serv (2 oz)	285	14	36	—
Elotes	1	220	11	26	—
Fajitas Beef	1 serv (4 oz)	245	12	3	—
Fajitas Chicken Dark	1 serv (4 oz)	236	11	2	—
Fajitas Chicken White	1 serv (4 oz)	191	6	3	—
Grilled Chicken Dark	1 serv (4.5 oz)	298	18	1	—
Grilled Chicken Dark No Skin	1 serv (3.4 oz)	170	7	1	—
Grilled Chicken White	1 serv (5 oz)	295	14	1	—
Grilled Chicken White No Skin	1 serv (3.8 oz)	167	3	tr	—
Guacamole	1 serv (1 oz)	48	4	2	—
Queso	1 serv (3 oz)	184	12	7	—
Refried Beans	1 serv (4 oz)	171	6	21	—
Sour Cream	1 serv (1 oz)	57	5	1	—
Spanish Rice	1 serv (4 oz)	181	5	30	—
Taco Bean & Cheese	1	292	12	35	—
Taco Black Bean	1	216	5	37	—
Taco Carne Guisada	1	202	8	20	—
Taco Crispy Beef	1	148	7	13	—

FOOD	PORTION	CALS	FAT	CARB	SUGAR
Taco Soft Chicken	1	217	9	21	—
Tortilla Corn	1 (6 in)	70	1	11	—
Tortilla Flour	1 (6 in)	129	3	22	—
Tortilla Soup	1 sm	249	8	26	—
Tortilla Soup	1 lg	371	13	32	—

TACO JOHN'S
DESSERTS

FOOD	PORTION	CALS	FAT	CARB	SUGAR
Apple Grande	1 serv	240	9	36	15
Choco Taco	1 serv	300	15	38	24
Churro	1 serv	230	11	31	19
Cinnamon Mini Swirl	1 piece	10	0	3	3

MAIN MENU SELECTIONS

FOOD	PORTION	CALS	FAT	CARB	SUGAR
Burrito Bean	1	380	12	53	1
Burrito Beefy	1	430	20	41	1
Burrito Chicken & Potato	1	460	19	54	1
Burrito Combination	1	400	16	47	1
Burrito Meat & Potato	1	490	23	55	1
Burrito Super	1	450	20	49	2
Crispy Taco	1 serv	180	10	13	0
Mexican Rice	1 serv	250	5	45	2
Nachos	1 serv	380	23	38	0
Potato Oles	1 lg	790	47	86	0
Potato Oles	1 sm	440	26	48	0
Potato Oles Bravo	1 serv	580	36	55	1
Potato Oles Super	1 serv	980	62	82	2
Potato Oles w/ Nacho Cheese	1 serv	550	35	52	0
Quesadilla Cheese	1	480	28	39	1
Quesadilla Chicken	1	540	29	41	1
Refried Beans	1 serv	400	14	50	2
Sierra Taco Beef	1	430	23	38	3
Sierra Taco Chicken	1	390	17	37	3
Softshell Taco	1	220	10	21	1

FOOD	PORTION	CALS	FAT	CARB	SUGAR
Softshell Taco Chicken	1	190	6	19	0
Super Nachos	1 serv	830	51	73	2
Super Nachos Chicken	1 serv	780	45	62	2
Taco Bravo	1 serv	340	14	30	1
Taco Burger	1	280	12	28	3
Texas Chili	1 serv	270	12	26	3
SALAD DRESSINGS AND TOPPINGS					
Bacon Ranch Dressing	1 serv (3 oz)	250	19	21	14
Barbecue Sauce	1 serv (2 oz)	70	0	15	9
Chipotle Cream Sauce	1 serv (3 oz)	450	45	6	3
Creamy Italian Dressing	1 serv (3 oz)	260	29	6	3
Guacamole	1 serv (2 oz)	90	9	6	2
Hot Sauce	1 serv (1 oz)	5	0	1	0
House Dressing	1 serv (3 oz)	140	15	5	2
Jalapenos	1 serv (2 oz)	15	1	3	1
Mild Sauce	1 serv (1 oz)	5	0	1	0
Nacho Cheese	1 serv (3 oz)	120	9	5	0
Pico De Gallo	1 serv (2 oz)	15	0	4	1
Ranch Dressing	1 serv (3 oz)	280	31	6	3
Salsa	1 serv (2 oz)	20	0	5	4
Sour Cream	1 serv (2 oz)	120	12	2	0
Super Hot Sauce	1 serv (1 oz)	10	0	2	1
SALADS					
Chicken Festiva w/o Dressing	1 serv	400	23	24	2
Chicken Taco w/o Dressing	1	530	27	45	5
Side w/o Dressing	1 serv	80	5	6	1
Taco w/o Dressing	1 serv	580	32	46	5
TACOTIME					
DESSERTS					
Cinnamon Crustos	1 serv	373	15	47	—
Fruit Filled Empanada	1 serv	250	9	37	—

FOOD	PORTION	CALS	FAT	CARB	SUGAR
MAIN MENU SELECTIONS					
Burrito Beef Bean & Cheese	1 serv	617	23	66	–
Burrito Casita	1 serv	647	31	54	–
Burrito Chicken & Black Bean	1 serv	400	18	45	–
Burrito Chicken BLT	1 serv	580	39	36	–
Burrito Crisp Bean	1 serv	427	18	53	–
Burrito Crisp Chicken	1	422	25	32	–
Burrito Crisp Meat	1 serv	552	30	39	–
Burrito Soft Bean	1	380	10	58	–
Burrito Soft Meat	1 serv	491	21	48	–
Burrito Veggie	1 serv	491	16	70	–
Burrito Big Juan Beef	1 serv	640	25	71	–
Burrito Big Juan Chicken	1 serv	620	24	69	–
Cheddar Fries	1 lg	704	48	54	–
Cheddar Fries	1 sm	352	24	27	–
Cheddar Melt	1 serv	205	11	17	–
Mexi-Fries	1 lg	532	34	54	–
Mexi-Fries	1 sm	266	17	27	–
Mexi-Rice	1 serv	159	2	30	–
Nachos	1 serv	680	38	61	–
Nachos Deluxe	1 serv	1048	57	91	–
Refritos Cheese Sauce Chips	1 serv	326	10	44	–
Stuffed Fries	1 lg	990	73	88	–
Stuffed Fries	1 sm	490	37	34	–
Taco Cheeseburger	1	633	36	48	–
Taco Crisp	1	295	17	16	–
Taco Soft	1 serv	316	15	23	–
Taco Soft ½ lb	1 serv	512	23	46	–
Taco Soft ½ lb Chicken	1 serv	387	16	41	–
Taco Super Soft	1 serv	510	23	50	–

FOOD	PORTION	CALS	FAT	CARB	SUGAR
SALAD DRESSINGS AND TOPPINGS					
1000 Island Dressing	1 serv (1 oz)	120	12	3	—
Green Sauce	1 serv (1 oz)	5	0	2	—
Original Hot Sauce	1 serv (1 oz)	10	0	2	—
Salsa Fresca	1 serv (1 oz)	65	0	16	—
SALADS					
Chicken Fiesta	1 serv	390	19	35	—
Taco	1 reg	479	28	30	—
Taco Salad Chicken	1 serv	370	21	27	—
Tostada	1 serv	628	33	48	—
TASTI D-LITE					
Vanilla	1 sm (4 oz)	40	tr	7	6
TGI FRIDAY'S					
Sizzling Chicken & Broccoli	1 serv	700	40	15	—
Sizzling NY Strip Steak w/ Blue Cheese & Broccoli	1 serv	684	36	15	—
TIM HORTONS					
BAGELS AND CREAM CHEESE					
Blueberry	1	200	2	59	10
Cinnamon Raisin	1	300	2	58	12
Cream Cheese Light	1.5 oz	90	7	3	3
Cream Cheese Plain	1.5 oz	140	14	1	1
Everything	1	300	2	57	8
Multigrain	1	300	3	58	8
Onion	1	295	2	58	8
Plain	1	290	2	57	8
Poppy Seed	1	300	3	58	8
Sesame Seed	1	300	3	57	7
Whole Wheat & Honey	1	300	2	59	11

FOOD	PORTION	CALS	FAT	CARB	SUGAR
BAKED SELECTIONS					
Biscuit Southern Country Cranberry	1	470	19	68	21
Biscuit Southern Country Raspberry	1	470	19	68	19
Cake Black Forest	1 serv	500	21	75	44
Cake Celebration	1 serv	500	16	85	56
Cake Chocolot Fantasy	1 serv	420	15	72	51
Cake Shadow	1 serv	430	19	63	43
Cookie Chocolate Chip	1	150	7	21	12
Cookie Macaroon	1	140	8	14	11
Cookie Oatcakes	1	190	10	22	10
Cookie Oatmeal Raisin	1	150	6	22	13
Cookie Peanut Butter	1	170	10	17	8
Cookie Peanut Butter Chocolate Chunk	1	170	10	18	11
Croissant Butter	1	210	11	25	3
Croissant Cheese	1	240	12	27	3
Danish Cherry Cheese	1	380	23	33	11
Donut Apple Fritter	1	300	14	40	14
Donut Chocolate Dip	1	230	10	33	11
Donut Chocolate Glazed	1	360	22	36	19
Donut Dutchie	1	280	13	39	18
Donut Filled Angel Cream	1	280	13	36	15
Donut Filled Blueberry	1	220	8	33	11
Donut Filled Boston Cream	1	230	8	36	13
Donut Filled Canadian Maple	1	230	8	36	13
Donut Filled Strawberry	1	220	8	33	10
Donut Honey Dip	1	230	10	32	10
Donut Honey Stick	1	280	15	34	13
Donut Maple Dip	1	250	10	36	15

FOOD	PORTION	CALS	FAT	CARB	SUGAR
Donut Old Fashion Glazed	1	270	12	39	22
Donut Old Fashion Plain	1	220	12	24	8
Donut Sour Cream Plain	1	280	18	25	11
Donut Sugar Twist	1	230	10	32	9
Muffin Blueberry Bran	1	300	9	51	21
Muffin Carrot Whole Wheat	1	410	22	52	24
Muffin Chocolate Chip	1	390	15	62	32
Muffin Low Fat Carrot	1	260	2	60	30
Muffin Low Fat Cranberry	1	260	2	60	30
Muffin Low Fat Honey	1	290	2	66	33
Muffin Oatbran Carrot 'n Raisin	1	340	11	57	26
Muffin Oatbran 'n Apple	1	350	12	58	24
Muffin Oatmeal Raisin	1	430	11	80	48
Muffin Raisin Bran	1	380	10	66	36
Muffin Wild Blueberry	1	330	11	54	27
Pie Apple	1 serv	540	31	62	26
Pie Banana Cream	1 serv	440	26	50	21
Pie Cherry	1 serv	570	31	70	35
Pie Chocolate Cream	1 serv	490	31	52	23
Tart Fresh Strawberry	1 serv	220	9	36	10
Tart Raisin Butter	1 serv	330	11	54	25
Tea Biscuit Plain	1	220	6	36	3
Tea Biscuit Raisin	1	250	6	47	15
Timbits Chocolate Glazed	1	70	3	9	5
Timbits Dutchie	1	60	2	10	5
Timbits Filled Banana Cream	1	45	1	8	2
Timbits Filled Lemon	1	50	2	9	3
Timbits Filled Spiced Apple	1	80	1	9	3

FOOD	PORTION	CALS	FAT	CARB	SUGAR
Timbits Filled Strawberry	1	50	1	9	3
Timbits Honey Dip	1	50	1	10	3
Timbits Old Fashion Plain	1	45	2	7	2
BEVERAGES					
Cafe Mocha	1 (10 oz)	250	10	34	3
Cappuccino English Toffee	1 (10 oz)	130	5	20	16
Cappuccino French Vanilla	1 (10 oz)	130	5	20	16
Cappuccino Iced	1 (16 oz)	430	23	54	52
Coffee Decaffeinated + Sugar & Cream	1 (10 oz)	80	4	10	10
Coffee + Sugar & Cream	1 (10 oz)	80	4	10	10
Hot Chocolate	1 (10 oz)	200	6	44	43
Tea + Sugar & Milk	1 (10 oz)	45	0	9	9
SANDWICHES					
Albacore Tuna Salad	1 serv	350	8	49	50
Black Forest Ham & Swiss	1 serv	640	27	53	4
Chunky Chicken Salad	1 serv	380	10	50	6
Fireside Roast Beef	1 serv	470	19	48	4
Garden Vegetable	1 serv	460	24	50	6
Harvest Turkey Breast	1 serv	470	18	53	4
SOUPS					
Barley & Wild Rice	1 serv	120	2	22	1
Chicken Noodle	1 serv	100	3	15	4
Chili	1 serv	320	9	32	10
Cream Of Broccoli	1 serv	190	7	27	9
Cream Of Mushroom	1 serv	195	10	21	4
Hearty Vegetable	1 serv	130	2	27	4
Minestrone	1 serv	125	2	25	4
Potato Bacon	1 serv	195	7	29	3
Vegetable Beef Barley	1 serv	110	2	14	5
T.J. CINNAMONS					
Cinnachips	1 bag (10 oz)	1130	50	157	—
Cinnamon Twist	1	260	13	33	—

FOOD	PORTION	CALS	FAT	CARB	SUGAR
Coffee Black	1 (12 oz)	0	0	0	0
Mocha Chill w/ Whipped Cream	1 (12.5 oz)	310	6	49	—
Mocha Chill w/o Whipped Cream	1 (12.5 oz)	260	4	48	—
Original Roll w/o Icing	1	500	17	81	—
Original Roll w/ Cream Cheese Icing	1	651	37	103	—
Pecan Sticky Roll	1	690	28	97	—

WHATABURGER
BAKED SELECTIONS

Cinnamon Roll	1	860	34	126	—

BEVERAGES

Shake Chocolate	1 sm (20 oz)	616	17	100	—
Shake Strawberry	1 sm (20 oz)	620	16	101	—
Shake Vanilla	1 sm (20 oz)	559	17	82	—

CHILDREN'S MENU SELECTIONS

Kid's Justaburger	1	306	15	27	—
Kid's Chicken Strips	1 serv	382	24	22	—

MAIN MENU SELECTIONS

Biscuit Buttermilk	1	300	16	34	—
Biscuit w/ Bacon	1	375	22	34	—
Biscuit w/ Bacon Egg & Cheese	1	476	29	35	—
Biscuit w/ Egg & Cheese	1	446	27	35	—
Biscuit w/ Sausage	1	517	35	34	—
Biscuit w/ Sausage Egg & Cheese	1	663	46	35	—
Biscuit w/ Sausage Gravy	1	491	33	47	—
Breakfast Platter w/ Bacon	1 serv	698	43	52	—
Breakfast Platter w/ Sausage	1 serv	840	56	52	—

FOOD	PORTION	CALS	FAT	CARB	SUGAR
Breakfast On A Bun Ranchero w/ Bacon	1	404	23	29	–
Breakfast On A Bun Ranchero w/ Sausage	1	546	36	29	–
Breakfast On A Bun w/ Bacon	1	398	23	28	–
Breakfast On A Bun w/ Sausage	1	540	36	28	–
Chicken Strips	2	382	24	22	–
Croutons Njoy Seasoned	1 pkg	35	2	4	–
French Fries	1 lg	514	26	66	–
French Fries	1 sm	257	13	33	–
Grape Jelly	1 pkg	35	0	9	–
Gravy White Peppered	1 serv	53	5	8	–
Hashbrown Sticks	1 serv	140	8	16	–
Honey	1 pkg	25	0	7	–
Hot Apple Pie	1	240	12	31	–
Justaburger	1	309	15	28	–
Ketchup	1 pkg	40	0	8	–
Margarine	1 pkg	23	3	0	–
Onion Rings	1 med	201	11	23	–
Pancake Syrup	1 pkg	120	0	31	–
Pancakes	1 serv	614	8	118	–
Pancakes w/ Bacon	1 serv	689	13	118	–
Pancakes w/ Sausage	1 serv	831	27	118	–
Picante Sauce	1 serv	5	0	1	–
Sandwich Egg	1	323	17	28	–
Sandwich Grilled Chicken	1	473	20	49	–
Sandwich Grilled Chicken w/o Bun	1	190	7	10	–
Sandwich Whatacatch	1	473	26	45	–
Sandwich Whatachick'n	1	523	21	63	–
Strawberry Jam	1 pkg	40	0	10	–

FOOD	PORTION	CALS	FAT	CARB	SUGAR
Taquito Bacon & Egg	1	387	22	25	—
Taquito Potato & Egg	1	382	20	33	—
Taquito Sausage & Egg	1	389	26	26	—
Taquito w/ Bacon Egg & Cheese	1	432	25	25	—
Taquito w/ Potato Egg & Cheese	1	427	24	33	—
Taquito w/ Sausage Egg & Cheese	1	434	27	26	—
Texas Toast	1 serv	328	15	42	—
Whataburger	1	607	30	53	—
Whataburger Double Meat	1	857	48	53	—
Whataburger Double Meat No Bun	1	520	36	4	—
Whataburger Jr.	1	315	16	29	—
Whataburger No Bun	1	270	18	4	—
Whataburger Triple Meat	1	1107	66	53	—
Whataburger w/ Bacon & Cheese	1	810	45	54	—
Whatacatch	2 pieces	814	65	38	—
SALAD DRESSINGS					
Low Fat Ranch	1 pkg	66	4	9	—
Low Fat Vinaigrette	1 pkg	35	2	6	—
Ranch	1 pkg	310	33	3	—
Thousand Island	1 pkg	150	13	11	—
SALADS					
Chicken Strips	1 serv	419	25	29	—
Chicken Strips w/ Cheddar Cheese	1 serv	600	39	32	—
Chicken Strips w/ Cheddar Cheese & Bacon	1 serv	675	45	33	—
Garden Salad	1	49	1	10	—

FOOD	PORTION	CALS	FAT	CARB	SUGAR
Garden w/ Cheddar Cheese	1 serv	218	15	10	—
Garden w/ Cheddar Cheese & Bacon	1 serv	293	20	11	—
Grilled Chicken	1 serv	229	7	19	—
Grilled Chicken w/ Cheddar Cheese	1 serv	398	21	19	—
Grilled Chicken w/ Cheddar Cheese & Bacon	1 serv	473	27	19	—

WHITE CASTLE
BEVERAGES

FOOD	PORTION	CALS	FAT	CARB	SUGAR
Shake Chocolate	16 oz	250	15	37	27
Shake Vanilla	16 oz	260	15	40	28

MAIN MENU SELECTIONS

FOOD	PORTION	CALS	FAT	CARB	SUGAR
Bacon Cheeseburger	1	200	13	12	0
Cheese Sticks	3	250	14	22	2
Cheeseburger	1	160	9	11	0
Chicken Rings	6	210	14	10	0
Double Cheeseburger	1	290	18	16	0
Double Hamburger	1	240	14	16	0
French Fries	1 sm	115	6	15	2
Hamburger	1	140	7	11	0
Onion Rings	6	260	13	31	4
Sandwich Breakfast	1	340	25	17	2
Sandwich Chicken	1	190	8	21	1
Sandwich Chicken Ring	1	180	8	20	2
Sandwich Fish	1	180	7	27	2

WINCHELL'S DONUTS

FOOD	PORTION	CALS	FAT	CARB	SUGAR
Chocolate Bar	1	240	16	29	—
Chocolate Round	1	240	16	29	—
Chocolate Twist	1	240	16	29	—
Croissant	1	260	17	28	—

FOOD	PORTION	CALS	FAT	CARB	SUGAR
Glazed Round	1	230	15	27	—
Glazed Twist	1	230	15	27	—
Iced Chocolate	1	230	15	28	—
Traditional	1	215	14	26	—

INDEX

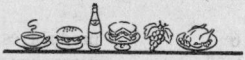

T = Table